BODY MRI HANDBOOK 2026

A Clinical Textbook Covering Hepatobiliary, Genitourinary, and Oncologic Diagnostic Interpretation for Radiology Residents

Ramon C. Henson, MD

Medical Disclaimer

This textbook is intended solely for educational and informational purposes and is designed to support the continuing professional development of licensed healthcare providers. The clinical content presented herein reflects information believed to be accurate and current at the time of publication; however, medicine evolves rapidly, and readers are advised that new research findings, updated clinical practice guidelines, and revised regulatory approvals may alter or supersede information contained in this work after its publication date.

Nothing in this publication constitutes medical advice, clinical guidance specific to any individual patient, or a substitute for the independent professional judgment of a licensed and qualified healthcare provider. No clinician-patient relationship is established, implied, or intended by the use of this textbook or any portion thereof. All clinical decisions, including but not limited to diagnosis, therapeutic selection, drug dosing, and patient monitoring, must be individualized based on thorough and direct assessment of the patient, the totality of current published evidence, applicable clinical practice guidelines, institutional protocols, and the informed professional judgment of the responsible clinician.

Drug information, dosages, treatment protocols, and therapeutic recommendations presented in this publication are offered for educational reference only and must be independently verified against current prescribing information, pharmacopeial references, and applicable regulatory approvals prior to clinical application. The author and publisher have made every reasonable effort to ensure the accuracy and completeness of the information presented; nevertheless, they expressly disclaim all liability for any adverse outcomes, clinical errors, patient harm, loss, or injury alleged to arise, directly or indirectly, from the use, misuse, or application of any information, recommendation, protocol, or clinical guidance contained in this publication.

TABLE OF CONTENT

PREFACE

Body MRI occupies a distinctive place in cross-sectional imaging. Unlike a single-organ subspecialty, it demands fluency across the liver, biliary tree, pancreas, spleen, adrenal glands, kidneys, prostate, uterus, ovaries, bowel, and mesentery, each governed by its own sequence requirements, its own differential diagnosis, and, increasingly, its own structured reporting system. A radiology resident reading a body MRI on call is expected to move seamlessly from recognizing a T2 hyperintense hepatic lesion to assigning an LI-RADS category to deciding whether the finding warrants biopsy, short-interval follow-up, or reassurance, all within the span of a single dictation. This textbook was written to support exactly that transition, from image to category to decision, as a single continuous act of clinical reasoning rather than three separate skills learned from three separate sources.

The chapters that follow are organized by organ system, moving from the physical and technical foundations of body MRI through the hepatobiliary and pancreatic system, the splenic, adrenal, and retroperitoneal compartment, the genitourinary tract, the female pelvis, the gastrointestinal and mesenteric compartment, and finally into whole-body and special-population applications. Each chapter integrates protocol guidance, pattern-based interpretation, and management reasoning into a single narrative, because in practice these are never separated: the sequence chosen determines what can be seen, what is seen determines the category assigned, and the category assigned determines what happens to the patient next.

How This Book Is Organized

Every chapter follows a consistent architecture: measurable learning objectives, a concise clinical overview, comprehensive coverage of the relevant Expanded Clinical Topic Structure elements (epidemiology, pathophysiology, clinical presentation, differential diagnosis, diagnostic workup, management, complications, and, where relevant, prevention, special populations, and patient counseling), narrative clinical cases that walk through real diagnostic reasoning, and clinical pearls, key points, and caution boxes that flag the pitfalls experienced readers learn to anticipate.

The Signal-to-Category Decision System

Woven through every chapter is this book's named proprietary feature: **The Signal-to-Category Decision System**. At every major diagnostic decision point, a branded five-part callout walks the reader from the imaging signal pattern itself, to the diagnostic category that pattern maps to, to the definitive clinical decision that category triggers, to the artifact or mimic that could be mistaken for it, and finally to a single high-yield anchor finding worth committing to memory. Every chapter closes with a Signal Synthesis Recap that consolidates the chapter's patterns into a single scannable review, and the book closes with **The Signal-to-Category Master Index**, a fully cross-referenced navigator of every pattern in the book, organized by organ system, for use during clinic, on call, or before a rotation.

A Note on Scope and Use

This handbook is written as a clinical reference, not an examination workbook. Its purpose is to build durable diagnostic judgment, the kind that holds up when a finding does not match a textbook description exactly, when two structured reporting systems seem to disagree, or when time pressure makes careful pattern recognition more important than ever. It is intended for the diagnostic radiology resident and body imaging fellow as a primary working reference, and for the practicing general radiologist as a comprehensive refresher on a subspecialty whose evidence base and structured reporting systems continue to evolve.

It is offered with the hope that it earns a place not on a shelf, but open beside the workstation.

CHAPTER 1: PRINCIPLES OF MR PHYSICS FOR BODY IMAGING

Learning Objectives

1. Explain the origin of the MR signal in terms of nuclear spin, precession, and the net magnetization vector, and relate this to why hydrogen is the clinically relevant nucleus in body imaging.
2. Differentiate T1 and T2 relaxation mechanisms and predict the signal behavior of common body tissues on T1-weighted, T2-weighted, and proton-density sequences.
3. Compare spin-echo, gradient-echo, and diffusion-weighted sequence families and select the appropriate sequence for a given body imaging question.
4. Describe how k-space is filled and reconstructed into an image, and predict the artifacts that result from specific k-space filling strategies.
5. Evaluate the trade-offs of field strength and coil selection in body MRI protocol design, and recognize chemical shift and susceptibility artifacts as they appear in practice.

Clinical Overview

Every diagnostic decision made from a body MRI examination rests on a physical process that begins long before an image reaches a workstation. The contrast that separates a benign hepatic cyst from a solid mass, the fat suppression that unmasks a lipid-poor adrenal adenoma, and the diffusion restriction that flags a small hepatocellular carcinoma are not arbitrary visual conventions; they are direct consequences of how hydrogen nuclei behave in a magnetic field and how that behavior is manipulated by pulse sequence design. A radiologist who understands this behavior reads protocols critically rather than passively, recognizes when an unusual appearance reflects a technical phenomenon rather than pathology, and can troubleshoot a nondiagnostic examination in real time rather than repeating it unnecessarily.

This chapter builds the physical foundation on which every subsequent organ-specific chapter depends. It is organized to move from the origin of the MR signal itself, through the pulse sequences that convert that signal into diagnostically useful contrast, through the spatial encoding process that assembles individual signal measurements into an image, and finally to the practical hardware decisions, field strength and coil selection, that determine image quality at the bedside. Two instances of this book's named proprietary feature are introduced here, applied for the first time to the artifact patterns that most often masquerade as pathology.

A recurring theme throughout this chapter, and throughout the book, is that image quality in body MRI is not a fixed property of the scanner but the product of a series of deliberate choices, sequence family, k-space strategy, field strength, coil configuration, each of which trades one form of image quality for another. A radiologist who treats a body MRI protocol as a fixed recipe will eventually encounter an examination degraded by motion, susceptibility, or inadequate coverage and will have no framework for understanding why, whereas a radiologist who understands the physical trade-offs underlying each acquisition choice can look at a degraded image and identify, often within seconds, which parameter should be adjusted on the next attempt. This diagnostic fluency, reading the acquisition as well as the anatomy, is what separates a technically competent reader from one who can troubleshoot a difficult examination in real time.

Fundamentals of Magnetic Resonance Signal Generation

Nuclear Spin, Precession, and the Net Magnetization Vector

The hydrogen nucleus, a single proton, possesses an intrinsic angular momentum called spin, which behaves as a small magnetic dipole. In the absence of an external field, the magnetic moments of the roughly ten to the twenty-second power hydrogen nuclei in a typical imaging voxel point in random directions, so their vector sum is effectively zero. When a patient is placed in the strong, static magnetic field of an MRI scanner, denoted B0, these moments preferentially align either parallel or antiparallel to B0, with a slight population excess in the lower-energy parallel orientation because thermal energy at body temperature is far greater than the energy difference between the two states. This small excess, on the order of a few nuclei per million, is what generates a net longitudinal magnetization vector, M0, aligned with B0. Because M0 arises from a probabilistic population difference rather than from every nucleus aligning identically, MR signal strength scales directly with field strength: doubling B0 roughly doubles the equilibrium magnetization and, correspondingly, the available signal, which is the physical basis for the diagnostic advantages of higher-field systems discussed later in this chapter.

Superimposed on this alignment is precession: each nucleus's magnetic moment rotates around the axis of B0 at a frequency proportional to field strength, described by the Larmor equation. At 1.5 tesla, hydrogen precesses at approximately sixty-four megahertz; at 3 tesla, at approximately one hundred twenty-eight megahertz. This precise, field-strength-dependent frequency is what allows a radiofrequency pulse tuned to that exact frequency to selectively excite hydrogen nuclei and tip the net magnetization vector away from its equilibrium alignment with B0. Because the Larmor frequency also varies slightly with local chemical environment, most notably between water-bound and fat-bound hydrogen, this same principle underlies both spatial encoding and the chemical shift phenomena discussed later in this chapter.

Longitudinal and Transverse Relaxation: T1 and T2

Once a radiofrequency pulse tips the net magnetization vector away from B0 into the transverse plane, two independent relaxation processes begin simultaneously, and their relative rates in different tissues are the entire basis of MR contrast. Because relaxation is a rate process rather than an instantaneous one, both T1 and T2 also vary with field strength, though in opposite directions and to different degrees, which is a second, distinct reason why body protocols cannot simply be copied unchanged between a 1.5-tesla and a 3-tesla system. T1 relaxation times lengthen with increasing field strength for most tissues, because the molecular tumbling frequencies that most efficiently drive T1 recovery become relatively less well matched to the higher Larmor frequency, while T2 relaxation times change comparatively little with field strength, since T2 decay depends primarily on local magnetic field inhomogeneities at the molecular level rather than on the absolute Larmor frequency itself. The practical consequence is that T1-weighted contrast between tissues, most importantly between an enhancing lesion and background parenchyma after gadolinium administration, is somewhat reduced at 3 tesla relative to 1.5 tesla unless repetition and echo times are deliberately adjusted to compensate, another instance of the field-strength trade-offs explored later in this chapter. T1 relaxation, also called spin-lattice relaxation, is the process by which the longitudinal component of magnetization recovers toward its equilibrium value as excited nuclei transfer energy back to the surrounding molecular lattice. Tissues in which molecular tumbling rates are close to the Larmor frequency, such as fat, relax efficiently and therefore recover longitudinal magnetization quickly, producing a short T1 and, correspondingly, high signal on T1-weighted images. Simple fluid, in which molecules tumble far faster than the Larmor frequency, relaxes inefficiently, producing a long T1 and low signal on T1-weighted sequences.

T2 relaxation, or spin-spin relaxation, describes the loss of coherence among the transverse magnetization vectors of individual nuclei as they experience slightly different local magnetic environments and gradually dephase relative to one another, independent of any energy loss to the lattice. Highly organized, water-rich tissue with restricted molecular motion, such as simple fluid, dephases slowly and therefore has a long T2, producing high signal on T2-weighted images; this is the physical basis for the bright appearance of cysts, edema, and ascites. Solid tissue with more heterogeneous local magnetic environments, including most tumors and fibrotic tissue, dephases more quickly, producing intermediate or lower T2 signal. T2-weighted imaging is therefore the workhorse sequence for detecting and characterizing fluid-containing and edematous processes throughout the body, while T1-weighted imaging is the workhorse for depicting fat, subacute hemorrhage, and proteinaceous content, and for assessing contrast enhancement.

KEY POINT: T1 and T2 are properties of tissue, not of the sequence; the sequence merely determines whether the acquired image is weighted to display differences in T1, differences in T2, or a combination of both. A single tissue can therefore appear dramatically different in signal intensity depending entirely on which relaxation property the chosen sequence emphasizes.

Pulse Sequences and Contrast Mechanisms in Body Imaging

Spin-Echo and Gradient-Echo Sequence Families

Spin-echo sequences use a ninety-degree excitation pulse followed by one or more one hundred eighty-degree refocusing pulses, which reverse the dephasing caused by fixed, static field inhomogeneities and thereby isolate true T2 decay from artifactual signal loss due to magnet imperfections and tissue susceptibility. Fast or turbo spin-echo variants, which acquire multiple lines of k-space per excitation using a train of refocusing pulses, are the mainstay of body T2-weighted imaging because they are relatively insensitive to motion-related dephasing and tolerate the moderate scan times required for adequate spatial resolution in the abdomen and pelvis. Gradient-echo sequences, by contrast, use a single excitation pulse of variable flip angle and refocus the signal using a gradient reversal rather than a radiofrequency pulse; because this technique does not correct for static field inhomogeneities, gradient-echo images are T2-star weighted rather than true T2-weighted, meaning they are considerably more sensitive to susceptibility effects. This sensitivity is a liability near metallic hardware or bowel gas but is exploited deliberately in techniques such as in-phase and opposed-phase imaging and in detecting blood degradation products and iron deposition.

In body imaging, gradient-echo sequences are also favored for their speed, which allows breath-hold acquisition and, critically, the rapid serial imaging required for dynamic contrast-enhanced sequences that capture the arterial, portal venous, and delayed phases of hepatic and renal enhancement. The choice between spin-echo and gradient-echo families is therefore rarely arbitrary: it reflects a deliberate trade-off between motion robustness and susceptibility sensitivity, and recognizing which family produced a given image is often the first step in explaining an unexpected signal finding.

Fat Suppression Techniques and Their Clinical Rationale

Because fat is bright on both T1- and T2-weighted sequences by virtue of its short T1 and, on fast spin-echo sequences, its relatively preserved T2 signal, unsuppressed fat signal can obscure adjacent pathology or mimic enhancement and hemorrhage. Chemical shift-based fat suppression techniques exploit the small but consistent difference in resonant frequency between fat- and water-bound protons, roughly three and a half parts per million, to selectively saturate or excite one species while leaving the other unaffected; these techniques are effective but degrade in the presence of field inhomogeneity, which is why fat suppression often fails at the periphery of the field of view or near air-tissue interfaces such as the bowel. Short tau inversion recovery, an alternative approach, instead nulls fat signal based on its short T1 relaxation time rather than its chemical shift, making it more uniform across a large field of view at the cost of also suppressing signal from any other short-T1 tissue, including subacute hemorrhage and gadolinium-enhanced structures, a limitation that matters when short tau inversion recovery is used after contrast administration.

The two-point Dixon technique, now standard on most modern body MRI protocols, instead acquires images with fat and water signal in phase and out of phase and combines them algebraically to generate separate fat-only and water-only images, along with in-phase and opposed-phase images, in a single acquisition. This approach is comparatively robust to field inhomogeneity and simultaneously provides the in-phase and opposed-phase contrast used to detect intracellular lipid, which is the physical basis for one of the most clinically important artifact-versus-pathology distinctions in body MRI.

Fat Suppression Technique	Physical Basis	Key Advantage	Key Limitation
Chemical fat saturation	Selective saturation at the fat resonant frequency	Preserves gadolinium and hemorrhage signal after saturation	Fails with field inhomogeneity, especially at field-of-view periphery
Short tau inversion recovery (STIR)	Nulls signal based on fat's short T1	Uniform suppression across a large field of view	Also nulls gadolinium enhancement and subacute hemorrhage

Two-point Dixon	Combines in-phase and opposed-phase acquisitions algebraically	Robust to inhomogeneity; yields four contrasts in one acquisition	Requires adequate field homogeneity for accurate water-fat separation at tissue boundaries

THE SIGNAL-TO-CATEGORY DECISION SYSTEM — Chemical Shift Artifact and the Lipid-Poor Adenoma Trap

The Signal Pattern: A well-defined adrenal nodule loses signal on opposed-phase images relative to in-phase images, and a thin, dark boundary line, the so-called India ink artifact, is visible outlining structures at fat-water interfaces on opposed-phase imaging throughout the abdomen.

Category Signature: Signal loss confined to the interior of a nodule that contains a mixture of fat and water within individual voxels indicates intravoxel lipid and is categorized as a benign, lipid-rich adenoma; a thin peripheral dark line at any fat-water boundary, including around organs, vessels, and normal fat planes, is instead a chemical shift boundary artifact and carries no diagnostic significance.

The Decision: A nodule demonstrating true intravoxel signal drop-out, quantified visually or by signal intensity index, can be confidently characterized as a lipid-rich adenoma without further imaging or biopsy; a peripheral India ink line alone, without internal signal loss, requires no action and should not be mistaken for a lesion margin or hemorrhage.

Trap Logic: The India ink artifact is easily mistaken for a true lesion capsule or for a rim of hemosiderin, particularly when it outlines a cyst or vessel adjacent to fat; the discriminating feature is that the artifact is present only at the interface, is one to two pixels wide, and shifts position slightly with changes in the frequency-encoding direction, whereas a true capsule or hemosiderin rim is present on both in-phase and opposed-phase images and does not shift.

Pattern Anchor: Signal loss inside a lesion on opposed-phase imaging means lipid and is diagnostic; a dark line only at its edge means chemical shift artifact and is nothing.

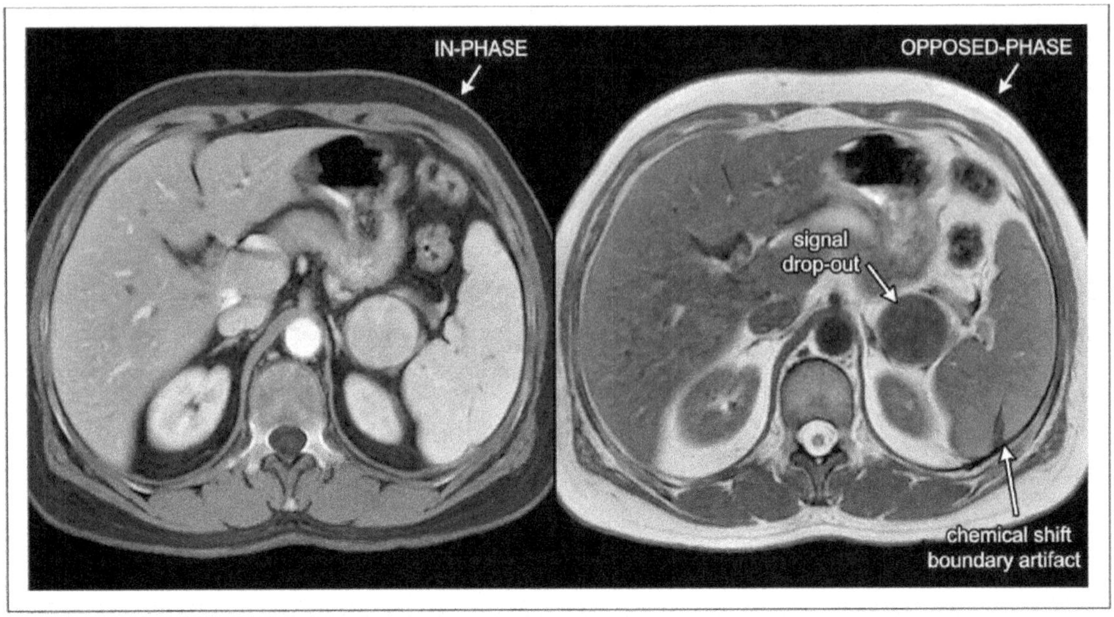

Figure 1.1: In-Phase and Opposed-Phase Signal Behavior of a Lipid-Rich Adrenal Adenoma

Diffusion-Weighted Imaging and the Apparent Diffusion Coefficient

Diffusion-weighted imaging measures the random, thermally driven Brownian motion of water molecules within tissue by applying paired diffusion-sensitizing gradients before signal readout; tissue in which water diffusion is restricted, most often because of high cellular density and correspondingly reduced extracellular space, loses less signal from these gradients and therefore appears relatively hyperintense at high b-values, while tissue with unrestricted diffusion, such as simple fluid, loses more signal and appears hypointense. Because this contrast depends on both diffusion restriction and underlying T2 signal, a phenomenon called T2 shine-through can cause a lesion with simply long T2, rather than true diffusion restriction, to appear falsely bright on a high b-value image alone. The apparent diffusion coefficient map, calculated from diffusion-weighted images acquired at two or more b-values, isolates the diffusion component from the T2 component: true restricted diffusion appears dark, or hypointense, on the apparent diffusion coefficient map, whereas T2 shine-through remains bright. This distinction is fundamental to nearly every malignancy-characterization pattern used later in this book, from focal liver lesions to prostate and adnexal masses, and a reader who cannot separate true restriction from shine-through will systematically overcall benign, fluid-containing lesions as malignant.

Steady-State Free Precession and Its Niche Applications in Body Imaging

Balanced steady-state free precession sequences occupy a distinct position among gradient-echo techniques: by fully rewinding all three gradient axes within each repetition and using a very short repetition time, they generate signal that depends on the ratio of T2 to T1 rather than on either relaxation time alone, producing images in which both fluid and flowing blood appear uniformly bright while most solid tissue appears comparatively dark. This contrast behavior makes balanced steady-state free precession less useful for the fat, lesion, and enhancement characterization that dominates most of this book, but it makes the technique extremely well suited to rapid anatomic surveys in which speed and motion insensitivity matter more than tissue-specific contrast, most notably single-shot sequences used for fetal and maternal anatomic survey during body MRI in pregnancy and rapid free-breathing cardiac cine and morphologic imaging. Because balanced steady-state free precession is highly sensitive to local field inhomogeneity, it is also prone to a characteristic banding artifact, seen as dark linear bands crossing the image where off-resonance effects cause destructive interference of the steady-state signal; these bands shift position when the center frequency is adjusted and should not be mistaken for a linear structural abnormality such as a septation or scar.

The choice of b-values, the numerical parameters that control the strength of the diffusion-sensitizing gradients, further shapes diagnostic performance. Low b-value images, typically in the range of zero to fifty seconds per square millimeter, retain substantial T2 signal and are useful chiefly for lesion detection and for generating the perfusion-related signal decay used in intravoxel incoherent motion modeling, but they are of limited value for lesion characterization because they do not adequately suppress signal from tissue with unrestricted diffusion. High b-value images, generally eight hundred to fifteen hundred seconds per square millimeter in abdominal protocols and up to two thousand in prostate-dedicated protocols, more effectively suppress unrestricted diffusion and increase conspicuity of truly restricted lesions, but at the cost of lower overall signal-to-noise ratio and increased susceptibility-related geometric distortion, particularly at 3 tesla. Because no single b-value is optimal for every purpose, most body protocols acquire at least three b-values, allowing both qualitative assessment of high b-value conspicuity and quantitative apparent diffusion coefficient calculation from the same acquisition, and the reader should always confirm which b-values were used before interpreting an apparent diffusion coefficient value in absolute terms, since apparent diffusion coefficient is itself dependent on the b-values from which it was derived and is not perfectly comparable across different protocols or institutions.

Spatial Encoding, k-Space, and Image Formation

Frequency and Phase Encoding

A radiofrequency pulse alone excites hydrogen nuclei uniformly throughout the imaging volume; spatial information is added by superimposing linear magnetic field gradients on top of B0 so that the Larmor frequency, and therefore the precise resonant frequency and phase of the returning signal, varies predictably with position. A slice-select gradient, applied during the excitation pulse, restricts excitation to a single slice by ensuring that only nuclei within a narrow range of positions along that gradient are resonant at the transmitted frequency. Within that slice, a frequency-encoding gradient applied during signal readout causes nuclei at different positions along one axis to precess, and therefore to emit signal, at slightly different frequencies, which can be separated by Fourier analysis. A phase-encoding gradient, applied briefly before readout and stepped through a range of strengths across repeated excitations, imparts a position-dependent phase shift along the perpendicular axis. Together, frequency and phase encoding allow every point in the image to be uniquely identified by the combination of frequency and phase of its contribution to the received signal.

Receiver bandwidth, the range of frequencies sampled during frequency encoding, has practical consequences that extend well beyond scan time. A narrow receiver bandwidth samples a smaller range of frequencies, which increases signal-to-noise ratio because less noise is admitted along with signal, and this is why narrow-bandwidth acquisitions are favored when signal is at a premium. The same narrow bandwidth, however, means that a given range of off-resonance frequencies, whether from chemical shift or from susceptibility-induced field distortion, is spread across a proportionally larger number of pixels along the frequency-encoding direction, which is why chemical shift artifact and susceptibility-related geometric distortion both worsen as receiver bandwidth is narrowed. Widening the receiver bandwidth compresses this same off-resonance range into fewer pixels, reducing chemical shift and distortion artifact at the cost of reduced signal-to-noise ratio, which is precisely the trade-off invoked in this chapter's second clinical case, where a wide-bandwidth fast spin-echo sequence was used specifically to shrink susceptibility artifact around a surgical clip enough to exclude a separate soft tissue process. Recognizing receiver bandwidth as a tunable parameter, rather than a fixed scanner setting, is what allows a radiologist to request a specific technical modification, rather than a simple repeat, when an examination is degraded by a bandwidth-related artifact.

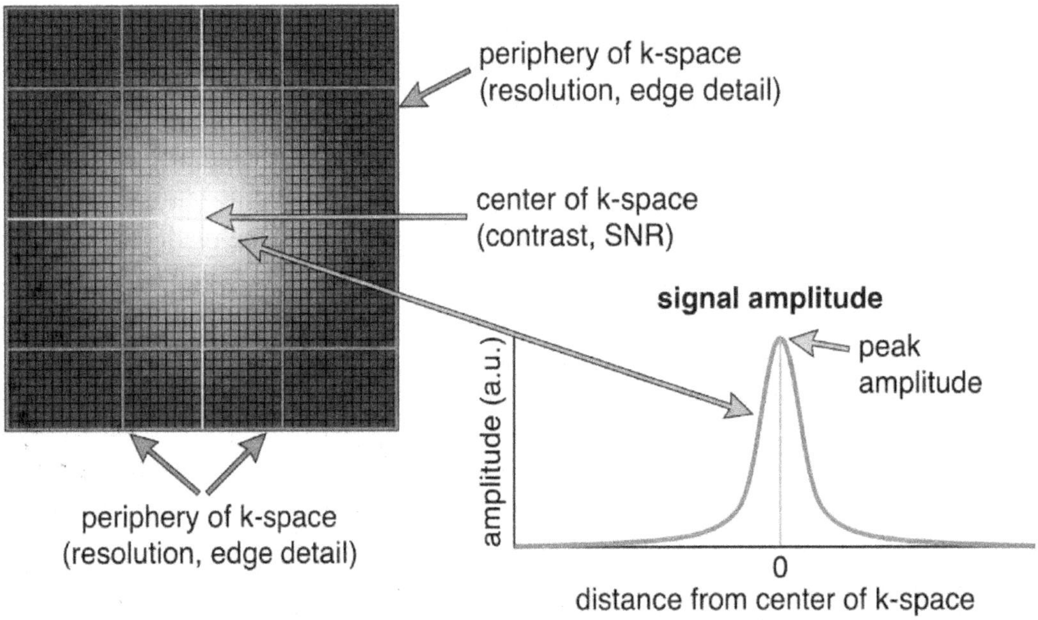

k-Space Filling Strategies and Their Trade-offs

Raw MR signal data are stored not as an image but as k-space, a matrix in which each point represents spatial frequency information rather than a direct spatial location; the center of k-space encodes overall image contrast and signal-to-noise, while the periphery encodes fine spatial detail and edge sharpness. An image is reconstructed from k-space by an inverse Fourier transform. Because different regions of k-space can be filled in different orders and at different rates, k-space filling strategy has direct clinical consequences. Sequences that fill the center of k-space early, a strategy exploited in single-shot and radial acquisitions, are relatively robust to motion because the contrast-determining data are acquired before significant patient movement can occur, which is why single-shot fast spin-echo sequences remain diagnostic even in patients who cannot suspend respiration. Conventional sequential k-space filling, by contrast, is more vulnerable to motion because data acquired at different points in the respiratory or cardiac cycle are combined into a single reconstruction, producing the ghosting and blurring artifacts discussed in the next chapter. Parallel imaging techniques, which use the differing spatial sensitivity profiles of multiple receiver coil elements to reconstruct a full image from an undersampled k-space, shorten acquisition time proportionally to the undersampling factor but reduce signal-to-noise ratio and, at high acceleration factors, can introduce characteristic wrap-around or noise-amplification artifacts concentrated toward the center of the image.

CAUTION: Aliasing, or wrap-around artifact, occurs when anatomy outside the prescribed field of view is nonetheless within the sensitive volume of the receiver coil; because phase encoding cannot distinguish position beyond one full cycle, this tissue is mismapped to the opposite side of the image. In body imaging this most often appears as a fold-over of the abdominal wall or contralateral shoulder onto the region of interest and should not be mistaken for a soft tissue mass.

Parallel Imaging, Acceleration, and Motion-Robust Acquisition Strategies

Parallel Imaging Reconstruction: SENSE and GRAPPA

Parallel imaging exploits the fact that each element of a multichannel receiver coil array has a distinct, spatially varying sensitivity profile, so that an undersampled k-space acquisition, one in which fewer phase-encoding steps are collected than would ordinarily be required, can still be reconstructed into a full image if the differing coil sensitivities are used to resolve the resulting ambiguity. Sensitivity encoding, commonly abbreviated SENSE, performs this reconstruction in the image domain: aliased images from each coil element, produced because the reduced phase-encoding sampling causes distant points in anatomy to fold onto one another, are unfolded using a previously measured map of each coil's spatial sensitivity. Generalized autocalibrating partially parallel acquisition, abbreviated GRAPPA, instead performs an analogous correction directly in k-space, synthesizing the missing phase-encoding lines from the acquired lines using coil-sensitivity information embedded in a small number of additional calibration lines acquired at the center of k-space. Both approaches shorten acquisition time in proportion to the acceleration factor selected, but both also reduce signal-to-noise ratio by an amount that depends on the acceleration factor and on the geometry of the coil array relative to the anatomy being imaged, a penalty quantified as the geometry factor, or g-factor. In practice, body MRI protocols rarely use acceleration factors much beyond two to three for this reason: signal-to-noise ratio in the abdomen is already comparatively limited relative to the brain or extremities, and aggressive acceleration produces diffuse image noise and, in regions of unfavorable coil geometry, focal noise amplification artifacts that can be mistaken for subtle pathology if the reader is unaware of the acquisition parameters used.

Compressed Sensing and Free-Breathing Acquisition Strategies

Compressed sensing extends the principle of undersampling further by exploiting the fact that most diagnostic MR images are sparse, or highly compressible, in an appropriate mathematical transform domain, meaning that far fewer independent data points are truly required to reconstruct a diagnostic-quality image than conventional Nyquist sampling would suggest. By acquiring k-space in a deliberately incoherent, pseudo-random pattern and reconstructing with an iterative algorithm that enforces both data consistency and sparsity, compressed sensing achieves acceleration factors considerably higher than parallel imaging alone can provide, and it is frequently combined with parallel imaging in current-generation body protocols. This combination has been particularly transformative for free-breathing dynamic contrast-enhanced imaging of the liver, in which continuous, golden-angle radial k-space acquisition throughout the respiratory cycle, reconstructed retrospectively into discrete respiratory or temporal bins, allows diagnostic-quality arterial phase imaging even in patients who cannot reliably suspend respiration, a population in whom conventional breath-hold dynamic imaging would otherwise be severely degraded by respiratory motion misregistration between phases. The trade-off, familiar by now, is computational: these reconstructions are more sensitive to patient motion that is irregular rather than periodic, and reconstruction artifacts can appear as streaking or temporal blurring that must be distinguished from true enhancement heterogeneity, reinforcing the chapter's central lesson that every acquisition strategy resolves one limitation by introducing a different one, and diagnostic confidence depends on recognizing which trade-off is in play for the sequence in front of you.

Field Strength, Coil Selection, and Signal Optimization

1.5 Tesla Versus 3 Tesla: Trade-offs for Body Imaging

Higher field strength increases baseline signal-to-noise ratio roughly in proportion to field strength, which can be reinvested as higher spatial resolution, faster acquisition, or both, and this advantage has made 3-tesla imaging increasingly standard for applications that demand fine spatial detail, such as prostate and rectal cancer staging. Higher field strength, however, also proportionally increases the frequency separation between fat and water protons, which worsens chemical shift artifact and, more importantly, shortens the tissue relaxation time constant T2-star, increasing susceptibility artifact near bowel gas, surgical clips, and other metal, a particular liability in the abdomen and pelvis where bowel gas is essentially universal. Radiofrequency energy deposition, quantified as specific absorption rate, also rises with the square of field strength, which can necessitate longer repetition times or reduced flip angles at 3 tesla and thereby offset some of the theoretical time savings. The choice of field strength in body imaging is therefore not simply a matter of using the newer or more powerful magnet; it is a deliberate trade-off between signal and resolution on one hand and susceptibility artifact and specific absorption rate limitations on the other, and protocol design should account for which factor dominates for a given clinical indication.

Specific absorption rate deserves particular attention in body protocol design because the abdomen and pelvis, unlike the brain, contain large volumes of conductive tissue and are frequently imaged with sequence trains that use multiple closely spaced refocusing pulses, both of which increase radiofrequency power deposition. Regulatory limits cap whole-body and partial-body specific absorption rate to protect against tissue heating, and when a prescribed sequence would exceed these limits, the scanner software automatically compensates, most commonly by lengthening repetition time, reducing the refocusing flip angle in turbo spin-echo sequences, or reducing the number of slices per acquisition, any of which can silently lengthen scan time or alter image contrast relative to what was intended. This becomes clinically relevant in larger patients and in specific absorption rate-sensitive populations such as pregnant patients, where protocols are deliberately modified in advance, discussed further in the chapter on body MRI in pediatric and pregnant patients, rather than left to automatic compensation at the time of scanning. A protocol that unexpectedly takes longer than usual, or that shows subtly different contrast than the same sequence obtained on a different patient, should prompt the reader to consider whether specific absorption rate-driven parameter adjustment, rather than a scanner malfunction, is the explanation.

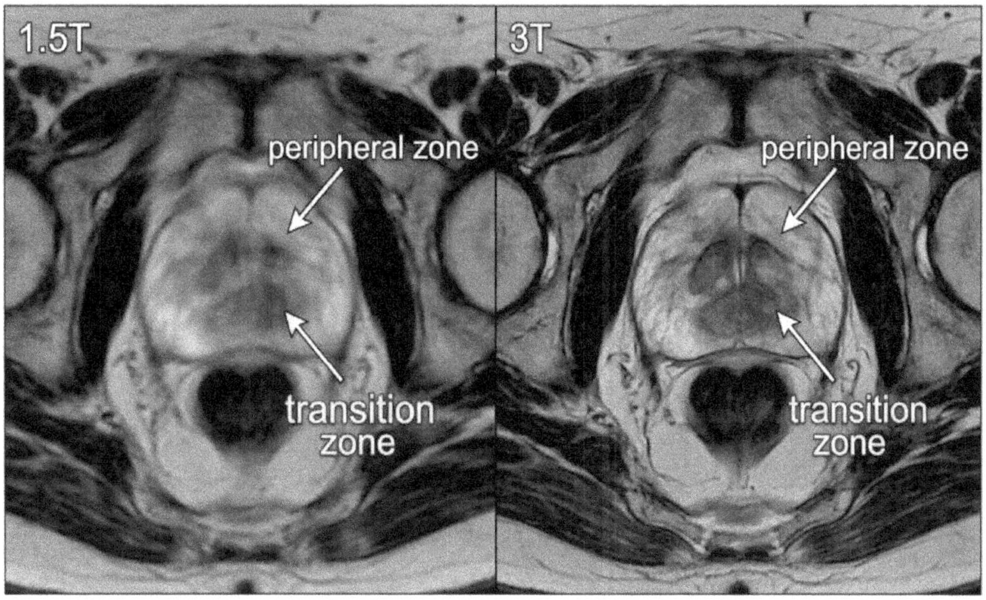

Coil Selection and Signal-to-Noise Ratio

Signal-to-noise ratio depends not only on field strength but on the proximity and design of the receiver coil, because signal reception falls off rapidly with distance from the coil element while background noise is comparatively distance-independent. Multichannel phased-array surface coils, positioned directly against the body surface, provide substantially higher local signal-to-noise ratio than the whole-body coil built into the magnet bore, and modern body protocols rely on combining the signal from many small, closely spaced coil elements both to maximize signal near the coil and to enable the parallel imaging acceleration described earlier in this chapter. Endorectal coils, used selectively in prostate imaging when very high spatial resolution of the peripheral zone is required, exploit this same distance-dependence to dramatic effect but introduce their own susceptibility and distortion artifacts near the coil itself and are used less routinely now that high-quality external phased-array imaging at 3 tesla has narrowed the resolution gap for most clinical indications.

THE SIGNAL-TO-CATEGORY DECISION SYSTEM — Susceptibility Artifact from Metallic Hardware and Surgical Clips

The Signal Pattern: A focal area of marked signal loss with adjacent geometric distortion and, on gradient-echo sequences in particular, a blooming pattern that extends well beyond the true size of the causative structure, most conspicuous near surgical clips, embolization coils, or orthopedic hardware.

Category Signature: This pattern is categorized as a technical susceptibility artifact rather than a soft tissue abnormality when its geometry is round or linear and matches a known prior surgical or interventional history, and when it is disproportionately more severe on gradient-echo than on spin-echo sequences at the same anatomic level.

The Decision: No further characterization is required for artifact confidently attributed to known hardware; if a discrepant clinical history or an asymmetric, expanding pattern raises concern for a separate process obscured by the artifact, a fast spin-echo sequence with a wide receiver bandwidth, or a dedicated metal artifact reduction sequence, should be obtained rather than accepting the gradient-echo appearance as definitive.

Trap Logic: Susceptibility artifact can obscure a genuine local recurrence or abscess adjacent to a surgical bed, and the temptation is to attribute all signal loss near known hardware to the hardware itself; the discriminating step is comparing the artifact's severity and geometry against sequences less sensitive to susceptibility, since a true soft tissue process will remain visible on those sequences while pure artifact will markedly diminish.

Pattern Anchor: When metal artifact and possible pathology overlap, switch to fast spin-echo with wide bandwidth before concluding the area cannot be assessed.

Clinical Case Presentations

Case 1. A 52-year-old woman undergoes MRI for characterization of an incidentally discovered right adrenal nodule found on a CT performed for unrelated abdominal pain. The radiologist reviewing the in-phase and opposed-phase gradient-echo images notes that the nodule loses signal intensity relative to the spleen on the opposed-phase sequence, and that this signal loss is present throughout the interior of the nodule rather than confined to a thin peripheral line. Recognizing this as intravoxel lipid signal drop-out rather than a chemical shift boundary artifact, the radiologist confidently characterizes the nodule as a lipid-rich adenoma, a benign finding requiring no further imaging. The report specifically documents the internal, rather than peripheral, distribution of signal loss to distinguish the finding from the India ink artifact that would otherwise be visible at the interface between the adrenal gland and surrounding retroperitoneal fat, and no follow-up imaging is recommended.

Case 2. A 68-year-old man with a remote history of cholecystectomy undergoes MRI for evaluation of vague right upper quadrant discomfort. Gradient-echo images through the gallbladder fossa demonstrate a focal area of signal loss with surrounding geometric distortion, corresponding to a surgical clip from the prior cholecystectomy. Because the referring clinician's note raises concern for a possible retained stone or abscess in this region, the radiologist does not simply attribute the finding to expected postsurgical artifact. Instead, a supplemental fast spin-echo sequence with widened receiver bandwidth is reviewed, on which the artifact is substantially smaller and no discrete fluid collection or soft tissue abnormality is identified adjacent to the clip. The final report distinguishes expected susceptibility artifact from the surgical clip from any residual pathology, reassures the referring clinician that no abscess or retained stone is present, and illustrates why a single gradient-echo sequence should never be the sole basis for excluding pathology immediately adjacent to metallic hardware.

Case 3. A 44-year-old man with a body mass index of forty-one is referred for MRI to characterize a hepatic lesion identified on ultrasound. The initial free-breathing dynamic contrast-enhanced series, acquired using a golden-angle radial acquisition with retrospective respiratory binning because the patient cannot reliably suspend respiration for the required duration, demonstrates streak-like artifact radiating from the aorta during the arterial phase images, raising concern among the technologist that the study may be nondiagnostic. Reviewing the images at the workstation, the radiologist recognizes the streaking as an expected consequence of angular undersampling inherent to the radial acquisition strategy at this patient's body habitus, most conspicuous near high-signal vascular structures during peak arterial enhancement, rather than a sign of true perfusion abnormality or motion misregistration. Because the streaking is symmetric around the aorta and does not correspond to a discrete parenchymal lesion, and because the liver parenchyma itself remains sufficiently free of artifact to characterize the lesion in question, which shows classic arterial phase hyperenhancement with portal venous washout, the radiologist proceeds to a confident diagnosis without repeating the sequence. The report notes the expected radial streak artifact explicitly, both to preempt any confusion on subsequent comparison examinations and to document that it was recognized and did not compromise lesion characterization, illustrating how understanding the specific acquisition strategy used, rather than treating every image as a generic photograph, is what allows a reader to distinguish an expected consequence of accelerated acquisition from a genuine diagnostic limitation.

THE SIGNAL-TO-CATEGORY DECISION SYSTEM — Foundational Artifact Recognition Arc

The Signal Pattern: This chapter introduced two recurring signal patterns that every subsequent chapter will build upon: intravoxel signal loss on opposed-phase imaging, and susceptibility-related signal loss and distortion near tissue interfaces or metal.

Category Signature: Internal, whole-lesion signal drop-out on opposed-phase imaging signifies lipid and a benign category; a thin peripheral dark line at any fat-water interface, or focal signal loss and distortion matched to known hardware geometry, signifies artifact and no category assignment is needed.

The Decision: Confident artifact recognition allows a lipid-rich adrenal adenoma to be characterized without follow-up and allows postsurgical susceptibility change to be dismissed without additional workup, while genuinely ambiguous cases are resolved by comparing gradient-echo findings against a less susceptibility-sensitive fast spin-echo sequence.

Trap Logic: The most common error across both patterns is treating a technical phenomenon as if it carries independent diagnostic weight, either overcalling a benign adenoma as indeterminate because of a misread India ink line, or dismissing genuine adjacent pathology because it lies near expected surgical artifact.

Pattern Anchor: Before signing out any signal loss on a body MRI, ask whether the pattern is internal to a lesion or confined to an interface or known hardware; that single distinction resolves the majority of artifact-versus-pathology questions in this book.

Summary and Key Concepts

MR signal originates from the small excess of hydrogen nuclei aligned with the static magnetic field, and its strength scales with field strength, which is why higher-field systems provide greater baseline signal-to-noise ratio.

T1 and T2 relaxation are intrinsic tissue properties; pulse sequence design determines which property is emphasized, which is why the same tissue can appear bright or dark depending entirely on the sequence used.

Spin-echo sequences correct for static field inhomogeneity and are relatively motion-robust; gradient-echo sequences are faster and enable dynamic contrast imaging but are inherently more sensitive to susceptibility artifact.

In-phase and opposed-phase imaging distinguishes true intravoxel lipid, a benign and diagnostically useful finding, from chemical shift boundary artifact, which carries no diagnostic weight and should never be mistaken for a lesion margin.

Diffusion-weighted imaging must always be interpreted alongside the apparent diffusion coefficient map to distinguish true restricted diffusion from T2 shine-through.

k-space filling strategy determines an acquisition's motion robustness; center-weighted and single-shot strategies tolerate motion far better than conventional sequential filling.

Field strength and coil selection trade signal-to-noise and resolution against susceptibility artifact and specific absorption rate, and protocol decisions should be tailored to which factor matters most for a given clinical question.

CHAPTER 2: BODY MRI PROTOCOL DESIGN AND SEQUENCE OPTIMIZATION

Learning Objectives

1. Apply the core principles of body MRI protocol design, including sequence selection, coverage, and the ordering of acquisitions within an examination.
2. Compare breath-hold, free-breathing, respiratory-triggered, and free-breathing radial acquisition strategies and select the appropriate approach for a given patient and clinical indication.
3. Explain the physiologic and technical basis of contrast bolus timing and predict the consequences of mistimed arterial phase acquisition.
4. Recognize the organ-specific protocol modifications required for hepatobiliary, pancreatic, renal, and pelvic MRI, and identify the most common protocol-related pitfalls in each.
5. Troubleshoot a suboptimal or nondiagnostic body MRI examination by identifying which protocol parameter is responsible and how it can be corrected.

Clinical Overview

A body MRI protocol is not a fixed template applied uniformly to every patient and every indication; it is a sequence of deliberate decisions, which sequences to acquire, in what order, with what coverage, timed against what physiologic event, that together determine whether the resulting examination answers the clinical question it was ordered to answer. The same physical principles introduced in the previous chapter, relaxation contrast, k-space filling strategy, field strength trade-offs, resurface here as practical protocol choices: a liver protocol built around dynamic contrast-enhanced imaging is only diagnostic if the arterial phase is timed correctly, a pancreatic protocol is only adequate if pancreatic-phase imaging is acquired before contrast redistributes into the interstitium, and a rectal cancer staging protocol is only interpretable if bowel peristalsis has been adequately suppressed. Protocol design is therefore inseparable from diagnostic interpretation; a radiologist who understands why a protocol is built the way it is can recognize immediately when a given examination has deviated from that design and can decide, often before the patient has left the scanner, whether the deviation is correctable.

Principles of Protocol Design in Body MRI

Matching Sequence Selection to the Clinical Question

Every body MRI protocol begins with the clinical indication, not with a generic organ-based template, because the sequences that best answer one question about an organ are frequently different from those that best answer another. A protocol built to characterize an incidentally discovered renal mass prioritizes precontrast imaging, corticomedullary and nephrographic phase dynamic imaging, and in-phase and opposed-phase sequences to assess for macroscopic and microscopic fat, while a protocol built to evaluate hematuria in the absence of a known mass instead prioritizes excretory-phase imaging of the collecting system and ureters, a fundamentally different acquisition strategy despite imaging the same organ. This principle, that the clinical question determines the protocol rather than the organ alone, recurs throughout the organ-specific chapters of this book and is the reason a single generic abdominal protocol, however comprehensive, is rarely the correct answer to every referral.

This principle extends to the choice of contrast agent itself. Extracellular gadolinium-based agents distribute into the vascular and interstitial space and are excreted renally, providing dynamic enhancement information without hepatocyte-specific delayed imaging, and remain the appropriate default for most abdominal and pelvic indications, including renal, pancreatic, and pelvic oncologic protocols. Hepatobiliary-specific agents, which are taken up by functioning hepatocytes and excreted in part into bile, add a hepatobiliary phase that provides incremental specificity for hepatocellular lesion characterization and for detecting biliary leaks, but come with a smaller bolus and different optimal injection rate, and their delayed hepatobiliary phase can be degraded in patients with significantly impaired hepatic function, in whom hepatocyte uptake is reduced and background liver-to-lesion contrast on the delayed phase falls proportionately. Selecting the correct contrast agent before the patient reaches the scanner, rather than defaulting reflexively to whichever agent is used most often in a given department, is therefore itself a protocol design decision with direct diagnostic consequences, not merely a matter of pharmacy stock or cost.

Sequence redundancy is a related and frequently underappreciated design principle: a well-designed protocol builds in at least one form of cross-check for its most diagnostically consequential findings, such as acquiring both in-phase and opposed-phase imaging so that a chemical shift artifact can always be distinguished from true lipid content, or acquiring both axial and coronal T2-weighted sequences so that an equivocal finding on one plane can be confirmed or refuted on another. This redundancy is not wasted acquisition time; it is what allows a radiologist to resolve the artifact-versus-pathology questions that recur throughout this book without requiring a separate follow-up examination, and protocols that omit this redundancy in the name of efficiency frequently generate more total imaging, through recalled or repeated studies, than they save.

Coverage, Slice Thickness, and Spatial Resolution Trade-offs

Coverage refers to the anatomic volume included in a given sequence, and it must be set deliberately rather than defaulted to a fixed range, because inadequate coverage is one of the most common and most easily preventable causes of a nondiagnostic examination. A liver protocol intended to evaluate for hepatocellular carcinoma in a cirrhotic patient must extend from the dome of the diaphragm through the lower pole of the kidneys to capture the entire liver as well as any extrahepatic disease, while a dedicated prostate protocol can restrict coverage to the true pelvis, allowing finer in-plane spatial resolution within the smaller field of view. This trade-off, that a fixed acquisition matrix divided across a smaller field of view yields smaller voxels and higher spatial resolution, while the same matrix divided across a larger field of view yields larger voxels and lower resolution, is the same fundamental trade-off between signal-to-noise ratio, spatial resolution, and acquisition time introduced in the previous chapter, now applied at the level of protocol design rather than pulse sequence physics. Slice thickness follows the same logic:

thinner slices improve through-plane resolution and reduce partial volume averaging of small structures, such as a subcentimeter pancreatic side-branch duct or a small adnexal lesion, but proportionally reduce signal-to-noise ratio per slice and increase total acquisition time, so slice thickness should be selected based on the smallest structure the protocol is specifically designed to detect or characterize.

Adapting Protocols for Patient-Specific Factors

Body habitus is among the most consequential patient-specific factors in protocol design, because signal-to-noise ratio falls with increasing distance from the receiver coil and with increasing tissue depth for radiofrequency penetration, so a standard protocol optimized for an average-sized patient frequently yields a noisier, lower-quality examination in a patient with a substantially larger body habitus. Compensating for this typically requires a deliberate combination of strategies rather than a single fix: increasing the number of signal averages to recover signal-to-noise ratio at the cost of longer acquisition time, widening the receiver bandwidth selectively where susceptibility rather than noise is the dominant concern, and, where available, selecting a larger-bore or wide-aperture magnet configuration that better accommodates coil placement. Conversely, in a very thin patient or a pediatric patient, the field of view and coil selection should be reduced accordingly to preserve spatial resolution rather than defaulting to an adult-sized field of view that wastes spatial resolution on empty space beyond the anatomy of interest. Patients with limited ability to remain still for a long examination, whether due to pain, altered mental status, or, in the pediatric population discussed in greater depth later in this book, developmental inability to cooperate, similarly require deliberate protocol truncation to the highest-yield sequences, sedation planning coordinated in advance, or substitution of faster, more motion-robust sequence variants even at some cost to spatial resolution, since a shorter, motion-free examination that answers the clinical question is diagnostically superior to a longer, more detailed protocol degraded by uncorrectable motion.

Breath-Hold, Free-Breathing, and Respiratory Compensation Strategies

Breath-Hold Acquisition and Its Limitations

Breath-hold acquisition remains the default strategy for most upper abdominal sequences because suspended respiration eliminates bulk respiratory motion during the acquisition window, producing sharp anatomic detail and reliable multiphase contrast timing. The principal limitation is patient-dependent: breath-hold sequences are typically designed around a fifteen- to twenty-second hold, and patients with poor pulmonary reserve, advanced age, sedation, or significant pain frequently cannot sustain a hold of this length without motion degrading the later portion of the acquisition, an especially consequential problem when the degraded portion corresponds to the peripheral, high-spatial-frequency regions of k-space that determine image sharpness. Coaching the patient before the sequence begins, including a practice breath-hold and clear instructions about the specific phase of respiration to hold, meaningfully improves compliance and should be regarded as a technical parameter of the protocol rather than a matter of bedside manner alone.

Supplemental oxygen, when appropriate and coordinated with the referring team, can meaningfully extend achievable breath-hold duration in patients with borderline pulmonary reserve by delaying the onset of air hunger, and some departments incorporate brief preoxygenation into the workflow for patients identified in advance as likely to struggle with prolonged holds. Beyond physiologic measures, the specific instruction given to the patient matters more than is often appreciated: instructing a patient simply to hold their breath, without specifying the depth or the point in the respiratory cycle at which to do so, produces inconsistent diaphragmatic position across sequential breath-holds, since patients tend to drift toward progressively shallower holds as an examination proceeds and fatigue accumulates, and this inconsistency is precisely what produces the interslice or intersequence misregistration discussed in the artifact pattern below. Standardizing the coaching instruction, most commonly asking the patient to hold at a comfortable, reproducible end-expiratory position rather than a maximal inspiratory one, and repeating that identical instruction verbatim before every hold, is a simple, no-cost intervention that measurably improves multiphase image registration.

Free-Breathing, Navigator-Triggered, and Radial Strategies

When breath-holding is unreliable, several alternative strategies substitute technical motion compensation for patient cooperation. Respiratory triggering uses an external bellows or navigator echo, a signal derived from the diaphragm or another moving structure, to acquire data only during a consistent portion of the respiratory cycle, typically end-expiration, at the cost of longer and less predictable total scan time because data acquisition pauses during the remainder of each respiratory cycle. Free-breathing radial acquisitions with retrospective motion correction, introduced in the previous chapter's discussion of compressed sensing, instead acquire data continuously throughout free respiration and sort or correct the data after acquisition, providing more predictable scan times and generally superior patient tolerance, particularly valuable for dynamic contrast-enhanced sequences in patients who cannot reliably breath-hold through multiple contrast phases. Averaging strategies, in which the same k-space line is acquired multiple times and combined, reduce the visual impact of motion by blurring rather than eliminating it, a reasonable compromise for sequences such as heavily T2-weighted single-shot imaging where mild blurring is better tolerated diagnostically than the ghosting artifact produced by uncorrected periodic motion.

THE SIGNAL-TO-CATEGORY DECISION SYSTEM — Respiratory Misregistration and the Pseudo-Lesion Trap

---

The Signal Pattern: A focal area of apparent signal discontinuity or a curvilinear band of artifactual signal change at the liver dome or splenic tip, most conspicuous on sequences acquired across multiple breath-holds of inconsistent depth.

Category Signature: A finding present on only one sequence, with a geometry that follows the diaphragmatic contour rather than a plausible lesion margin, and that is absent when the corresponding anatomic level is reviewed on an adjacent sequence acquired at a different point in the respiratory cycle, is categorized as respiratory misregistration artifact rather than a true parenchymal abnormality.

The Decision: No further characterization is needed once misregistration is confirmed by comparing the suspicious region across all available sequences and, if necessary, requesting a repeat acquisition with a coached, reproducible breath-hold depth; a finding that persists in the same location and geometry across independently acquired sequences should instead be worked up as a true lesion.

Trap Logic: Misregistration artifact is most treacherous when it occurs at a fixed anatomic location across an entire examination because the reader may reasonably assume that reproducibility implies a true finding; the discriminating step is confirming reproducibility of a genuine lesion's signal characteristics across sequences of different contrast weighting, not merely reproducibility of its location, since artifact tied to the diaphragm recurs at the same location regardless of underlying tissue contrast.

Pattern Anchor: A subcapsular hepatic or splenic abnormality that changes contour or disappears when compared across sequences taken at different breath-hold depths is misregistration, not pathology.

Figure 2.1: Aortic Time-Intensity Curve for Contrast Bolus Timing

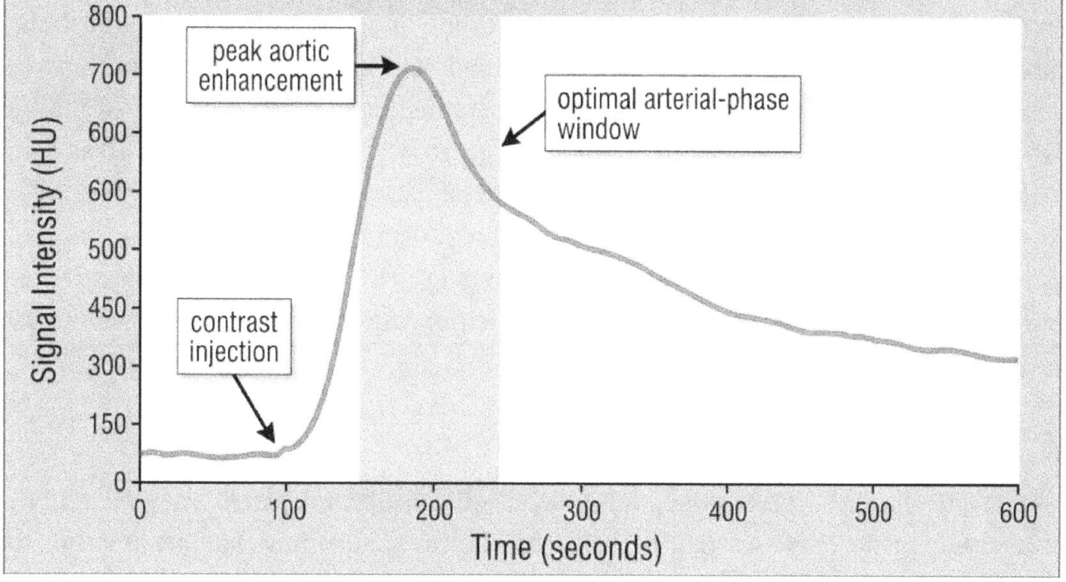

Contrast Timing and Dynamic Phase Acquisition

Bolus Tracking and Test Bolus Techniques

Because the interval between contrast injection and peak arterial enhancement varies with cardiac output, injection rate, and venous access, fixed-delay arterial phase timing is unreliable across the range of patients encountered in clinical practice, particularly in patients with reduced cardiac output, in whom contrast arrival is delayed, or hyperdynamic circulation, in whom it is accelerated. Bolus tracking techniques monitor signal intensity in the aorta in real time during contrast injection using a low-resolution monitoring sequence and automatically trigger the diagnostic arterial-phase acquisition once a predefined signal threshold is reached, adapting the timing to each patient's individual circulation. Test bolus techniques instead inject a small preliminary volume of contrast before the diagnostic bolus, measure the time to peak aortic enhancement from this test injection, and use that measured delay to time the subsequent diagnostic acquisition; this approach is more predictable but adds contrast volume and total examination time. Both techniques share the same underlying goal, replacing a fixed assumption about circulation time with a patient-specific measurement, and understanding which technique produced a given arterial phase image helps explain occasional timing failures, such as a test bolus performed with a different injection rate than the diagnostic bolus, which can introduce a systematic timing error.

Consequences of Mistimed Arterial Phase Imaging

Arterial phase timing is not a matter of technical elegance alone; it directly determines diagnostic accuracy for the vascular enhancement patterns that define hepatocellular carcinoma, renal cell carcinoma, and numerous other body malignancies. An arterial phase acquired too early, before peak hepatic arterial inflow, understates the true degree of arterial enhancement a lesion will ultimately demonstrate and can cause a truly hypervascular lesion to appear only mildly or equivocally enhancing, a false-negative pattern that risks missing a lesion that meets categorical criteria for malignancy on a properly timed acquisition. An arterial phase acquired too late allows contrast to have already begun washing out of a hypervascular lesion and redistributing into surrounding parenchyma, producing a so-called pseudo-washout appearance in which normal background parenchymal enhancement has caught up to, or even exceeds, lesion enhancement, mimicking the washout pattern otherwise considered a specific sign of malignancy in an entirely different, spurious way. Because both timing errors can alter categorical assignment under frameworks such as LI-RADS, discussed in detail in the hepatobiliary chapters of this book, recognizing the visual signature of mistimed arterial phase acquisition, most reliably the appearance of the hepatic and portal veins on the same acquisition, incompletely enhancing in a correctly timed true arterial phase, fully enhancing in a late arterial or early portal venous acquisition, is an essential quality-control skill for any reader of body MRI.

Dual and Delayed Phase Imaging Considerations

Beyond the arterial phase, portal venous and delayed or equilibrium phase imaging serve distinct and complementary diagnostic purposes that protocol design must accommodate separately. Portal venous phase imaging, acquired roughly sixty to seventy seconds after contrast injection, provides the strongest parenchymal enhancement and is generally the most sensitive phase for detecting hypovascular lesions, such as most pancreatic adenocarcinomas and many hepatic metastases, which enhance less than surrounding parenchyma and are therefore best seen against a maximally enhanced background. Delayed or equilibrium phase imaging, acquired at three to five minutes, captures the washout behavior that is central to hepatocellular carcinoma characterization and also allows detection of delayed enhancement patterns characteristic of certain fibrous or desmoplastic lesions, such as cholangiocarcinoma, which characteristically shows progressive, rather than washout, enhancement into the delayed phase. Because these two phases interrogate fundamentally different pathophysiology, a protocol that substitutes one for the other, for instance omitting true delayed imaging in favor of a second portal venous acquisition to save time, quietly sacrifices the specific diagnostic information that only delayed-phase washout or progressive enhancement can provide, an omission that is not always apparent to the interpreting radiologist unless the protocol's phase timing is explicitly documented and reviewed.

Figure 2.2 — Optimal Breath-Hold Coaching Sequence for Multiphase Hepatic Imaging

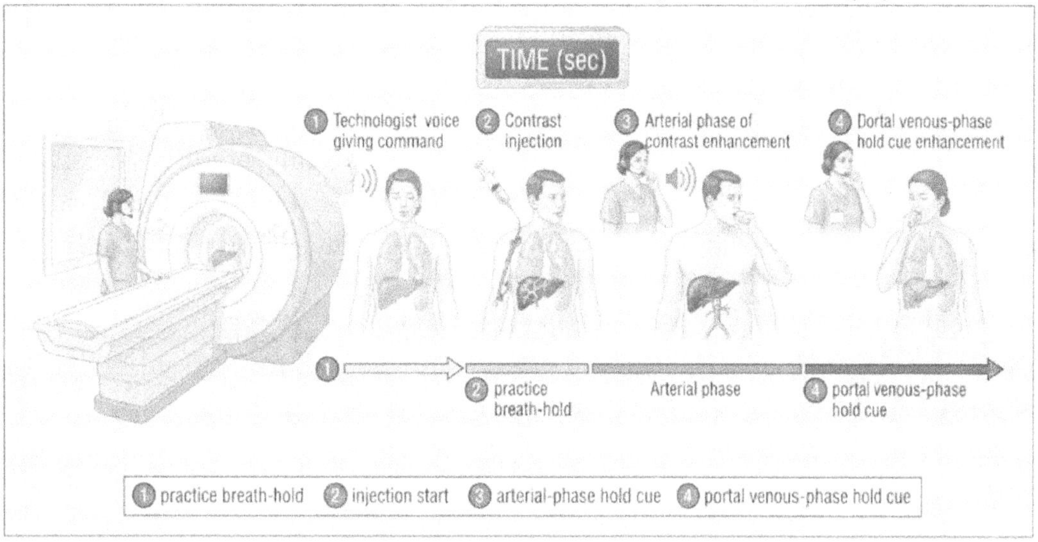

Figure 2.2 — Optimal Breath-Hold Coaching Sequence for Multiphase Hepatic Imaging

Sequence Ordering, Total Examination Time, and Efficiency

Sequencing Acquisitions to Protect Diagnostic Priorities

The order in which sequences are acquired within an examination is itself a protocol design decision, because patient fatigue, motion, and, in sedated or critically ill patients, physiologic instability all tend to accumulate over the course of a long examination, so the sequences most critical to the primary clinical question should generally be acquired while the patient is freshest and most cooperative rather than left until the end as an afterthought. In a liver protocol built around dynamic contrast-enhanced imaging, the precontrast and immediate postcontrast dynamic phases are timed against the contrast bolus and cannot be delayed, which fixes their position in the sequence and requires that all other, non-time-critical sequences, such as additional T2-weighted or diffusion-weighted imaging, be scheduled either before contrast administration or in the intervals between critical dynamic phases, so that the fixed-timing sequences are never at risk of being rushed or omitted because of accumulated delay earlier in the examination. Diffusion-weighted imaging deserves particular scheduling attention because, unlike most other sequences, it is generally unaffected by the presence of extracellular gadolinium contrast and can therefore be acquired at essentially any point in the protocol, giving the technologist flexibility to place it wherever it best fills an otherwise idle interval, such as during the delay before a hepatobiliary phase.

Total Examination Time as a Quality Variable

Total examination time is often treated purely as an operational or scheduling concern, but it is also a direct determinant of diagnostic quality, because longer examinations proportionally increase the cumulative probability of patient motion, discomfort, and, in claustrophobic or anxious patients, premature termination before all diagnostically necessary sequences are complete. Protocol designers must therefore weigh the incremental diagnostic value of each additional sequence against this cumulative risk; a protocol that adds a marginal sequence of limited incremental value at the cost of five additional minutes may paradoxically reduce overall diagnostic yield if that additional time meaningfully increases the likelihood that the patient cannot tolerate the full examination. This trade-off is the underlying rationale for abbreviated protocols used in specific clinical contexts, such as hepatocellular carcinoma surveillance in patients at only modest risk, where a shortened sequence set focused on the highest-yield contrasts, typically T2-weighted, diffusion-weighted, and limited dynamic imaging, preserves most of the diagnostic sensitivity of a full diagnostic protocol while substantially reducing total table time, patient burden, and cost, an approach increasingly supported by outcomes data in appropriately selected surveillance populations.

Organ System	Time-Critical Sequences	Flexible-Timing Sequences	Common Scheduling Error
Liver (dynamic protocol)	Precontrast, arterial, portal venous, delayed dynamic phases	T2-weighted, diffusion-weighted, in/opposed-phase	Diffusion-weighted imaging acquired after contrast in a protocol requiring precontrast diffusion baseline
Pancreas	Pancreatic parenchymal phase (earlier than hepatic arterial phase)	Precontrast T1, MRCP	Pancreatic phase timed identically to hepatic arterial phase, missing true peak pancreatic enhancement
Prostate	Diffusion-weighted and dynamic contrast-enhanced sequences	T2-weighted high-resolution sequences	Patient motion accumulating before diffusion-weighted imaging is acquired late in a long protocol
Rectum	T2-weighted high-resolution sequences after adequate distension	Diffusion-weighted imaging	High-resolution T2 acquired before antiperistaltic agent has taken effect

Organ-Specific Protocol Considerations and Common Pitfalls

Hepatobiliary and Pancreatic Protocol Considerations

Hepatobiliary protocols typically include a hepatobiliary phase, acquired ten to twenty minutes after administration of a hepatobiliary-specific gadolinium contrast agent, during which normal functioning hepatocytes take up and excrete contrast into bile canaliculi while most malignant hepatocellular lesions, lacking normal hepatocyte transporter function, do not, producing a pattern of relative lesion hypointensity that adds diagnostic specificity beyond dynamic phase imaging alone. This delayed phase requires deliberate protocol planning, including scheduling of other sequences to fill the intervening delay productively, and its diagnostic value depends on adequate patient cooperation with a final breath-hold potentially twenty minutes after the patient's last successful hold, by which point fatigue can meaningfully degrade image quality if not anticipated. Pancreatic protocols place unusual emphasis on a distinct pancreatic parenchymal phase, timed earlier than the hepatic arterial phase because the pancreas enhances earlier than the liver, and on thin-section, fat-suppressed T1-weighted imaging, because the pancreas's intrinsically high T1 signal relative to surrounding structures makes fat suppression essential for lesion conspicuity, a technical detail easily overlooked if a pancreatic examination is protocoled as a generic abdominal study rather than a dedicated pancreatic examination.

Magnetic resonance cholangiopancreatography sequences add a further layer of protocol-specific requirement: heavily T2-weighted, either thick-slab single-shot or thin-section three-dimensional acquisitions rely entirely on the intrinsic T2 contrast between static or slow-moving fluid within the bile ducts and pancreatic duct and the surrounding solid tissue, without any contrast agent, and are therefore exquisitely sensitive to any factor that degrades fluid signal or introduces motion, including inadequate fasting, which allows gastric and duodenal fluid to obscure the ampullary region, and incomplete breath-holding on three-dimensional acquisitions, which are more susceptible to motion blurring than single-shot two-dimensional sequences because of their longer acquisition time. A dedicated cholangiopancreatography protocol should therefore always specify an adequate fasting interval, typically four to six hours, and should include both a rapid single-shot sequence, which tolerates poor breath-holding, and, when feasible, a higher-resolution three-dimensional sequence, so that the examination is not left entirely dependent on a single acquisition technique's particular vulnerabilities.

Renal, Pelvic, and Bowel Protocol Considerations

Renal mass protocols require precontrast imaging as an essential, non-optional component, because enhancement is assessed by direct comparison of precontrast and postcontrast signal intensity in the same lesion, an assessment that is impossible if precontrast imaging was omitted under the assumption that postcontrast imaging alone would suffice. Pelvic protocols, particularly for prostate, rectal, and gynecologic oncologic staging, depend heavily on antiperistaltic premedication and bladder and bowel preparation, since peristalsis and excessive bladder or rectal distension both degrade the fine anatomic detail on which local staging depends; a rectal cancer staging examination performed without adequate rectal distension by water or gel, for instance, can significantly understate the conspicuity of the mesorectal fascia, a structure whose involvement is central to surgical planning. Bowel protocols for suspected inflammatory bowel disease require oral contrast administered in sufficient volume and with sufficient time before scanning to achieve adequate small bowel distension, without which bowel wall thickening from inadequate distension can be difficult to distinguish from true inflammatory wall thickening, a distinction covered in detail in the gastrointestinal imaging chapters of this book.

Gynecologic and rectal oncologic staging protocols share a further requirement not always appreciated outside dedicated pelvic imaging practice: high-resolution T2-weighted imaging must be planned in a true short-axis orientation relative to the structure being staged, perpendicular to the endocervical canal for cervical cancer or perpendicular to the long axis of the rectal tumor for rectal cancer, rather than in a fixed body-axial plane, because local staging depends on accurately depicting the relationship between tumor and adjacent structures, the parametrium in cervical cancer or the mesorectal fascia in rectal cancer, in cross-section, and a fixed axial plane obtained without regard to the tumor's or organ's actual orientation can systematically misrepresent the depth and extent of local invasion. Planning these oblique planes correctly requires the technologist to review a preliminary large-field-of-view localizer sequence before prescribing the dedicated high-resolution sequences, an additional planning step that is easy to omit under time pressure but that determines whether the resulting images are actually usable for the staging purpose the examination was ordered to serve.

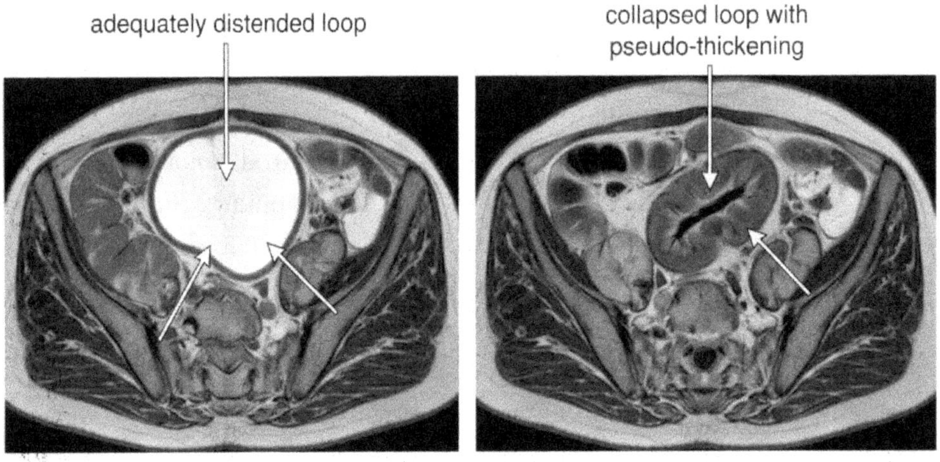

Figure 2.3: Adequately versus Inadequately Distended Small Bowel Loop on MR

Figure 2.3: Adequately versus Inadequately Distended Small Bowel Loop on MR Enterography

THE SIGNAL-TO-CATEGORY DECISION SYSTEM — Incomplete Bowel Distension Mimicking Wall Thickening

The Signal Pattern: A segment of small or large bowel appears to demonstrate mural thickening with mild mucosal enhancement on a single sequence, without the layered wall stratification or adjacent mesenteric changes typically accompanying true active inflammation.

Category Signature: Apparent thickening confined to a nondistended, collapsed bowel loop, particularly one that appears normal in caliber on an adjacent sequence or at a slightly different table position, is categorized as a distension-related pseudo-thickening artifact rather than a true inflammatory or neoplastic process.

The Decision: No further workup is required for a collapsed loop that normalizes on a well-distended sequence; persistent, reproducible wall thickening present across multiple sequences and distension states, especially when accompanied by mesenteric hyperemia or fat stranding, should instead be evaluated as active disease using the criteria detailed in the bowel MRI chapter.

Trap Logic: Distal ileal loops and the sigmoid colon are particularly prone to transient collapse during long bowel protocols, and a single collapsed loop occurring in a patient with known inflammatory bowel disease is easily overcalled as an active segment; the discriminating step is always confirming the same segment on a second sequence or a delayed acquisition before assigning disease activity.

Pattern Anchor: Never characterize bowel wall thickening on a single sequence without confirming that the segment was adequately distended; when in doubt, look for the same loop on another sequence before committing to a diagnosis of active disease.

Clinical Case Presentations

Case 1. A 61-year-old man with cirrhosis undergoes surveillance MRI for hepatocellular carcinoma. The dynamic series demonstrates a two-centimeter hepatic observation that appears only mildly hyperenhancing relative to background liver on the labeled arterial phase image, insufficient by itself to meet criteria for definite arterial phase hyperenhancement. Reviewing the arterial phase image critically, the radiologist notes that the hepatic and portal veins are almost fully enhanced, a finding more consistent with a late arterial or early portal venous phase than a true early arterial phase, and correlates this with the bolus-tracking trigger log, which shows a longer than expected delay between trigger threshold and acquisition start. Recognizing that the labeled arterial phase is very likely mistimed, the radiologist reviews the observation's appearance on the portal venous phase and washout imaging, where it demonstrates unambiguous washout and a capsule appearance, sufficient to establish a confident LI-RADS 5 categorization despite the equivocal arterial phase, and the report specifically notes the timing concern so that a subsequent examination can be adjusted accordingly.

Case 2. A 35-year-old woman with known Crohn disease undergoes MR enterography for assessment of disease activity prior to a medication change. On the initial review, a mid-ileal loop appears to show wall thickening with mild mucosal hyperenhancement, raising concern for an active segment not previously described. Before finalizing this as new disease activity, the radiologist checks the same anatomic region on the coronal single-shot sequence acquired at a slightly later point in the examination and finds the loop to be well distended with a normal, thin wall, confirming that the initial appearance reflected transient underdistension rather than true inflammation. The final report describes the terminal ileum, the segment of primary clinical concern, using only the well-distended sequences, and explicitly notes that the mid-ileal loop in question was reassessed and found to be normal once adequately distended, preventing an incorrect impression of disease progression that could otherwise have altered the patient's treatment plan.

Case 3. A 58-year-old man with painless jaundice is referred for MRI and magnetic resonance cholangiopancreatography to evaluate for a suspected pancreatic head mass. The initial thick-slab single-shot cholangiopancreatography images are markedly degraded by fluid-filled stomach and duodenum overlying the expected location of the ampulla, obscuring the distal common bile duct, and the technologist notes that the patient reports having eaten a light breakfast approximately two hours before the examination rather than observing the intended four-to-six-hour fasting interval. Recognizing that the degraded ampullary detail reflects inadequate fasting rather than a technical failure of the sequence itself, the radiologist requests a repeat three-dimensional cholangiopancreatography acquisition after an additional oral antiperistaltic agent and a period of further fasting, which substantially clears the overlying fluid signal and reveals an abrupt, shouldered stricture of the distal common bile duct with associated upstream ductal dilation, a pattern concerning for malignant obstruction. The final report documents both the initial technical limitation and the corrective step taken, ensuring that the referring surgical team understands the ductal findings were confirmed on adequately prepared imaging rather than relying on the initially degraded sequence.

THE SIGNAL-TO-CATEGORY DECISION SYSTEM — Protocol Quality-Control Arc

---

The Signal Pattern: This chapter's two patterns, respiratory misregistration at organ margins and distension-dependent bowel wall pseudo-thickening, share a common signature: an apparent abnormality present on one sequence or acquisition state that fails to reproduce under a different technical condition.

Category Signature: A finding that changes geometry, disappears, or normalizes when the same anatomy is reviewed under a different breath-hold, distension state, or timing condition is categorized as a technical artifact of protocol execution rather than true pathology.

The Decision: Confirming reproducibility across sequences before committing to a diagnosis, and requesting a targeted repeat acquisition when reproducibility cannot be established, resolves the great majority of these apparent findings without unnecessary follow-up imaging or biopsy.

Trap Logic: The shared trap across this chapter is treating a single sequence as sufficient evidence for a diagnosis; both patterns are only correctly resolved by deliberately cross-checking the finding against a second sequence acquired under different technical conditions.

Pattern Anchor: Before finalizing any equivocal finding at an organ margin or within bowel, confirm it is present on more than one sequence acquired under different breath-hold or distension conditions.

Summary and Key Concepts

Protocol design begins with the clinical question, not a generic organ template; the same organ requires different sequences depending on what the referring clinician needs answered.

Coverage, slice thickness, and spatial resolution are interdependent choices that trade signal-to-noise ratio and acquisition time against diagnostic detail, and should be set deliberately for the indication at hand.

Breath-hold acquisition remains the default for upper abdominal imaging but fails in patients with poor pulmonary reserve; free-breathing, navigator-triggered, and compressed-sensing radial strategies substitute technical motion compensation for patient cooperation.

Bolus tracking and test bolus techniques replace a fixed assumption about circulation time with a patient-specific measurement, and understanding which technique was used explains many otherwise puzzling timing failures.

Mistimed arterial phase imaging can produce false-negative hypoenhancement or a pseudo-washout appearance that mimics malignant washout; the enhancement state of the hepatic and portal veins is a reliable clue to true acquisition timing.

Hepatobiliary, pancreatic, renal, pelvic, and bowel protocols each carry organ-specific requirements, precontrast imaging for renal masses, antiperistaltic premedication for pelvic staging, adequate distension for bowel imaging, whose omission is a common and preventable cause of nondiagnostic examinations.

An apparent abnormality that changes or disappears when compared across sequences acquired under different technical conditions should be presumed artifactual until proven otherwise by reproducibility across multiple acquisitions.

CHAPTER 3: CONTRAST AGENTS, MR SAFETY, AND PATIENT PREPARATION

Learning Objectives

1. Classify gadolinium-based contrast agents by chemical structure and stability, and relate agent class to the risk of gadolinium retention and nephrogenic systemic fibrosis.
2. Apply current renal risk-stratification practice to determine whether and how a gadolinium-based agent should be administered in a patient with impaired renal function.
3. Recognize the clinical spectrum of acute contrast reactions, grade their severity, and outline the corresponding management pathway.
4. Distinguish MR-safe, MR-conditional, and MR-unsafe devices and describe the screening process required before a patient with an implant or device enters the MR environment.
5. Apply practical strategies for patient preparation, including claustrophobia management and positioning, that improve examination completion and diagnostic quality.

Clinical Overview

Contrast administration and MR safety screening are not administrative prerequisites that precede the diagnostic portion of a body MRI examination; they are clinical decisions in their own right, each carrying its own risk-benefit calculation, its own decision thresholds, and its own failure modes that can compromise an examination as thoroughly as a technical protocol error. A radiologist who defers entirely to a standardized screening form or a fixed contrast dosing convention, without understanding the physiology and safety reasoning behind those conventions, is poorly equipped to handle the patient who does not fit the standard pathway, the patient with borderline renal function, the patient with an older-generation cardiac device, or the patient whose anxiety threatens to end the examination before it begins.

This chapter addresses three interlocking domains that together determine whether a body MRI examination can proceed safely and be completed diagnostically: the pharmacology and safety profile of gadolinium-based contrast agents, the physical and procedural safety requirements of the MR environment itself, and the practical, non-technical work of preparing a patient to tolerate the examination. Two instances of the Signal-to-Category Decision System are applied here to the acute contrast reaction and to implant safety classification, extending the pattern-recognition framework introduced in the first two chapters from diagnostic image interpretation to clinical decision-making at the point of care.

Gadolinium-Based Contrast Agents: Classification and Pharmacokinetics

Chelate Structure and Thermodynamic and Kinetic Stability

Free gadolinium ion is toxic, interfering with calcium-dependent cellular processes and precipitating as insoluble salts in tissue, so every clinically used gadolinium-based contrast agent binds the gadolinium ion within an organic chelate designed to keep it sequestered from the time of injection through renal excretion. Chelates are broadly divided by molecular architecture into linear agents, in which the chelating ligand wraps around the gadolinium ion in an open, flexible configuration, and macrocyclic agents, in which the ligand forms a rigid, preorganized cage that encloses the ion more completely. This structural difference translates directly into stability: macrocyclic agents demonstrate substantially higher thermodynamic and kinetic stability, meaning they are less likely to release free gadolinium ion in vivo, both because the bound state is more energetically favorable and because the rigid cage structure dissociates more slowly even when challenged by competing endogenous ions such as zinc, copper, and calcium, a process called transmetalation that can occur over the course of the agent's circulation and excretion. Ionic agents, whether linear or macrocyclic, carry an additional layer of stability compared to nonionic agents of the same structural class because the ionic charge itself impedes transmetalation, though this distinction matters less in current practice than the linear-versus-macrocyclic distinction, which is now the primary axis along which agent selection and gadolinium retention risk are considered.

Relaxivity, the measure of how effectively a given agent shortens T1 relaxation time per unit concentration, is a separate property from stability and determines the signal-generating efficiency of an agent independent of its safety profile; two agents with markedly different stability can have similar relaxivity, and two agents with similar stability can differ meaningfully in relaxivity, so agent selection in practice reflects a combination of both properties rather than either alone. Higher-relaxivity agents allow equivalent diagnostic enhancement at a lower administered dose, which is clinically relevant both because lower dose reduces any dose-dependent safety consideration and because some higher-relaxivity agents are specifically formulated with weak, transient protein-binding interactions that further amplify their effective relaxivity in blood without meaningfully affecting their overall stability or excretion pathway, a distinction that occasionally causes confusion when relaxivity and stability are conflated as though they were the same property.

Extracellular and Hepatobiliary-Specific Agent Pharmacokinetics

Extracellular agents distribute rapidly from the vascular space into the interstitial space of most tissues, following simple two-compartment pharmacokinetics, and are excreted essentially unchanged by glomerular filtration, with a normal elimination half-life on the order of ninety minutes to two hours in a patient with normal renal function; this straightforward pharmacokinetic behavior is what makes dynamic phase timing, discussed in the previous chapter, predictable and reproducible. Hepatobiliary-specific agents follow a more complex, dual-pathway pharmacokinetic profile: a variable fraction of the injected dose, typically in the range of five to fifty percent depending on the specific agent, is taken up by functioning hepatocytes through organic anion transporter-mediated active transport and subsequently excreted into bile, while the remainder follows conventional renal excretion, and it is this hepatocyte-specific fraction that produces the diagnostically valuable hepatobiliary phase discussed in the preceding chapter. Because hepatocyte transporter expression and function can be reduced by significant hepatic parenchymal disease, the fraction of dose undergoing biliary excretion, and therefore the intensity and timing of hepatobiliary phase enhancement, is itself a rough physiologic indicator of hepatic function, a relationship exploited increasingly in the assessment of diffuse liver disease covered in a later chapter of this book.

Contrast Dosing and Injection Technique

Standard extracellular agent dosing is generally weight-based, on the order of zero point one to zero point two millimoles per kilogram depending on the specific agent and indication, and should be confirmed against current departmental dosing protocols and the specific agent's labeling rather than assumed from memory, since dosing conventions and approved indications vary meaningfully between agents and between jurisdictions. Hepatobiliary-specific agents are typically dosed lower on a per-kilogram basis than extracellular agents, reflecting both their dual excretion pathway and the fact that diagnostic hepatobiliary phase enhancement does not require the same peak vascular concentration that dynamic arterial phase imaging depends on. Injection rate and technique matter nearly as much as dose: a rapid, tightly bolused injection, typically delivered through a power injector at two to three milliliters per second followed immediately by a saline flush to clear the injection line and push the full contrast bolus into central circulation, is essential for the compact, well-defined bolus geometry that dynamic phase timing techniques described in the previous chapter depend on, and a slow, hand-injected bolus, or one without an adequate saline flush, produces prolonged, smeared contrast arrival that degrades arterial-phase image quality regardless of how precisely bolus tracking or test bolus timing was performed. Adequate intravenous access, generally a twenty-gauge or larger catheter placed in an antecubital vein when power injection at higher flow rates is planned, should be confirmed before contrast administration begins, since an inadequate catheter is a common, entirely preventable cause of extravasation, discussed further below, or of a failed or inadequate bolus.

Agent Class	Chelate Structure	Relative Stability	Typical Clinical Role
Macrocyclic, ionic or nonionic	Rigid, preorganized cage	Highest thermodynamic and kinetic stability	Preferred agent class for reduced renal function or anticipated repeated dosing
Linear, ionic	Open, flexible chelate with ionic charge	Intermediate stability	Selectively used where specific pharmacokinetic properties are advantageous
Linear, nonionic	Open, flexible chelate without ionic charge	Lowest stability among standard classes	Largely restricted or withdrawn from use in higher-risk populations at many institutions
Hepatobiliary-specific (typically linear)	Variable, agent-specific	Agent-specific; dual renal and biliary excretion	Reserved for indications requiring a hepatobiliary phase

Nephrogenic Systemic Fibrosis and Renal Risk Stratification

Pathophysiology and Historical Context of Nephrogenic Systemic Fibrosis

Nephrogenic systemic fibrosis is a rare but severe fibrosing disorder of skin and, in advanced cases, internal organs, characterized histologically by dermal proliferation of fibrocytes and deposition of collagen and mucin, producing progressive skin thickening, tethering, and joint contracture that can be profoundly disabling. The disorder was linked, in the mid-2000s, specifically to gadolinium exposure in patients with severely impaired renal function, in whom markedly prolonged elimination half-life allows far more time for transmetalation and free gadolinium release than occurs in patients with normal renal clearance, and the great majority of confirmed cases were subsequently traced to administration of less stable linear agents, several of which have since been withdrawn from use in the specific higher-risk populations discussed below or from the market entirely in many jurisdictions. This causal link, established through careful pharmacovigilance and case-control study rather than through a single definitive mechanism proven at the molecular level, remains the foundational example, discussed in every body MRI training program, of how contrast agent stability and patient-specific pharmacokinetics interact to produce a serious adverse outcome, and it is the reason renal function assessment is treated as a mandatory, non-negotiable step before gadolinium administration rather than a formality.

Current Renal Screening and Risk-Stratified Agent Selection

Current practice stratifies patients by estimated glomerular filtration rate and by the presence of acute kidney injury, since nephrogenic systemic fibrosis risk correlates more strongly with markedly reduced or absent renal clearance than with mild to moderate chronic impairment. Patients with an estimated glomerular filtration rate persistently at or above approximately thirty milliliters per minute per 1.73 square meters, without acute kidney injury, are generally considered to carry a very low risk with any currently marketed agent at standard clinical dosing, and most departments do not require additional precaution beyond routine agent selection in this population. Patients with more severely reduced estimated glomerular filtration rate, acute kidney injury of any severity, or those on dialysis represent the population in whom nephrogenic systemic fibrosis risk is concentrated, and in this group current practice favors exclusive use of a macrocyclic agent, administered at the lowest dose consistent with diagnostic image quality, with the risk-benefit discussion documented and, where dialysis is already part of the patient's care, timing of dialysis relative to contrast administration considered, though dialysis itself is not a fully protective measure against nephrogenic systemic fibrosis and should not be used to justify unrestricted contrast administration in this population. Because these thresholds and agent-specific recommendations are periodically revised as new pharmacovigilance data accumulate, protocols should always be checked against the department's current, guideline-concordant contrast policy rather than committed to memory as a fixed, unchanging rule.

Screening Questionnaires and Point-of-Care Renal Function Assessment

Practical renal risk stratification begins with a structured screening questionnaire administered before every contrast-enhanced examination, capturing known chronic kidney disease, dialysis status, solitary kidney, prior nephrotoxic exposure, and recent hospitalization or acute illness that might herald acute kidney injury even in a patient with previously normal renal function. In outpatients without risk factors identified on screening, many departments do not require a same-day laboratory estimated glomerular filtration rate, relying instead on a recent value on file or on the absence of risk factors identified through questionnaire; inpatients, patients with any positive screening response, and patients presenting emergently without prior records generally do require a current, same-day or recent estimated glomerular filtration rate before contrast is administered, since renal function can change acutely in the inpatient and emergency setting in ways that a screening questionnaire alone cannot reliably detect. This tiered approach balances thoroughness against efficiency, reserving mandatory laboratory confirmation for the populations in whom acute or previously undocumented renal impairment is genuinely plausible, rather than imposing a uniform laboratory requirement on every patient regardless of risk profile.

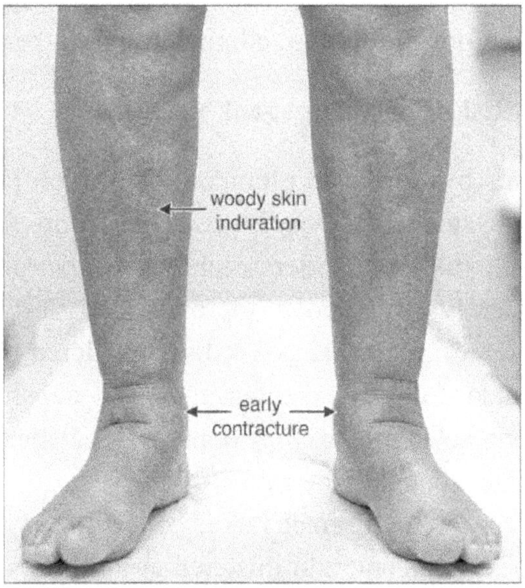

Figure 3.1

Distinguishing Gadolinium Safety Considerations From Iodinated Contrast Nephrotoxicity

A persistent point of confusion among referring clinicians and even some radiologists is conflating the renal safety considerations of gadolinium-based agents with the distinct, better-established phenomenon of contrast-induced nephropathy associated with iodinated contrast media used in computed tomography. Contrast-induced nephropathy is a direct nephrotoxic effect on renal tubular cells, dose-dependent and most consequential in patients with pre-existing renal impairment undergoing intra-arterial or high-dose intravenous iodinated contrast administration; gadolinium-based agents at standard MRI dosing are not associated with a comparable direct nephrotoxic mechanism, and the entire nephrogenic systemic fibrosis concern operates through a fundamentally different pathway, gadolinium retention and dissociation in tissue, rather than direct tubular injury. This distinction matters practically because a patient appropriately deemed too high-risk for iodinated contrast at CT because of concern for contrast-induced nephropathy is not automatically at equivalent risk from an appropriately selected, macrocyclic gadolinium-based agent at MRI, and reflexively declining a clinically indicated contrast-enhanced MRI in such a patient, out of a mistaken extension of iodinated contrast precautions, can deprive the patient of a diagnostically superior examination without a correspondingly justified safety rationale.

Gadolinium Deposition, Adverse Reactions, and Contrast Safety Protocols

Gadolinium Brain and Tissue Deposition in Patients With Normal Renal Function

Distinct from nephrogenic systemic fibrosis, a separate body of evidence accumulated over the past decade has demonstrated that trace amounts of gadolinium can be detected in the brain, bone, and other tissues of patients with entirely normal renal function following repeated gadolinium-based contrast administration, with deposition occurring to a measurably greater degree after linear agents than after macrocyclic agents, again reflecting the underlying stability difference between chelate classes. No causal link between this trace tissue deposition and any specific clinical symptom or disease has been established in patients with normal renal function, and regulatory and professional society guidance has therefore not restricted gadolinium use in this population but has generally reinforced two prudent practices: preferential use of macrocyclic agents, particularly in patients anticipated to require multiple contrast-enhanced examinations over their lifetime, such as those with chronic conditions requiring MRI surveillance, and use of the lowest dose of contrast that achieves the diagnostic purpose of the examination, avoiding reflexive administration of contrast for indications where a noncontrast or single-phase protocol would suffice.

Contrast Extravasation and Local Tissue Injury

Extravasation, the inadvertent deposition of contrast into the soft tissues surrounding the injection site rather than into the vascular lumen, occurs in a small but consistent minority of power-injected examinations and, while gadolinium-based agents are generally less tissue-toxic than iodinated contrast media when extravasated, larger-volume extravasations can still produce local swelling, pain, and, rarely, compartment syndrome-like presentations requiring surgical evaluation, particularly when a large volume is deposited in a confined fascial compartment such as the volar forearm. Immediate recognition, prompted by patient-reported pain or burning at the injection site during power injection, or by the technologist's observation of localized swelling, should prompt immediate cessation of the injection, elevation of the affected extremity, and clinical assessment of the extent of extravasation, generally with close outpatient follow-up for small-volume extravasations and more urgent surgical consultation for large-volume extravasations or those associated with signs of neurovascular compromise. Because the diagnostic examination itself may need to be aborted, delayed, or completed with a reduced or supplemental dose depending on how much of the intended bolus was successfully delivered intravascularly, extravasation management is not purely a safety concern but also a factor that can directly affect whether the resulting images are diagnostically adequate, and this should be explicitly considered before deciding whether to proceed with image acquisition.

Recognizing and Grading Acute Contrast Reactions

Acute reactions to gadolinium-based contrast agents are considerably less common than reactions to iodinated contrast media but occur across a similar clinical spectrum, from mild, self-limited symptoms such as transient nausea, warmth, or a few scattered hives, through moderate reactions involving more diffuse urticaria, facial or laryngeal edema without airway compromise, or bronchospasm, to severe, life-threatening reactions involving hypotension, significant airway compromise, or cardiovascular collapse. Correctly grading reaction severity in real time is the single most important determinant of appropriate management, because undertreating a moderate reaction risks progression to a severe one, while reflexively escalating a mild, self-limited reaction to aggressive pharmacologic treatment exposes the patient to unnecessary medication risk. The great majority of reactions, mild and even many moderate reactions, are self-limited or respond promptly to conservative measures and close observation, and the physiologic distinction between a true anaphylactoid contrast reaction and a vasovagal response, which can superficially resemble a reaction through pallor, diaphoresis, and hypotension but is instead mediated by increased vagal tone rather than mast cell degranulation, is a critical and frequently underemphasized discrimination in real-time management.

Patients with a documented history of a prior moderate or severe contrast reaction, whether to a gadolinium-based or an iodinated agent, warrant a deliberate premedication and risk-mitigation strategy before any subsequent contrast-enhanced examination, since prior reaction history is among the strongest predictors of a repeat reaction. Standard premedication regimens typically combine a corticosteroid, administered on a fixed schedule beginning many hours before the examination to allow adequate anti-inflammatory effect, with an antihistamine administered closer to the time of the examination, though the specific agents, doses, and timing intervals vary between institutional protocols and should be confirmed against current departmental guidance rather than assumed. Premedication meaningfully reduces but does not eliminate the risk of a repeat reaction, and a patient who has been premedicated should still be monitored with the same vigilance as any other patient receiving contrast, since a small but real minority of premedicated patients with a strong reaction history will nonetheless experience a breakthrough reaction, and premedication should never be treated as a substitute for having emergency response resources immediately available throughout the injection and observation period.

Documentation following any contrast reaction, regardless of severity, should specify the reaction grade, the treatment administered, the time course of symptom onset and resolution, and the specific contrast agent and dose given, since this record directly informs the premedication and agent-selection decision for every subsequent contrast-enhanced examination the patient may require. A vague chart notation such as simply noting an allergic reaction, without grading or specifying the treating agent, forces every subsequent radiologist to either default to maximal precaution, which can mean unnecessarily denying a low-risk patient a clinically indicated examination, or to underestimate a genuinely severe prior reaction, either of which is avoidable with a complete, specific initial record.

Figure 3.2: Contrast Administration Monitoring Setup and Emergency Equipment Positioning

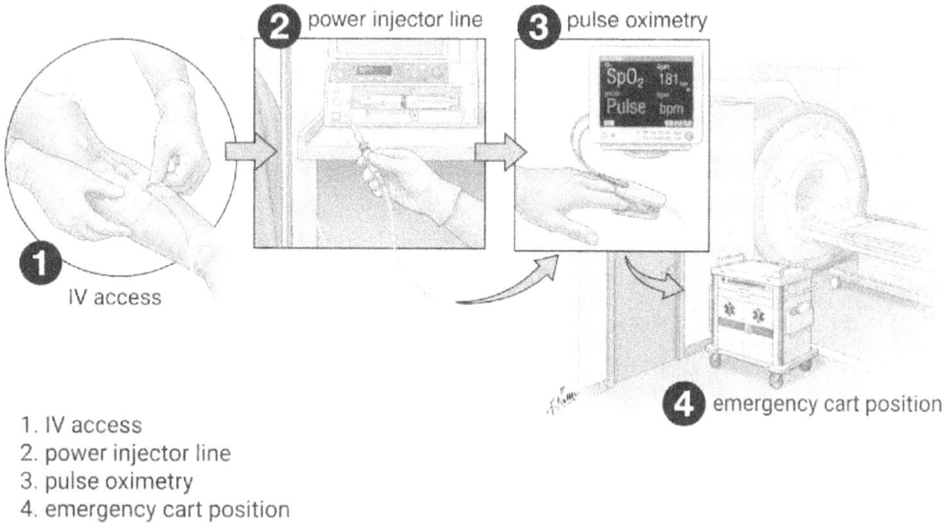

THE SIGNAL-TO-CATEGORY DECISION SYSTEM — Grading the Acute Contrast Reaction

The Signal Pattern: A patient develops cutaneous, respiratory, or hemodynamic symptoms within minutes of gadolinium-based contrast injection, ranging from a few scattered hives and mild pruritus to diffuse urticaria, wheezing, facial edema, or hypotension with tachycardia or bradycardia.

Category Signature: Symptoms limited to mild, transient cutaneous findings without respiratory or hemodynamic involvement are categorized as a mild reaction; diffuse urticaria, mild bronchospasm, or facial edema without airway compromise are categorized as moderate; and any airway compromise, significant bronchospasm, or hypotension with altered mental status or hemodynamic instability is categorized as severe.

The Decision: Mild reactions generally require only observation and reassurance; moderate reactions warrant pharmacologic treatment matched to the specific symptom, antihistamine for urticaria, bronchodilator for bronchospasm, and closer monitoring; severe reactions require immediate activation of the department's emergency response protocol, including epinephrine, airway management resources, and, when hemodynamic instability is present, intravenous fluids and continuous monitoring, without delay for further observation.

Trap Logic: A vasovagal reaction, marked by pallor, diaphoresis, nausea, and hypotension typically accompanied by bradycardia rather than tachycardia, is easily mistaken for a severe anaphylactoid reaction; the discriminating feature is heart rate, since true anaphylactoid reactions are characteristically associated with tachycardia and compensatory or direct cardiovascular effects, while vagally mediated events are characteristically bradycardic, and management of the two differs substantially, with vasovagal reactions responding to leg elevation and supportive care rather than epinephrine.

Pattern Anchor: Hypotension with tachycardia after contrast points toward a true reaction requiring escalation; hypotension with bradycardia points toward a vasovagal event requiring supportive care, not epinephrine.

MR Safety: Implants, Devices, and the Ferromagnetic Environment

The Static Field, Gradient Fields, and Radiofrequency Energy as Distinct Hazards

The MR environment presents three physically distinct hazards, each with its own mechanism and its own implications for implant and device safety. The strong static magnetic field exerts translational and rotational force on any sufficiently ferromagnetic object, which is the mechanism behind projectile injuries from loose ferromagnetic items and behind torque or displacement forces on certain implanted devices, and this force does not diminish once the patient or object is inside the bore; it is present throughout the entire time the object remains within the field. Rapidly switching gradient fields, used for spatial encoding as described in the first chapter, can induce electrical currents in any conductive loop, including looped monitoring cables, and, in patients with certain electrically active implants, can potentially induce unintended stimulation or device malfunction. Radiofrequency energy deposited during imaging, quantified as specific absorption rate and discussed in the previous chapter's discussion of field strength trade-offs, can cause localized tissue heating, an effect dramatically amplified around conductive materials that behave as antennas, including certain wires, leads, and, notoriously, any conductive loop formed inadvertently by a patient's own body position or by looped cabling in contact with skin. Understanding these three distinct mechanisms explains why a given implant might be safe with respect to one hazard, magnetic displacement, for instance, while remaining hazardous with respect to another, radiofrequency-induced heating along a lead.

MR-Safe, MR-Conditional, and MR-Unsafe Classification

Devices and implants are formally classified using standardized terminology: MR-safe items pose no known hazard in any MR environment and require no special labeling review, MR-unsafe items pose a known, unacceptable hazard in any MR environment and are absolutely contraindicated, and MR-conditional items, the largest and most clinically important category, have been demonstrated safe under a specific, explicitly defined set of conditions, which may include limits on field strength, specific absorption rate, gradient slew rate, and, for certain devices, required positioning or programming changes before scanning. The critical practical implication of the MR-conditional category is that safety is never a property of the device in isolation; it is a property of the device operated within its labeled conditions on a specific scanner, and a device labeled MR-conditional at 1.5 tesla is not automatically safe at 3 tesla, nor is a device conditional under one manufacturer's labeling automatically presumed safe simply because a superficially similar device from another manufacturer carries conditional labeling. Screening staff must therefore identify the specific make and model of any implanted device, consult the current manufacturer labeling or an authoritative implant safety reference for that specific device, and confirm that the intended scanner and sequence parameters fall within the labeled conditions before the patient enters the MR environment, a process that cannot be shortcut by relying on a patient's verbal assurance that a device is safe or on outdated information from a prior examination at a different facility.

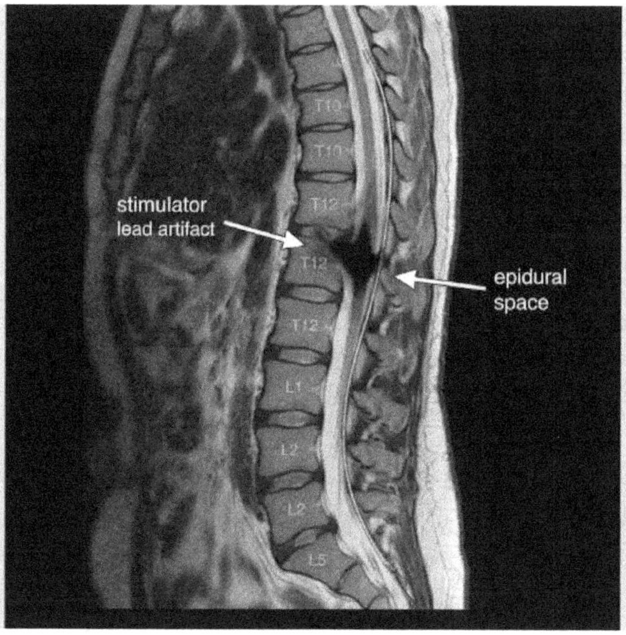

Ferromagnetic Screening Beyond Implanted Devices

Implant and device screening addresses only one component of the MR safety environment; ferromagnetic screening of the patient's own person and of everything brought into the scanner room, including staff, ancillary equipment, and any object accompanying the patient, is an equally essential and distinct safety domain. Loose ferromagnetic objects, from wheelchairs and oxygen tanks to hairpins, coins, and, in emergent settings, unsecured medical equipment, are the mechanism behind projectile injuries, which occur when such an object is drawn toward the bore with force proportional to both its ferromagnetic content and the static field strength at its location, and the risk is not confined to obviously metallic objects; some medical equipment and even certain clothing components contain ferromagnetic elements not apparent on casual inspection. This is why standard practice designates the MR environment in zones of progressively restricted access, with the innermost zone, the scanner room itself, accessible only after every person and object has passed dedicated ferromagnetic screening, typically including both a verbal and written screening questionnaire and, in most modern departments, a handheld or walk-through ferromagnetic detection system, and why exceptions are never made for emergent situations, since an oxygen tank or piece of resuscitation equipment brought into the scanner room without screening represents one of the most severe and well-documented mechanisms of catastrophic MR safety injury, precisely because the emergent context creates pressure to bypass the screening step that exists specifically to prevent this outcome.

THE SIGNAL-TO-CATEGORY DECISION SYSTEM — Screening the Implanted Cardiac Device

The Signal Pattern: A patient presenting for body MRI reports a cardiac pacemaker or implantable cardioverter-defibrillator, and the screening form or device identification card lists a specific manufacturer and model number.

Category Signature: Devices verified against current manufacturer labeling as MR-conditional at the intended field strength, with documented programming or monitoring requirements met, are categorized as safe to proceed; devices that cannot be identified, that lack documentation, or that are confirmed MR-unsafe are categorized as contraindicated pending further evaluation.

The Decision: For a confirmed MR-conditional device, coordinate with electrophysiology or the device manufacturer's representative to implement the required conditional settings, typically including a magnet mode or fixed-rate programming, before scanning and continuous cardiac monitoring throughout, followed by device interrogation and reprogramming afterward; for a device that cannot be positively identified, the examination should not proceed until identification is obtained, regardless of time pressure from the requesting clinical team.

Trap Logic: An older device model, implanted years before a facility adopted a given screening protocol, is easily assumed to carry the same conditional status as a newer device from the same manufacturer family; the discriminating step is verifying the specific model number against current labeling every time, since older device generations are frequently MR-unsafe or subject to more restrictive conditions than their newer successors despite superficial similarity in appearance or manufacturer.

Pattern Anchor: No cardiac device proceeds to scanning based on a patient's verbal report alone; the specific model number must be verified against current labeling before every examination, without exception.

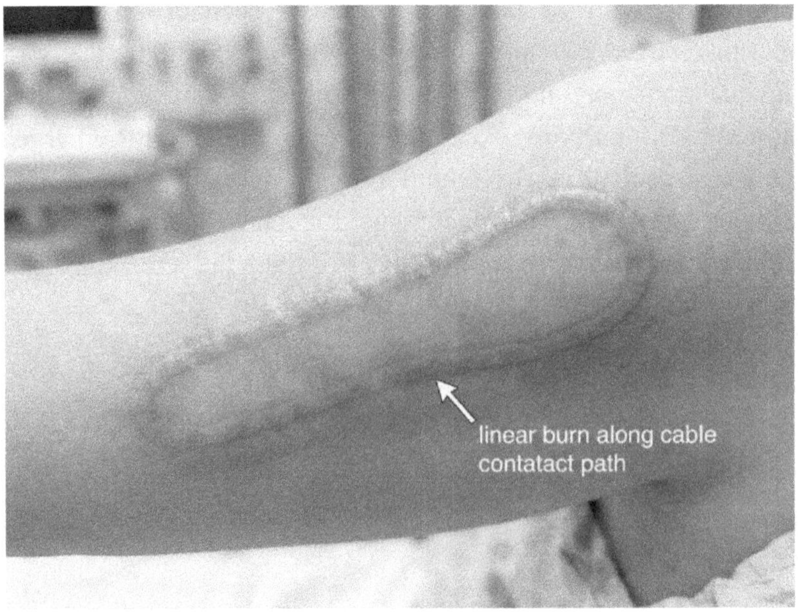

Patient Preparation and Claustrophobia Management

Practical Strategies for Claustrophobia and Anxiety

Clinically significant claustrophobia or anxiety severe enough to threaten examination completion is common enough in body MRI practice, given typical examination durations of thirty to forty-five minutes or more, that departments benefit from a structured, tiered approach rather than an ad hoc response at the time of difficulty. Simple, low-cost measures, including a thorough explanation of what the patient will experience, feet-first positioning where the clinical protocol allows it so the patient's head remains outside the bore for at least part of the examination, prism glasses or a mirror that allows the patient to see out of the bore, blindfolding for patients who find the visual confinement more distressing than the physical confinement, and continuous verbal reassurance through the intercom during the examination, resolve the majority of mild to moderate anxiety without pharmacologic intervention. For patients with more severe claustrophobia identified in advance, either through direct patient report or through a documented history of prior incomplete MRI examinations, scheduling an anxiolytic premedication in coordination with the referring clinician, arranging for a support person to remain in the scanner room when institutional policy permits, or scheduling the examination on a wide-bore magnet configuration when available, are all reasonable proactive strategies that reduce the likelihood of an incomplete or motion-degraded examination far more effectively than attempting to manage severe anxiety reactively once the patient is already in the bore and in distress.

Positioning, Immobilization, and Pre-Scan Instructions

Beyond anxiety management, deliberate attention to positioning and immobilization meaningfully reduces motion artifact independent of any pulse sequence-level compensation strategy discussed in earlier chapters. Padding and immobilization devices placed to gently restrict the specific anatomic region under examination, rather than the whole body indiscriminately, reduce voluntary and semi-voluntary movement without adding to patient discomfort, and clear, specific pre-scan instructions, particularly for breath-hold coaching as discussed in the previous chapter and for instructing patients to remain still even during the noisy gradient switching of the scan itself, meaningfully improve compliance when delivered before the patient enters the bore rather than shouted over an intercom mid-sequence. Bladder and bowel preparation instructions, relevant to the pelvic protocols discussed in the previous chapter, should likewise be communicated clearly at the time of scheduling rather than left to be discovered as inadequate once the patient is already positioned on the table, since a patient who has not followed preparation instructions because they were never adequately communicated cannot reasonably be expected to have complied, and repeating an entire examination for a preventable preparation failure is a poor use of both the patient's time and departmental resources.

Special Considerations in Pediatric and Cognitively Impaired Patients

Pediatric patients and cognitively impaired adults require preparation strategies that extend beyond the anxiety-management techniques described above, since neither population can always be expected to understand or comply with verbal instruction alone, regardless of how clearly it is delivered. Age- and developmentally appropriate preparation, including child-life specialist involvement, simulated mock scanning sessions before the actual examination, and, when necessary, sedation or general anesthesia coordinated with an anesthesia team, are standard components of a pediatric body MRI program, and the specific protocol modifications required for pediatric patients, including field-of-view, coil selection, and sequence adjustments to accommodate smaller body habitus and, in sedated patients, altered breathing patterns, are addressed in detail in the chapter on body MRI in pediatric and pregnant patients later in this book. Cognitively impaired adults, including patients with dementia or acute delirium, similarly may require a caregiver present for reassurance, simplified real-time instructions repeated frequently rather than delivered once at the outset, or, when agitation precludes a diagnostic examination despite these measures, a coordinated decision with the referring team about whether sedation, an alternative imaging modality, or deferral of the examination best serves the patient, since a coerced or physically restrained attempt at MRI in a severely agitated patient rarely produces diagnostic images and carries its own safety risk to both the patient and staff.

Clinical Case Presentations

Case 1. A 67-year-old woman with stage 4 chronic kidney disease, estimated glomerular filtration rate of eighteen milliliters per minute per 1.73 square meters, is referred for MRI to characterize a renal mass. Given her severely reduced renal function, the ordering nephrologist and the radiologist discuss the risk-benefit balance directly rather than proceeding automatically. Because renal mass characterization in this case genuinely requires contrast-enhanced imaging to assess for enhancement, the diagnostic feature that distinguishes a solid renal mass from a complex cyst, the team elects to proceed with a macrocyclic agent at the lowest dose consistent with diagnostic quality, documents the risk-benefit discussion in the chart, and confirms the patient is not on a fixed hemodialysis schedule that would allow timing adjustment. The examination proceeds without incident, and the report specifically documents the agent class and dose administered, both for the patient's ongoing record and to inform any future imaging decisions in this same patient.

Case 2. During a routine screening breast and abdominal MRI for a patient with a strong family history of malignancy, the patient develops diffuse urticaria and mild facial flushing approximately three minutes after contrast injection, without wheezing, stridor, or a measurable drop in blood pressure. The technologist immediately stops the injection, and the covering radiologist, assessing the patient at bedside, correctly categorizes this as a moderate reaction based on the diffuse cutaneous involvement without respiratory or hemodynamic compromise. Diphenhydramine is administered per the department's standing protocol, the patient is observed for thirty minutes with resolution of symptoms, and the examination is not resumed that day; the reaction, its grading, and the treatment given are documented in detail, and the patient's chart is flagged for premedication and closer monitoring should future contrast-enhanced imaging be required.

Case 3. A 54-year-old man presents for lumbar spine and abdominal MRI and reports during screening that he has a spinal cord stimulator of some kind implanted years earlier at another institution, but he does not know the manufacturer or model, and no device card is available. Despite time pressure from a same-day add-on request, the screening technologist declines to proceed and instead contacts the implanting facility's records department to obtain the specific device identification. The device is ultimately identified as an older-generation spinal cord stimulator that is not MR-conditional under any labeling, and the examination is deferred entirely pending discussion with the patient's pain management specialist about device explantation or an alternative imaging modality. This case is documented specifically to reinforce, for the whole screening team, that verbal device description alone is never sufficient grounds to proceed, regardless of scheduling pressure.

THE SIGNAL-TO-CATEGORY DECISION SYSTEM — Contrast and Device Safety Arc

The Signal Pattern: This chapter's two patterns, the acute contrast reaction and the implanted device screening question, both present as an ambiguous clinical signal requiring rapid, correct categorization under real-time pressure rather than at leisure during image interpretation.

Category Signature: Reaction severity is categorized by the specific combination of cutaneous, respiratory, and hemodynamic findings present, with heart rate direction distinguishing true reaction from vasovagal event; device safety is categorized as conditional-and-verified, contraindicated, or unknown-and-not-yet-cleared based on positively identified manufacturer labeling, never on verbal report.

The Decision: Correct categorization drives an immediate, specific action, observation, targeted pharmacologic treatment, or emergency escalation for reactions; proceed, defer pending identification, or contraindicate for devices, and in both domains the decision should never default to proceeding under uncertainty.

Trap Logic: The shared trap across both patterns is mistaking a superficially similar but mechanistically distinct presentation, a vasovagal event for a true reaction, or an older device generation for its safely labeled successor, for the pattern it resembles rather than the pattern it actually is.

Pattern Anchor: When uncertain whether a reaction is vasovagal or true anaphylactoid, check the heart rate; when uncertain whether a device is safe, verify the specific model against current labeling before proceeding, every time.

Summary and Key Concepts

Macrocyclic gadolinium-based agents are more thermodynamically and kinetically stable than linear agents, resulting in lower rates of transmetalation and free gadolinium release, and are preferentially used in patients at elevated risk, including those with reduced renal function.

Nephrogenic systemic fibrosis risk is concentrated in patients with severely reduced estimated glomerular filtration rate or acute kidney injury, and current practice restricts gadolinium use in this population to macrocyclic agents at the lowest diagnostic dose.

Trace gadolinium tissue deposition occurs even in patients with normal renal function, more so with linear than macrocyclic agents, without an established clinical consequence, but reinforces the practice of using the lowest effective dose and preferring macrocyclic agents for patients anticipated to require repeated contrast studies.

Acute contrast reactions are graded mild, moderate, or severe based on the specific combination of cutaneous, respiratory, and hemodynamic findings, and heart rate direction helps distinguish a true reaction from a vasovagal event, which requires different management.

The MR environment presents three distinct hazards, static field forces, gradient-induced currents, and radiofrequency heating, and a device's safety with respect to one hazard does not guarantee safety with respect to another.

MR-conditional device safety is specific to make, model, field strength, and labeled scan conditions; it is never established by verbal patient report and must be reverified against current manufacturer labeling for every examination.

Proactive claustrophobia management, positioning, and clear pre-scan preparation instructions meaningfully reduce the incidence of incomplete or motion-degraded examinations and are far more effective than reactive management once distress has already developed.

CHAPTER 4: ARTIFACT RECOGNITION AND MITIGATION IN BODY MRI

Learning Objectives

1. Recognize the appearance of cardiac, vascular pulsation, and peristaltic motion artifacts and apply appropriate technical strategies to mitigate each.
2. Identify truncation, Gibbs ringing, and partial volume artifacts and distinguish them from true structural abnormality.
3. Recognize radiofrequency interference, zipper artifacts, and dielectric shading, and relate each to its underlying technical cause.
4. Distinguish flow-related artifacts, including flow voids, flow-related enhancement, and phase-contrast aliasing, from true vascular or parenchymal pathology.
5. Apply a systematic, stepwise approach to troubleshooting an unfamiliar or ambiguous image artifact encountered in clinical practice.

Clinical Overview

The preceding three chapters introduced artifact recognition piecemeal, chemical shift and susceptibility artifact alongside the physics that produces them, respiratory misregistration and bowel distension artifact alongside protocol design, radiofrequency and static-field hazards alongside patient safety. This chapter consolidates and extends that foundation into a dedicated, systematic treatment of the remaining major artifact categories encountered in body MRI, and, more importantly, builds the diagnostic habit of artifact troubleshooting itself: given an unfamiliar or ambiguous image appearance, how does an experienced reader work backward from the artifact's geometry and behavior to its underlying technical cause, and from that cause to a specific corrective action.

Artifact recognition is not a peripheral skill practiced only when something looks obviously wrong; the majority of artifacts in body MRI are subtle enough to be genuinely mistaken for pathology by a reader who has not internalized their characteristic signatures, and the consequences of that error run in both directions, unnecessary follow-up imaging or biopsy when artifact is overcalled as disease, and missed pathology when a genuine finding is dismissed as artifact without adequate scrutiny. Two further instances of the Signal-to-Category Decision System are introduced in this chapter, applied to vascular pulsation ghosting and to dielectric shading, two of the most commonly encountered and most commonly misread artifact patterns in routine abdominal and pelvic MRI.

Motion Artifacts: Cardiac, Vascular Pulsation, and Peristaltic Sources

Cardiac and Vascular Pulsation Ghosting

Pulsatile motion of the aorta and other major vessels displaces the vessel wall by a small but consistent amount with each cardiac cycle, and because this displacement occurs at a frequency unrelated to the phase-encoding steps of a conventional two-dimensional acquisition, the resulting inconsistency in the phase-encoded signal from the pulsating vessel is spread across the entire image along the phase-encoding direction, producing a series of discrete ghost images of the vessel, evenly spaced and progressively fainter, propagating away from the true vessel position. This ghosting most commonly involves the aorta in upper abdominal imaging and can superimpose directly onto the liver, pancreas, or adjacent structures, where a ghost can mimic a focal lesion, particularly on single-phase or non-dynamic sequences where there is no opportunity to compare the suspicious finding against a differently timed acquisition. Because ghosting propagates specifically along the phase-encoding direction, one of the most practical and immediate diagnostic maneuvers when a suspicious focus is identified near a major vessel is to check the phase-encoding direction recorded for that sequence and confirm whether the finding lies along a line connecting the vessel to the edge of the field of view in that specific direction, a geometric relationship that true pathology does not share.

The spacing between successive ghosts along the phase-encoding direction is itself predictable from the acquisition parameters, since ghost position is determined by the ratio of the physiologic motion frequency to the phase-encoding repetition rate, and this relationship can be used deliberately as a confirmatory check: an experienced reader who suspects ghosting can estimate the expected ghost spacing from the sequence's repetition time and the patient's approximate heart rate, and confirm that the suspicious foci fall at the predicted intervals, a quantitative cross-check that adds confidence beyond visual pattern recognition alone, particularly useful when only two or three ghosts are visible rather than the full, easily recognized series.

Voluntary and Bulk Patient Motion

Distinct from the periodic, physiologic motion sources discussed above, voluntary or semi-voluntary bulk patient motion, shifting position, coughing, or reflexive movement in response to discomfort or the acoustic noise of gradient switching, produces a less predictable pattern of image degradation, typically appearing as generalized blurring or a more chaotic, non-periodic ghosting pattern rather than the regular, evenly spaced ghosts characteristic of cardiac or respiratory motion. Because this type of motion is inherently less predictable, technical correction strategies such as gating or saturation bands are largely ineffective against it, and mitigation instead depends primarily on the patient preparation and immobilization strategies discussed in the previous chapter, along with judicious use of motion-robust acquisition strategies, single-shot sequences and radial or propeller-type k-space trajectories that are inherently more tolerant of intermittent bulk motion than conventional sequential k-space filling. When bulk motion has already degraded a completed sequence, the most reliable remedy is simply repeating the acquisition after addressing the underlying cause, whether that is inadequate immobilization, unaddressed pain, or unrecognized anxiety, since no post-processing correction reliably recovers diagnostic quality from severe, non-periodic bulk motion once the raw data has already been corrupted by it.

Technical Strategies for Pulsation and Peristaltic Motion Suppression

Several technical strategies mitigate pulsation ghosting, each intervening at a different point in the underlying mechanism. Swapping the phase-encoding direction so that it runs anterior-to-posterior rather than right-to-left, or vice versa, redirects the resulting ghost artifact away from the region of greatest clinical interest, a simple and frequently used first-line adjustment. Cardiac gating or triggering, analogous to the respiratory triggering discussed in the previous chapter, synchronizes data acquisition to a consistent point in the cardiac cycle, most commonly using a peripheral pulse oximetry signal as a practical surrogate for a true electrocardiographic trigger in body imaging, eliminating the cycle-to-cycle inconsistency that produces ghosting at the cost of longer, less predictable acquisition time. Saturation bands, additional radiofrequency pulses applied to suppress signal from tissue outside the region of diagnostic interest before it can contribute to the acquired data, are commonly placed anterior to the aorta specifically to reduce the signal available to ghost forward into the imaged anatomy. Peristaltic motion of the bowel is addressed differently, primarily through pharmacologic antiperistaltic premedication, discussed in the previous chapter's pelvic protocol section, since peristalsis is a physiologic process not amenable to gating or saturation band strategies in the same way vascular pulsation is.

THE SIGNAL-TO-CATEGORY DECISION SYSTEM — Aortic Pulsation Ghosting Mimicking a Pancreatic or Hepatic Lesion

---

The Signal Pattern: A focal area of altered signal intensity is identified in the pancreas, left hepatic lobe, or another structure adjacent to the aorta, arranged in a line extending from the aorta toward the edge of the image along a single direction.

Category Signature: A finding whose position lies precisely along the phase-encoding direction from a pulsatile vessel, and which recurs as a series of progressively fainter, evenly spaced foci rather than a single discrete focus, is categorized as pulsation ghosting artifact; a finding without this geometric relationship, or one that persists in the same location and configuration on a sequence with a different phase-encoding direction, is categorized as a true focal abnormality.

The Decision: Ghosting artifact confirmed by its characteristic geometry requires no further workup; a finding that persists across sequences with different phase-encoding directions, or that does not align with the expected ghosting geometry from an adjacent pulsatile vessel, should be evaluated as a genuine lesion using the organ-specific criteria detailed in later chapters.

The Trap Logic: Ghosting artifact is most dangerous when it is faint and solitary rather than displaying its full, multiply-repeated pattern, which can occur when only the first, brightest ghost is conspicuous against background tissue; the discriminating step in this circumstance is checking the recorded phase-encoding direction for the sequence and confirming that the finding aligns with a line drawn from the aorta in that specific direction.

Pattern Anchor: Any focal finding adjacent to the aorta that lies along the phase-encoding direction should be presumed ghosting until proven otherwise by persistence on a sequence with a different phase-encoding direction.

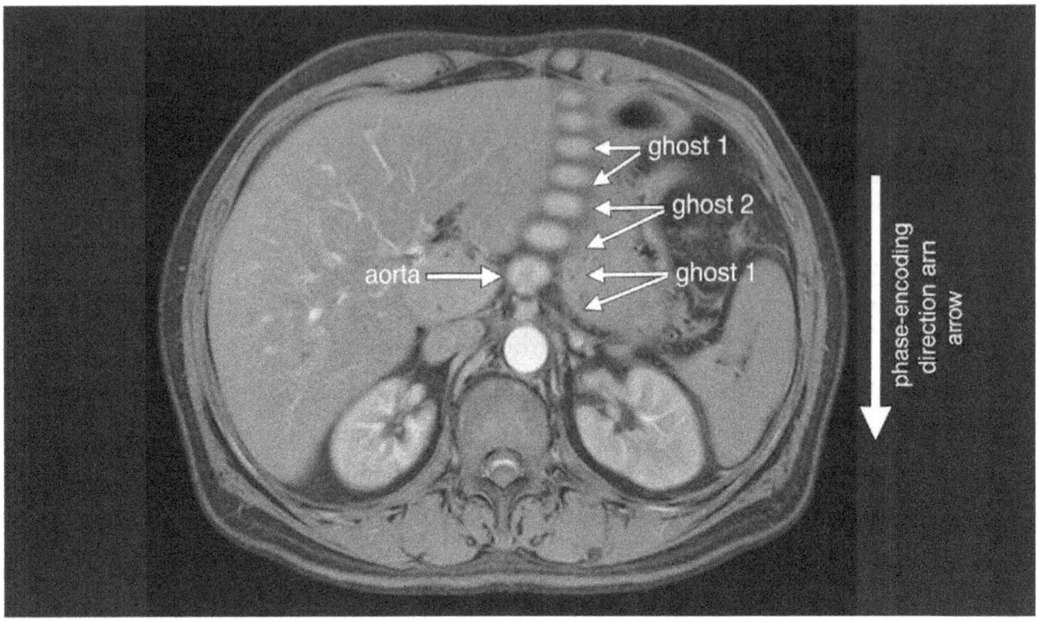

Truncation, Gibbs Ringing, and Partial Volume Artifacts

Truncation and Gibbs Ringing at High-Contrast Interfaces

Because k-space is sampled over a finite range rather than to infinity, the Fourier reconstruction of any sharp, high-contrast tissue boundary inevitably includes a series of alternating bright and dark bands parallel to that boundary, a phenomenon called truncation or Gibbs ringing, most conspicuous at interfaces with the greatest signal difference, such as between cerebrospinal fluid and spinal cord on sagittal spine imaging, or, in body imaging, at the interface between high-signal fluid or fat and adjacent low-signal structures, including the wall of the bladder, gallbladder, or a large cyst. The number and conspicuity of these bands is directly related to k-space coverage, meaning lower spatial resolution acquisitions, in which fewer high-spatial-frequency k-space lines are sampled, demonstrate more pronounced ringing than higher-resolution acquisitions of the same anatomy, which is why Gibbs ringing is often more apparent on rapidly acquired single-shot sequences than on higher-resolution, longer-acquisition three-dimensional sequences of the same structure. Recognizing Gibbs ringing as a fine, regularly spaced band pattern parallel to a genuine high-contrast interface, rather than a discrete structural abnormality such as a septation, dissection flap, or wall thickening, prevents the artifact from being overcalled as a structural finding, particularly within the bladder or gallbladder lumen, where a Gibbs ringing band can superficially resemble a thin septation or a small polyp.

Gibbs ringing can be reduced, though not entirely eliminated, by increasing the acquisition matrix, which extends k-space coverage and correspondingly narrows the width of the ringing bands until they become subvisual, or by applying a k-space apodization filter during reconstruction, which deliberately tapers the contribution of the outermost, highest-spatial-frequency k-space lines to reduce ringing at the cost of a modest, generally acceptable reduction in true spatial resolution. Because these are reconstruction-level and acquisition-level trade-offs rather than free corrections, most body MRI protocols accept some residual Gibbs ringing as a normal feature of clinically practical acquisition times, and the diagnostic solution in practice is recognition rather than elimination: knowing that a fine, regularly spaced band pattern immediately adjacent to a high-contrast interface is expected and clinically insignificant, rather than attempting to protocol every sequence at a resolution high enough to make the artifact disappear entirely, which would come at an impractical cost in acquisition time for most routine indications.

The Magic Angle Effect Near Tendons and Ligaments

Collagen-rich structures with a highly ordered fibrillar architecture, most notably tendons and ligaments encountered at the periphery of pelvic and musculoskeletal-adjacent body MRI fields of view, normally demonstrate very low signal on all conventional sequences because their restricted molecular motion produces extremely short T2 relaxation. When such a structure is oriented at approximately fifty-five degrees relative to the main magnetic field, a geometric relationship called the magic angle, the dipolar interactions responsible for this rapid T2 decay are transiently averaged toward zero, producing an artifactual increase in signal intensity on short echo time sequences that can mimic tendinosis, partial tearing, or other true tendon pathology. This effect is most pronounced on sequences with short echo times and diminishes markedly on sequences with longer echo times, since the underlying T2 of the tissue, even at the magic angle, remains far shorter than that of true pathologic tissue edema or degeneration; comparing the questionable focus of increased signal across a short and a long echo time sequence, where true pathology remains relatively hyperintense on both while a magic angle artifact largely resolves on the longer echo time sequence, is the standard discriminating maneuver, and confirming the anatomic orientation of the tendon or ligament in question relative to the main field, most reliably done on a scout or localizer image, provides an additional geometric confirmation.

Partial Volume Averaging

Partial volume averaging occurs whenever a single voxel contains more than one tissue type, in which case the signal recorded for that voxel represents a weighted average of the contributions from each tissue rather than a pure representation of either, and its practical consequence in body imaging is most often the underestimation of small lesion size or the blurring of a small lesion's true signal characteristics toward those of adjacent normal tissue, particularly problematic for lesions smaller than approximately twice the slice thickness, which are almost never adequately characterized on a single slice without partial volume contamination from immediately adjacent tissue. This is a primary rationale for the thin-section imaging emphasized in several organ-specific protocols throughout this book, since reducing slice thickness reduces the proportion of a small lesion's volume that is averaged together with adjacent normal parenchyma, and for the practice of evaluating a small lesion across multiple contiguous slices rather than relying on its appearance on a single slice alone, since the slice demonstrating the least partial volume contamination, typically the one passing closest to the lesion's true center, provides the most representative characterization.

Partial volume averaging also has specific quantitative consequences beyond size and signal characterization: apparent diffusion coefficient measurements obtained from a lesion smaller than the acquisition's effective resolution will be systematically biased toward the value of adjacent normal tissue, a phenomenon that can cause a small, truly restricted malignant lesion to demonstrate a falsely elevated apparent diffusion coefficient more consistent with a benign process, simply because the measurement voxel captures a substantial proportion of surrounding, non-restricted tissue alongside the lesion itself. This bias is one of the more consequential and less appreciated practical limitations of quantitative apparent diffusion coefficient interpretation in small lesions throughout this book, and it reinforces why apparent diffusion coefficient values should always be interpreted in conjunction with qualitative high b-value signal and conventional anatomic sequences, rather than treated as an isolated, purely quantitative threshold, particularly for lesions approaching the spatial resolution limits of the acquisition.

Radiofrequency Interference, Zipper Artifacts, and Dielectric Effects

External Radiofrequency Interference and Zipper Artifacts

The MR scanner room is shielded specifically to exclude external radiofrequency energy at frequencies near the Larmor frequency, since any such energy reaching the receiver coil is indistinguishable from true MR signal and will be reconstructed into the image at the spatial location corresponding to its frequency, typically producing a characteristic narrow band or stripe of noise, called a zipper artifact, running across the entire image in the frequency-encoding direction at a position corresponding to the interfering frequency. Zipper artifacts most commonly result from a breach in room shielding integrity, a door left open during acquisition, a piece of unshielded electronic equipment brought into the room, or, less commonly, a failing shield component requiring engineering service, and their appearance, a thin, sharply defined line crossing the entire image regardless of the anatomy present, is rarely confused with true pathology once recognized, though a zipper artifact superimposed directly over a region of clinical interest can obscure genuine findings and may require the acquisition to be repeated after the interference source is identified and eliminated.

Practical troubleshooting of a zipper artifact begins with confirming that the finding is genuinely a straight line spanning the entire image at a fixed position along the frequency-encoding direction, distinguishing it from other linear artifacts such as the coil-interface seam sometimes visible where two elements of a phased-array coil meet, which is typically less sharply defined and does not extend fully across the image. Once confirmed, the technologist should systematically exclude common interference sources before resuming scanning: verifying the scanner room door is fully closed and the radiofrequency shielding seal is intact, confirming no unshielded electronic device, including certain patient monitoring equipment, mobile phones, or improperly rated infusion pumps, has been brought into the room, and, if the artifact persists despite excluding these common causes, escalating to a service engineer to assess for a genuine shielding or hardware fault, since a persistent zipper artifact with no identifiable environmental cause can indicate a developing equipment problem that will affect every subsequent examination until corrected.

Dielectric Effects and B1 Field Inhomogeneity at Higher Field Strength

At 3 tesla, the wavelength of the radiofrequency excitation pulse becomes comparable to the physical dimensions of the human torso, and this creates constructive and destructive interference patterns within the body itself, an effect governed by the dielectric properties of tissue and most pronounced in regions of high water content and large cross-sectional area, such as the pelvis and abdomen in patients with a larger body habitus. The practical consequence is spatially nonuniform excitation, commonly manifesting as a region of artifactually increased or decreased signal intensity, often centrally located within the abdomen or pelvis, a pattern sometimes called central brightening or, when signal is instead reduced, central shading, neither of which corresponds to any true difference in underlying tissue composition. Because this effect scales with field strength and with the dielectric properties of the specific tissue present, it is more pronounced at 3 tesla than at 1.5 tesla and more pronounced in patients with ascites or other large fluid collections, which have particularly high dielectric constants, than in patients without such fluid.

Beyond the dielectric padding solution introduced later in this section, modern 3-tesla scanners increasingly incorporate hardware and software mitigation built directly into the system, most notably multi-transmit or parallel transmit technology, in which radiofrequency energy is transmitted through multiple independent channels rather than a single transmit source, allowing the relative phase and amplitude of each channel to be adjusted, a process called radiofrequency shimming, to actively compensate for the destructive interference pattern responsible for dielectric shading before it degrades the image. Where available, radiofrequency shimming substantially reduces the need for supplemental dielectric padding and is generally applied automatically as part of routine 3-tesla protocol calibration, though it does not eliminate the effect entirely in the largest-habitus patients or those with the most pronounced fluid collections.

THE SIGNAL-TO-CATEGORY DECISION SYSTEM — Dielectric Shading Mimicking Diffuse Parenchymal Disease

---

The Signal Pattern: A broad, poorly marginated region of altered signal intensity, either brighter or darker than expected, involving a substantial portion of the pelvis or central abdomen, without a discrete margin and without a corresponding abnormality on a differently weighted sequence.

Category Signature: A broad signal alteration that is geographic rather than anatomic, meaning it does not respect organ boundaries or known anatomic planes, that is more pronounced centrally within the field of view, and that occurs in a large-habitus patient or one with a large fluid collection imaged at 3 tesla, is categorized as dielectric shading artifact rather than diffuse parenchymal disease.

The Decision: Confirmed dielectric shading requires no further workup and should be explicitly distinguished in the report from true diffuse disease; if genuine diagnostic uncertainty remains, repeating the affected sequence with dielectric padding, a specialized high-permittivity pad placed adjacent to the patient to locally correct the B1 field, or acquiring the sequence at 1.5 tesla instead, will typically resolve the artifact and confirm its technical origin.

The Trap Logic: Dielectric shading is most treacherous in the liver and pelvic organs, where it can mimic diffuse hepatic steatosis, edema, or infiltrative disease on a single sequence; the discriminating step is checking whether the signal alteration respects the expected anatomic boundaries and margins of the organ in question, since true diffuse parenchymal disease, even when extensive, still conforms to organ contour, whereas dielectric shading crosses organ boundaries in a geographic distribution unrelated to anatomy.

Pattern Anchor: A broad signal abnormality that ignores organ boundaries and is most pronounced centrally in a large-habitus patient at 3 tesla should be presumed dielectric artifact until confirmed otherwise by a corrective repeat acquisition.

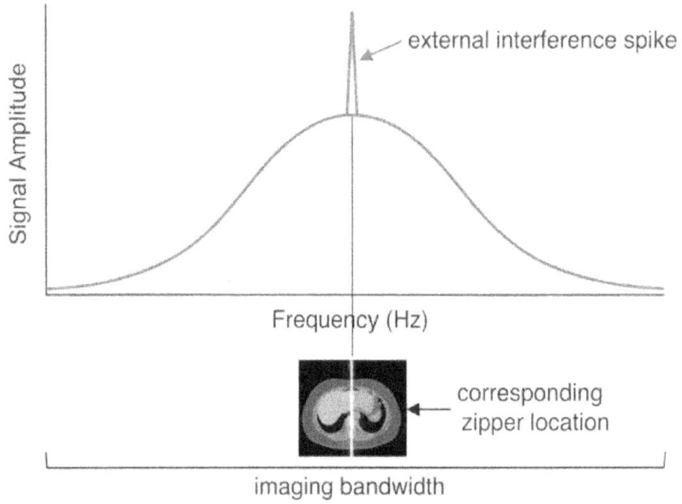

Figure 4.2: Radiofrequency Spectrum Diagram Illustrating the Origin of a Zipper Artifact

Flow-Related Artifacts and Their Diagnostic Pitfalls

Flow Voids and Flow-Related Enhancement

Rapidly flowing blood, most notably within the aorta and inferior vena cava, frequently appears as a signal void on spin-echo sequences because protons excited within the vessel at the time of the initial radiofrequency pulse have typically flowed out of the imaging slice before the refocusing pulse and signal readout occur, so no coherent signal remains to be recorded, a phenomenon exploited deliberately in some vascular imaging techniques but one that can be mistaken for a filling defect, thrombus, or dissection if not recognized as an expected consequence of normal, rapid laminar flow. Conversely, on gradient-echo sequences, particularly those using a short repetition time, unsaturated blood flowing into the imaging slice from outside can appear paradoxically hyperintense relative to stationary tissue, a phenomenon called flow-related enhancement or the time-of-flight effect, because inflowing blood has not been subjected to the repeated excitation pulses that progressively saturate stationary tissue signal within the slice; this effect is exploited intentionally in unenhanced MR angiography but can otherwise create confusing bright signal within a vessel that might be misinterpreted as enhancing thrombus or a flow-related pseudolesion if the sequence type and flow direction are not considered.

Figure 4.3 — Diagnostic Imaging: Dielectric Shading Artifact on Pelvic MRI at 3 Tesla

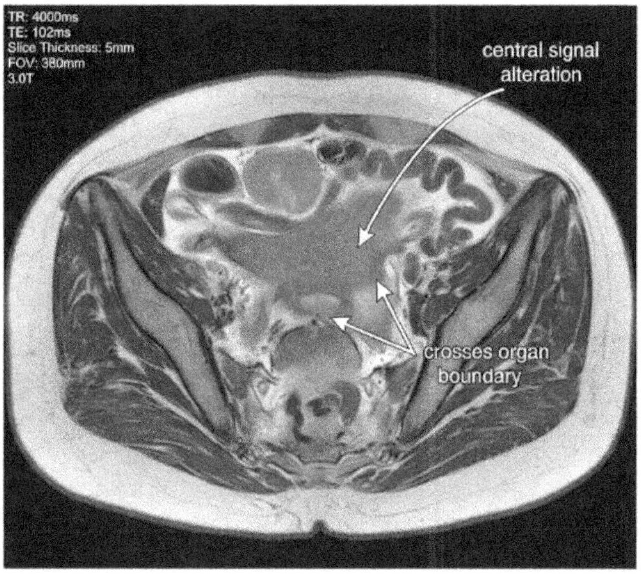

A related, specifically named phenomenon, the entry-slice effect, describes the same underlying mechanism, unsaturated inflowing spins appearing hyperintense relative to saturated stationary tissue, but occurs specifically on multi-slice spin-echo acquisitions at the entry slice where blood first enters the imaging volume, and it can be distinguished from true intraluminal pathology by its characteristic confinement to the first one or two slices at the edge of the acquired volume, with normal, expected flow void reappearing on subsequent interior slices as the blood becomes progressively saturated after passing through several successive excitation pulses. Even-echo rephasing, encountered on multi-echo spin-echo sequences, produces a related but distinct pattern in which slow, laminar flow that appears as signal loss on odd echoes paradoxically regains signal on even echoes because the phase dispersion accumulated by the first refocusing pulse is exactly canceled by an identical, oppositely directed dispersion accumulated before the second; recognizing this specific echo-dependent signal pattern, rather than interpreting the even-echo signal recovery as evidence of a mural nodule or clot lysis, prevents an artifactual finding from being escalated into an incorrect diagnosis of partial or resolving thrombosis.

Slow Flow, Turbulence, and Phase-Contrast Artifacts

Slow or turbulent flow, encountered in dilated or aneurysmal vessels, at the site of a stenosis, or within the portal venous system in patients with portal hypertension, behaves less predictably than the rapid laminar flow described above and can produce intermediate, heterogeneous signal within the vessel lumen that superficially resembles thrombus, particularly on a single sequence; the distinguishing step in this circumstance is comparing the vessel's appearance across multiple sequences with different flow sensitivities, including a dedicated flow-sensitive or angiographic sequence when genuine uncertainty exists, since true thrombus maintains a consistent signal pattern across flow-sensitive and flow-insensitive sequences while artifactual signal related to slow or turbulent flow characteristically changes appearance between them. Phase-contrast and other flow-quantification techniques, used selectively in body MRI for applications such as portal venous flow assessment, carry their own artifact, velocity aliasing, in which flow velocity exceeding the technique's selected velocity-encoding range wraps around to an artifactually reversed or understated value, analogous in principle to the spatial aliasing discussed in the first chapter of this book but occurring in the velocity domain rather than the spatial domain, and correctable by selecting a higher velocity-encoding range and repeating the measurement.

Artifact	Characteristic Appearance	Primary Cause	First-Line Mitigation
Vascular pulsation ghosting	Evenly spaced, fainter repeating foci along phase-encoding direction	Pulsatile vessel motion inconsistent across phase-encoding steps	Swap phase-encoding direction; saturation band; cardiac gating
Gibbs ringing	Fine parallel bands at high-contrast interfaces	Finite k-space sampling of a sharp boundary	Increase acquisition matrix; k-space apodization filter
Magic angle effect	Focal T1/short-echo hyperintensity in tendon or ligament near 55 degrees to B0	Dipolar interaction averaging at the magic angle	Compare short and long echo time sequences
Zipper artifact	Sharp line across entire image at fixed frequency position	External radiofrequency interference or shielding breach	Confirm door seal and exclude unshielded equipment; repeat acquisition
Dielectric shading	Broad geographic signal alteration crossing organ boundaries	B1 field inhomogeneity at high field strength in large or fluid-rich patients	Dielectric padding; radiofrequency shimming; consider 1.5 tesla
Even-echo rephasing	Slow-flow signal loss on odd echoes, signal recovery on even echoes	Cancellation of phase dispersion between successive refocusing pulses	Recognize echo-dependent pattern; correlate with flow-sensitive sequence

A Systematic Approach to Artifact Troubleshooting

A Stepwise Framework for an Unfamiliar Artifact

When an unfamiliar or ambiguous signal abnormality is encountered, a systematic troubleshooting sequence resolves the great majority of cases more reliably than an unstructured attempt to pattern-match against remembered examples. The first step is geometric: does the finding's shape, orientation, or position correspond to a known technical direction or structure, the phase-encoding direction, the position of an adjacent pulsatile vessel, the boundary of a high-contrast interface, or the field-of-view edge, rather than to a plausible anatomic or pathologic structure. The second step is behavioral: does the finding persist, change, or disappear when compared across sequences with different technical parameters, different phase-encoding direction, different breath-hold or distension state, different field strength or receiver bandwidth, since true pathology is reproducible across technical variation while most artifacts are not. The third step is contextual: does the finding's appearance match a specific, named artifact pattern given the clinical and technical context, a large-habitus patient at 3 tesla, a patient with a known implant, an examination performed without adequate fasting or bowel preparation, since many artifacts are specifically associated with identifiable risk factors that, once recognized, immediately narrow the differential. When these three steps do not resolve the ambiguity, escalation to a technologist review of the raw acquisition parameters, a repeat targeted sequence, or, when necessary, correlation with another imaging modality is a reasonable and appropriate next step rather than committing to an uncertain interpretation in either direction.

Documenting Artifact-Limited Examinations in the Report

When an examination is degraded by artifact that cannot be fully corrected, whether because a patient could not tolerate a repeat acquisition, because the artifact source could not be eliminated in real time, or because the diagnostic question can still be adequately answered despite the limitation, the report should explicitly state which specific artifact affected which specific sequence or anatomic region, and, when relevant, whether that limitation affects the confidence of a specific reported finding. A vague, generic disclaimer noting only that motion artifact was present, without specifying its severity, distribution, or diagnostic impact, provides little practical guidance to the referring clinician about whether the findings can be relied upon, whereas a specific statement, for example that dielectric shading limited assessment of the anterior bladder wall but did not affect evaluation of the primary rectal tumor, allows the referring team to correctly calibrate their confidence in the specific findings that matter most for management. This same discipline of specific, rather than generic, documentation applies equally to the confirmed-artifact cases throughout this chapter, where explicitly stating that a finding was confirmed as artifact, and by what specific method, protects both the patient from unnecessary downstream workup and the interpreting radiologist from an ambiguous record that could be misread by a future reader unfamiliar with the reasoning applied at the time.

Figure 4.4: Dielectric Pad Placement for B1 Field Correction at 3 Tesla

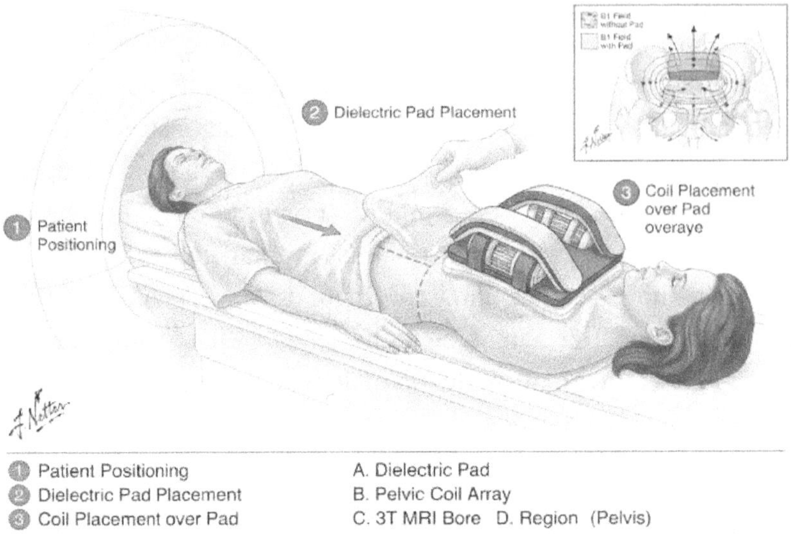

Clinical Case Presentations

Case 1. A 45-year-old woman undergoes MRI for evaluation of a known pancreatic cystic lesion. On the axial T1-weighted gradient-echo dynamic series, a small, round focus of low signal is noted in the pancreatic body, raising initial concern for a second, previously undescribed lesion. Before characterizing this as a new finding, the radiologist notes that the focus lies directly along a line extending from the adjacent splenic artery in the anterior-to-posterior direction, which was the recorded phase-encoding direction for this sequence, and that an identical focus is absent on a T2-weighted sequence acquired with a different phase-encoding direction. Recognizing this as vascular pulsation ghosting from the splenic artery rather than a true second lesion, the radiologist excludes it from the report, documents the single known cystic lesion using its established measurements, and avoids an unnecessary escalation in follow-up recommendations that an incorrectly characterized second lesion would otherwise have triggered.

Case 2. A 71-year-old man with a body mass index of thirty-eight undergoes pelvic MRI at 3 tesla for staging of a newly diagnosed rectal cancer. The initial high-resolution T2-weighted sequences demonstrate broad, geographic signal alteration crossing from the bladder wall into the adjacent rectal wall and mesorectal fat, without a discrete margin, that could be misread as diffuse tumor infiltration extending well beyond the known primary lesion. Recognizing this pattern as consistent with dielectric shading given the patient's body habitus and the field strength used, the technologist repeats the affected sequence with a dielectric pad positioned over the pelvis, which substantially reduces the signal alteration and reveals a normal-caliber, sharply marginated bladder wall and a rectal tumor confined to a smaller, well-defined segment, allowing accurate T-staging that would otherwise have been artifactually overstated.

Case 3. A 29-year-old man with cirrhosis and known portal hypertension undergoes MRI to evaluate for portal vein thrombosis prior to possible transplant evaluation. The initial spin-echo sequence demonstrates heterogeneous, intermediate signal within the main portal vein that could represent thrombus. Rather than finalizing this interpretation from a single sequence, the radiologist reviews a dedicated flow-sensitive gradient-echo sequence obtained as part of the same protocol, on which the portal vein demonstrates uniform flow-related signal without a discrete filling defect, consistent with slow but patent flow rather than thrombus. The final report specifically documents that the intermediate signal on the spin-echo sequence reflected slow-flow artifact rather than true thrombus, based on its resolution on flow-sensitive imaging, allowing the transplant evaluation to proceed without an incorrect contraindication being raised.

Case 4. A 33-year-old woman undergoes pelvic MRI for evaluation of chronic pelvic pain, and the high-resolution T2-weighted images demonstrate an area of increased signal within a segment of the sacrospinous ligament near the field-of-view periphery, raising initial concern for ligamentous injury or inflammatory change. Because the finding is encountered incidentally at the edge of a pelvic protocol not specifically designed to evaluate ligamentous structures, the radiologist compares the region on the available short and long echo time sequences within the same examination and finds that the signal alteration is present on the short echo time sequence but largely resolves on the longer echo time acquisition, and confirms on the sagittal localizer that the ligament segment in question courses at an oblique angle consistent with proximity to the magic angle relative to the main field. Recognizing this pattern as magic angle artifact rather than true ligamentous pathology, the radiologist excludes it from the impression and notes that no dedicated ligamentous abnormality is identified, avoiding an unnecessary referral for a structure that was never actually pathologic.

THE SIGNAL-TO-CATEGORY DECISION SYSTEM — Artifact Troubleshooting Arc

The Signal Pattern: This chapter's patterns share a common structure: an apparent abnormality whose true origin is technical rather than pathologic, revealed by geometry, reproducibility across technical variation, or clinical context rather than by its appearance on a single sequence alone.

Category Signature: A finding is categorized as artifact when its geometry matches a known technical direction or structure, when it fails to reproduce across sequences with varied technical parameters, or when it occurs in a clinical context specifically associated with a named artifact pattern; a finding that persists across all of these checks is categorized as true pathology.

The Decision: Confirmed artifact requires no further workup and should be explicitly excluded from the differential in the report; genuine uncertainty after systematic troubleshooting warrants a targeted repeat acquisition or technologist consultation rather than a guessed interpretation.

The Trap Logic: Every pattern in this chapter is most dangerous when only partially expressed, a solitary ghost rather than the full ghosting series, subtle rather than obvious dielectric shading, intermediate rather than frankly artifactual flow signal, since partial expression is what allows an artifact to masquerade convincingly as a true, if atypical, finding.

Pattern Anchor: Before committing to a diagnosis for any equivocal finding, run it through geometry, reproducibility, and clinical context; artifact fails at least one of these three checks, while true pathology passes all three.

Summary and Key Concepts

Vascular pulsation ghosting propagates along the phase-encoding direction from a pulsatile vessel and can be mitigated by swapping phase-encoding direction, cardiac gating, or saturation bands; its geometric relationship to the causative vessel is the key to recognizing it.

Gibbs ringing produces regularly spaced bands parallel to high-contrast interfaces and increases with lower spatial resolution; partial volume averaging blurs the true signal and size of small lesions and is mitigated by thin-section imaging.

Zipper artifacts indicate external radiofrequency interference, most often a shielding breach, and appear as a sharp line across the image at a position corresponding to the interfering frequency.

Dielectric shading, most pronounced at 3 tesla in large-habitus patients or those with large fluid collections, produces broad, geographic signal alteration that crosses anatomic boundaries and can mimic diffuse parenchymal disease.

Flow voids and flow-related enhancement are expected consequences of normal blood flow on spin-echo and gradient-echo sequences respectively, and should not be mistaken for thrombus or a flow-related pseudolesion.

Slow or turbulent flow can mimic thrombus on a single sequence; comparing the vessel's appearance across flow-sensitive and flow-insensitive sequences resolves the great majority of these cases.

A systematic troubleshooting approach, evaluating geometry, reproducibility across technical variation, and clinical context, resolves most unfamiliar or ambiguous artifacts more reliably than unstructured pattern matching.

CHAPTER 5: DIFFUSE LIVER DISEASE, STEATOSIS, AND HEPATIC FIBROSIS

Learning Objectives

1. Classify hepatic steatosis by underlying etiology and explain the pathophysiologic basis of chemical shift-based fat quantification techniques.
2. Apply proton density fat fraction measurement to grade hepatic steatosis and recognize the technical pitfalls that can bias this measurement.
3. Describe the pathophysiology of progressive hepatic fibrosis and relate specific morphologic and functional imaging findings to fibrosis stage.
4. Apply MR elastography to hepatic fibrosis staging and recognize the physiologic confounders that can falsely elevate or depress measured liver stiffness.
5. Recognize the MRI appearance of hepatic iron overload and distinguish primary hereditary hemochromatosis from secondary iron overload states.

Clinical Overview

Diffuse liver disease, unlike the focal hepatic lesions addressed in the following chapter, is characterized by pathologic processes distributed throughout the hepatic parenchyma rather than confined to a discrete mass, and its assessment depends on a different set of imaging tools: quantitative fat and iron measurement rather than lesion characterization, and stiffness measurement rather than enhancement pattern. These processes are not academic curiosities; hepatic steatosis affects a substantial proportion of the adult population in developed countries, and progressive hepatic fibrosis, whatever its underlying cause, is the final common pathway toward cirrhosis, portal hypertension, and hepatocellular carcinoma risk, the last of which is addressed in detail in the following chapter on focal liver lesions and the LI-RADS framework.

Body MRI has become the noninvasive reference standard for quantifying both hepatic fat content and hepatic fibrosis, substantially reducing reliance on liver biopsy for these specific purposes, and this chapter builds the physiologic and technical foundation for that role: how fat and iron alter the MR signal in ways that can be quantified rather than merely described qualitatively, and how fibrosis alters the mechanical properties of liver tissue in ways that MR elastography can measure directly. Two instances of the Signal-to-Category Decision System are applied here, to fat quantification in the presence of confounding iron deposition, and to elastography-based fibrosis staging in the presence of confounding inflammation or venous congestion.

Hepatic Steatosis: Pathophysiology and Classification

Pathophysiology of Triglyceride Accumulation in Hepatocytes

Hepatic steatosis develops when the rate of hepatocyte triglyceride accumulation, driven by increased delivery of free fatty acids from peripheral adipose tissue lipolysis, increased hepatic de novo lipogenesis, or both, exceeds the liver's capacity to export triglyceride as very low-density lipoprotein or to oxidize fatty acids through mitochondrial beta-oxidation, resulting in progressive accumulation of macrovesicular fat droplets within hepatocytes. This metabolic imbalance is most commonly driven by insulin resistance, in which impaired insulin signaling both increases peripheral lipolysis and promotes hepatic de novo lipogenesis simultaneously, which is why hepatic steatosis is so strongly linked epidemiologically to obesity, type 2 diabetes, and the broader metabolic syndrome, a relationship reflected in the terminology shift from nonalcoholic fatty liver disease to metabolic dysfunction-associated steatotic liver disease, now the preferred nomenclature in current guidelines because it centers the metabolic pathophysiology rather than defining the condition negatively by the absence of alcohol use.

Simple steatosis, in which triglyceride accumulation occurs without significant hepatocyte injury or inflammation, was historically considered a relatively benign, non-progressive condition, but a substantial minority of affected patients progress to steatohepatitis, in which accumulated intrahepatocyte lipid, particularly toxic lipid intermediates such as free fatty acids and ceramides rather than inert triglyceride itself, drives mitochondrial dysfunction, oxidative stress, and hepatocyte injury manifesting histologically as ballooning degeneration, lobular inflammation, and, critically, the stellate cell activation that initiates the fibrotic cascade detailed later in this chapter. This progression from simple steatosis to steatohepatitis to fibrosis is the central clinical concern driving the intensive quantitative MRI surveillance described throughout this chapter, since simple steatosis alone carries a comparatively favorable prognosis while steatohepatitis with progressive fibrosis is the pathway responsible for essentially all of the cirrhosis and hepatocellular carcinoma risk ultimately attributable to metabolic dysfunction-associated liver disease, which is why fat quantification and fibrosis staging are performed together rather than fat fraction being treated as a sufficient endpoint on its own.

From Steatosis to Steatohepatitis: Multiple-Hit Pathophysiology

Contemporary pathophysiologic models describe the progression from simple steatosis to steatohepatitis as a multiple-hit process rather than a single causal step, in which insulin resistance and the resulting hepatic lipid accumulation constitute a first, sensitizing hit that renders hepatocytes more vulnerable to subsequent injurious exposures, including oxidative stress from dysfunctional lipid metabolism itself, gut-derived endotoxin reaching the liver through an altered intestinal microbiome and increased intestinal permeability, and genetic and epigenetic factors that modulate individual susceptibility to progression, most notably variants in the PNPLA3 gene, which is associated with both greater steatosis severity and a substantially increased risk of progression to fibrosis independent of body mass index or diabetes status. This multiple-hit framework explains a clinically important observation that MRI quantification captures well: two patients with numerically identical proton density fat fraction values can nonetheless carry substantially different risk of progression to steatohepatitis and fibrosis, since fat fraction alone measures only the degree of triglyceride accumulation, the first hit, without capturing the presence or absence of the additional inflammatory and genetic factors that determine whether progression actually occurs, which is part of the rationale for pairing fat quantification with elastography-based fibrosis assessment rather than relying on either measurement in isolation.

Etiologic Classification and Risk Factors

Beyond the metabolic dysfunction-associated pathway, which accounts for the large majority of hepatic steatosis encountered in current clinical practice, alcohol-associated liver disease produces a histologically similar pattern of hepatocyte fat accumulation through a distinct mechanism, direct hepatotoxic effects of ethanol metabolism on mitochondrial fatty acid oxidation and on the cellular redox state, and the two etiologies frequently coexist in the same patient, complicating attribution of steatosis severity to a single cause. Less common causes include drug-induced steatosis, associated with medications such as methotrexate, tamoxifen, and certain antiretroviral agents, and a range of inherited metabolic disorders that impair fatty acid oxidation or lipoprotein assembly, generally presenting in childhood or with a distinctive clinical context that distinguishes them from the far more common metabolic dysfunction-associated pattern. Because the imaging appearance of steatosis is nonspecific to its underlying cause, correlating the degree and distribution of fat quantified by MRI with the clinical context, body mass index, diabetes status, alcohol history, and medication list, remains essential to appropriate interpretation and management guidance, since MRI itself cannot definitively distinguish between these etiologies.

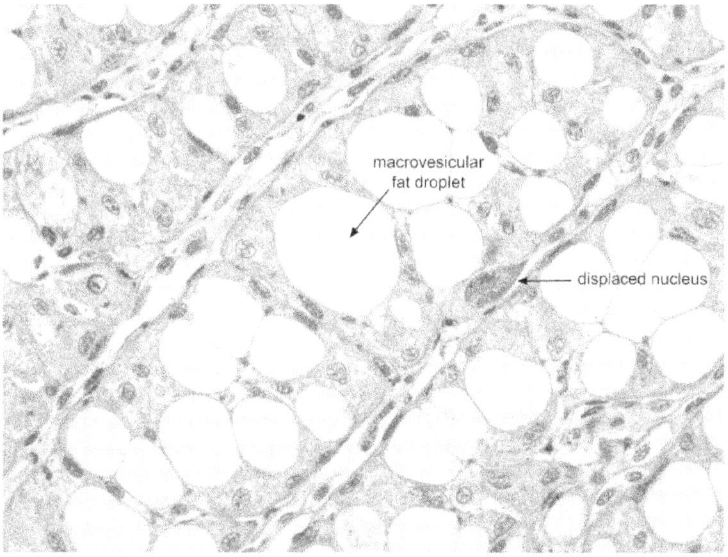

Where alcohol-associated liver disease and metabolic dysfunction-associated steatotic liver disease coexist, a combination increasingly recognized in clinical practice and now formally designated as a distinct overlap category in current nomenclature, the imaging findings of steatosis and fibrosis are essentially indistinguishable from either pure entity, and MRI's contribution in this setting shifts from etiologic discrimination toward accurate quantification of current disease severity, information that remains clinically actionable and prognostically important regardless of the precise proportional contribution of each etiologic factor. A careful, structured alcohol history, ideally obtained using a validated screening instrument rather than an informal question embedded in a general history, therefore remains an essential complement to MRI quantification in every patient undergoing diffuse liver disease evaluation, since the therapeutic implications, alcohol cessation counseling and referral in addition to metabolic intervention, differ meaningfully from management of metabolic dysfunction-associated disease alone, even though the imaging appearance itself provides no reliable means of separating the two contributions.

MRI Techniques for Fat Quantification

Proton Density Fat Fraction and the Confounder-Corrected Approach

Proton density fat fraction, the current reference-standard MRI biomarker for hepatic steatosis, is defined as the proportion of the total mobile proton signal within a voxel that arises from fat protons rather than water protons, and its calculation depends on the multi-echo chemical shift technique introduced in the first chapter of this book, extended here to correct for several confounding factors that a simple two-point in-phase and opposed-phase calculation does not adequately address. Because fat itself contains multiple distinct chemical species, olefinic, methylene, and methyl protons among others, each with a slightly different resonant frequency, a single-peak fat model systematically underestimates true fat fraction at high fat content; confounder-corrected proton density fat fraction techniques instead use a multi-peak spectral model that accounts for this chemical complexity, along with correction for T1 bias, since fat and water have different T1 relaxation times that would otherwise differentially weight their signal contributions, and correction for T2-star decay, which, left uncorrected, is confounded by the very iron deposition discussed later in this chapter.

Accurate fat fraction measurement also depends on careful attention to region-of-interest placement and acquisition technique that is easy to overlook when the calculation itself is performed automatically by scanner software. Regions of interest should be placed within homogeneous parenchyma, avoiding large intrahepatic vessels, the immediate subcapsular liver margin where susceptibility effects from the adjacent lung base or bowel gas can introduce measurement error, and any focal hepatic lesion, whose fat or iron content, if present, would otherwise be averaged into a measurement intended to characterize the background parenchyma rather than the lesion itself. Because fat distribution can be heterogeneous, particularly in early or patchy steatosis, sampling multiple regions of interest across different hepatic segments, rather than relying on a single measurement, and averaging or reporting the range of values obtained, provides a more representative characterization of overall hepatic fat burden than a single, potentially unrepresentative sample, a practice increasingly standard in dedicated hepatic MRI protocols and specifically recommended when segmental fat distribution appears visually heterogeneous on the source images.

Grading Steatosis and Its Clinical Correlation

Proton density fat fraction values are generally interpreted using threshold-based grading, with values below approximately five percent considered within the normal range, five to seventeen percent considered mild steatosis, seventeen to twenty-two percent moderate, and above twenty-two percent severe, though the precise numeric thresholds vary slightly between validation studies and should be interpreted as approximate rather than rigidly fixed boundaries. These quantitative grades correlate reasonably well with histologic steatosis grading obtained by liver biopsy, which is what has allowed proton density fat fraction to substantially reduce, though not eliminate, the clinical need for biopsy specifically to grade steatosis severity, reserving biopsy instead for indications requiring histologic assessment of inflammation, ballooning degeneration, or fibrosis stage that quantitative MRI fat and stiffness measurement together cannot fully substitute for in every clinical scenario. Because proton density fat fraction is a continuous, reproducible quantitative measurement rather than a categorical visual assessment, it is particularly well suited to longitudinal monitoring of steatosis in response to weight loss, pharmacologic therapy, or bariatric surgery, a use case increasingly common in metabolic dysfunction-associated steatotic liver disease management and one in which qualitative visual assessment of fat signal would be far less sensitive to clinically meaningful interval change.

THE SIGNAL-TO-CATEGORY DECISION SYSTEM — Iron-Confounded Fat Quantification

The Signal Pattern: A proton density fat fraction map generated using a standard confounder-corrected technique yields an unexpectedly low or discordant fat fraction value in a patient with strong clinical risk factors for steatosis, or the underlying source images show unusually rapid signal decay across increasing echo times.

Category Signature: A discordantly low or unreliable fat fraction value accompanied by an elevated R2-star or T2-star decay rate, reflecting coexistent hepatic iron deposition, is categorized as an iron-confounded measurement requiring cautious interpretation; a fat fraction value obtained with normal T2-star decay and full multi-peak, multi-confounder correction applied is categorized as a reliable, directly interpretable measurement.

The Decision: When significant iron deposition is identified, the R2-star or T2-star map itself should be reported alongside the fat fraction value, both because iron overload is a clinically significant finding in its own right, addressed later in this chapter, and because the fat fraction value in this setting should be interpreted with the awareness that severe iron overload can still introduce some residual quantification error even with confounder correction applied, warranting correlation with the clinical context rather than acceptance of the numeric value in isolation.

Trap Logic: A radiologist unfamiliar with T2-star confounding may report an artifactually low or falsely reassuring fat fraction in a patient with concurrent iron overload as evidence against clinically significant steatosis; the discriminating step is always reviewing the R2-star or T2-star map alongside the fat fraction map before finalizing a steatosis grade, since the two measurements are acquired from the same data set and should always be interpreted together, never the fat fraction map in isolation.

Pattern Anchor: Never finalize a proton density fat fraction grade without checking the corresponding R2-star or T2-star value for confounding iron deposition.

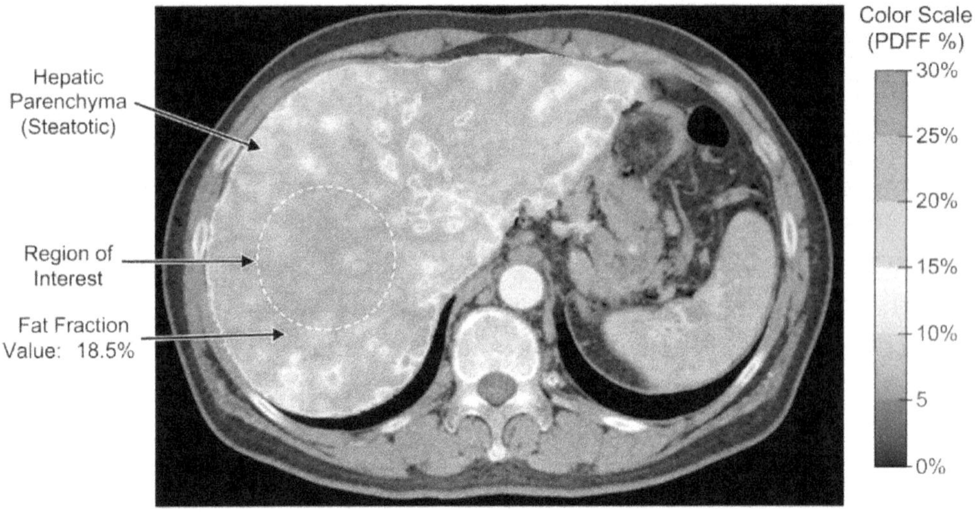

Figure 5.2: Proton Density Fat Fraction Map Demonstrating Moderate Hepatic Steatosis

Hepatic Fibrosis and Cirrhosis: Pathophysiology and Staging

The Pathophysiology of Progressive Fibrosis

Chronic hepatocellular injury, whatever its cause, activates hepatic stellate cells, normally quiescent, vitamin A-storing perisinusoidal cells that transform into proliferative, collagen-producing myofibroblast-like cells in response to sustained inflammatory signaling, and it is this stellate cell activation, rather than the initiating injury itself, that drives progressive deposition of fibrous extracellular matrix within the hepatic parenchyma. Early fibrosis is typically periportal or pericentral in distribution depending on the underlying etiology and pattern of injury, but as fibrosis progresses, bridging fibrous septa form between portal tracts and central veins, progressively distorting normal hepatic architecture, and the end stage of this process, cirrhosis, is defined by the combination of diffuse fibrosis with regenerative nodule formation, a structural reorganization that fundamentally alters both the liver's mechanical properties, the basis for elastography-based staging discussed below, and its vascular architecture, producing the portal hypertension responsible for many of cirrhosis's most serious clinical complications.

Histopathologic Fibrosis Staging Systems and Their Imaging Correlates

Histologic fibrosis staging systems, most widely the METAVIR system originally developed for chronic viral hepatitis and now applied more broadly, describe fibrosis on an ordinal scale from F0, no fibrosis, through F1 and F2, portal fibrosis with few or several bridging septa, to F3, numerous bridging septa without frank cirrhosis, and F4, established cirrhosis, and it is this histologic staging framework against which quantitative MRI elastography stiffness thresholds have been validated in the biopsy-correlation studies that established current clinical practice. Understanding this correlation is important for correctly communicating MRI-derived fibrosis stage to referring clinicians, who are frequently more familiar with METAVIR or the related Ishak staging system from prior biopsy reports than with elastography stiffness values in isolation, and reporting an MRI elastography result alongside its approximate histologic stage equivalent, rather than as a kilopascal value without clinical translation, substantially improves the report's practical utility for guiding management decisions such as variceal screening or hepatocellular carcinoma surveillance initiation, both of which are typically triggered by a histologic or histologic-equivalent stage of F3 or F4 rather than by the numeric stiffness value alone.

Morphologic Imaging Signs of Advancing Fibrosis and Cirrhosis

Beyond quantitative stiffness measurement, conventional morphologic MRI findings remain clinically valuable indicators of advancing fibrosis and established cirrhosis, and recognizing them is often the first clue that prompts more detailed fibrosis assessment. Nodular hepatic contour, best appreciated on high-resolution T1- or T2-weighted images of the liver surface, reflects the combination of regenerative nodules and intervening fibrous septa characteristic of cirrhotic architecture, and relative segmental volume redistribution, typically caudate lobe and lateral segment hypertrophy with right lobe atrophy, reflects differential fibrotic involvement and altered portal venous flow distribution across hepatic segments. Secondary signs of portal hypertension, splenomegaly, portosystemic venous collaterals, and ascites, while not direct measures of hepatic fibrosis itself, are important corroborating findings that should prompt careful assessment for cirrhosis even when the liver's contour and volume distribution are not yet dramatically abnormal, since these secondary signs can occasionally precede obvious morphologic change in the liver itself, particularly in the earlier stages of decompensation.

Regenerative and dysplastic nodules, distinct from the frank hepatocellular carcinoma addressed in the following chapter, are additional morphologic findings encountered in the cirrhotic liver, representing a biologic continuum from benign regenerative tissue through low-grade and high-grade dysplasia to frank malignancy, and while detailed nodule-by-nodule characterization is the focus of the LI-RADS framework covered in the next chapter, recognizing that a cirrhotic liver frequently contains numerous small nodules of uncertain or indeterminate significance is essential context for this chapter's diffuse disease assessment, since the presence of innumerable small nodules is itself a morphologic sign of advanced cirrhotic remodeling worth noting in the report even when no single nodule meets criteria for dedicated LI-RADS categorization.

MR Elastography and Other Techniques for Fibrosis Assessment

The Physical Basis of MR Elastography

MR elastography quantifies tissue stiffness directly by generating low-frequency mechanical shear waves within the liver, typically using an external passive driver placed against the patient's abdominal wall and connected to an active driver that produces continuous acoustic vibration during acquisition, and then imaging the propagation of these waves through hepatic tissue using a specialized phase-contrast MRI sequence sensitized to the microscopic tissue displacement caused by the passing wave. Because shear wave propagation speed increases with tissue stiffness, a fundamental physical relationship rather than an empirical correlation, the measured wave speed can be converted directly into a quantitative shear stiffness value, typically expressed in kilopascals, that increases progressively and reproducibly across the spectrum from normal liver through advancing fibrosis stages to cirrhosis, providing a genuinely mechanical, rather than indirect or surrogate, measurement of the structural change fibrosis produces.

Staging Thresholds and Clinical Application

Liver stiffness measured by MR elastography correlates closely with histologic fibrosis stage across validated threshold ranges, with normal liver typically measuring below approximately two point five kilopascals and cirrhosis typically exceeding five kilopascals, with intermediate fibrosis stages falling at intermediate stiffness values, though, as with proton density fat fraction thresholds, exact numeric cutoffs vary somewhat between published validation studies and equipment vendors and should be applied using the specific thresholds validated for the technique and platform in use at a given institution. This quantitative, reproducible staging capability has meaningfully reduced reliance on liver biopsy for fibrosis staging in chronic liver disease management, and because the measurement is noninvasive and can be repeated without procedural risk, MR elastography is now used routinely for longitudinal monitoring of fibrosis progression or regression in response to treatment of the underlying liver disease, whether that is antiviral therapy for chronic viral hepatitis, weight loss and metabolic intervention for metabolic dysfunction-associated steatotic liver disease, or alcohol cessation for alcohol-associated liver disease.

THE SIGNAL-TO-CATEGORY DECISION SYSTEM — Elastography Stiffness Confounded by Inflammation or Congestion

The Signal Pattern: Measured liver stiffness on MR elastography is unexpectedly elevated relative to the degree of fibrosis suggested by other clinical and imaging findings, or an elevated stiffness value is obtained in a patient with a clinical presentation more consistent with acute hepatitis or right heart failure than chronic fibrosing liver disease.

Category Signature: Elevated stiffness in the setting of markedly elevated serum transaminases, a clinical picture of acute hepatitis, or imaging and clinical findings of hepatic venous congestion such as dilated hepatic veins and inferior vena cava in a patient with known heart failure, is categorized as a confounded stiffness measurement rather than a true reflection of fibrosis stage; stiffness elevation in a patient with a stable, chronic clinical picture and no evidence of acute inflammation or venous congestion is categorized as a reliable fibrosis stage indicator.

The Decision: When acute inflammation or venous congestion is suspected as a confounder, elastography should be deferred or repeated after the confounding process resolves, acute hepatitis has settled, or heart failure has been treated, rather than the stiffness value being used to assign a fibrosis stage during the acute or congested state, since doing so risks substantially overstaging a patient's true chronic fibrosis burden.

Trap Logic: The most consequential error is applying standard fibrosis-stage stiffness thresholds without first confirming clinical stability, since both acute hepatic inflammation and passive venous congestion can elevate measured stiffness by a degree comparable to one or more full fibrosis stages independent of any true change in fibrous content; the discriminating step is always correlating the stiffness value with concurrent liver function tests and, when relevant, cardiac and hepatic venous imaging findings before finalizing a stage.

Pattern Anchor: An elevated elastography stiffness value in a patient with acute transaminase elevation or known heart failure should prompt deferral and clinical correlation, not immediate fibrosis staging.

Complementary Quantitative Techniques: Diffusion-Weighted Imaging and T1 Mapping

Beyond elastography, several additional quantitative MRI techniques provide complementary, if generally less validated, information about hepatic fibrosis. Diffusion-weighted imaging apparent diffusion coefficient values tend to decrease progressively with advancing fibrosis, reflecting the combination of increased extracellular fibrous matrix restricting water mobility and altered microvascular perfusion, though apparent diffusion coefficient's diagnostic performance for fibrosis staging is generally inferior to elastography, with greater overlap between adjacent fibrosis stages and greater susceptibility to the technical confounders discussed in the first chapter of this book, limiting its role to a supportive rather than primary staging tool. T1 mapping, particularly extracellular volume fraction calculated from pre- and post-contrast T1 measurements in a manner directly analogous to techniques long established in cardiac MRI, provides a measurement more specifically tied to the extracellular fibrous matrix itself rather than to the combined mechanical and cellular changes captured by elastography stiffness, and has shown promising correlation with histologic fibrosis in emerging research, though it has not yet achieved the same level of clinical validation, standardization, or widespread availability as MR elastography, and is used at present as a research and selectively applied clinical tool rather than a routine component of every diffuse liver disease protocol.

Hepatic Iron Overload and Its MRI Assessment

Primary and Secondary Iron Overload

Hereditary hemochromatosis, most commonly caused by mutations in the HFE gene affecting hepcidin regulation, results in inappropriately increased intestinal iron absorption that progressively deposits excess iron predominantly within hepatocytes, producing a pattern of primarily parenchymal, relatively pancreas- and spleen-sparing iron deposition in earlier stages, which can progress to hepatic fibrosis, cirrhosis, and, notably, a distinctly elevated risk of hepatocellular carcinoma independent of fibrosis stage if untreated. Secondary iron overload, by contrast, most commonly results from repeated red blood cell transfusion in patients with chronic transfusion-dependent conditions such as thalassemia major or myelodysplastic syndrome, and follows a different anatomic distribution, initially depositing iron within the reticuloendothelial system, predominantly Kupffer cells in the liver and macrophages in the spleen and bone marrow, before spilling over into hepatocytes and other parenchymal cells only once reticuloendothelial iron storage capacity is exceeded, a distinction that helps differentiate the two entities on imaging even before genetic or transfusion history is available.

Monitoring treatment response is a central longitudinal application of quantitative iron imaging in both primary and secondary overload. In hereditary hemochromatosis managed with therapeutic phlebotomy, serial R2-star or T2-star measurement provides an objective, noninvasive means of confirming that hepatic iron concentration is declining toward target levels without requiring repeated biopsy, and can help determine when maintenance-phase, less frequent phlebotomy is appropriate in place of the more intensive induction-phase schedule used at diagnosis. In transfusion-dependent secondary overload managed with iron chelation therapy, quantitative MRI iron assessment, performed at both the liver and, using a related but distinct T2-star technique, the heart, since cardiac iron deposition follows a different time course than hepatic deposition and carries its own distinct and serious risk of iron-related cardiomyopathy, has become a standard component of chelation therapy monitoring across major transfusion-dependent hematologic conditions, guiding chelator dose adjustment in a way that serum ferritin, a comparatively crude and acute-phase-reactant-confounded surrogate marker, cannot achieve with comparable precision or organ specificity.

MRI Quantification of Hepatic Iron Content

Iron is strongly paramagnetic and produces local magnetic field inhomogeneity at the microscopic level that accelerates T2 and T2-star signal decay in a manner directly proportional to tissue iron concentration, the same physical principle underlying the R2-star confounder discussed earlier in this chapter, now applied deliberately as the primary quantification technique for hepatic iron content rather than treated as an unwanted confounder. Multi-echo gradient-echo sequences acquired across a range of echo times allow calculation of a T2-star or R2-star map, from which hepatic iron concentration can be estimated using validated calibration curves relating decay rate to biopsy-proven liver iron concentration, providing a noninvasive alternative to the liver biopsy historically required to quantify iron overload severity and guide the decision to initiate iron chelation or therapeutic phlebotomy. Because severe iron overload produces extremely rapid signal decay, sequences must include sufficiently short minimum echo times to accurately characterize the most severely affected patients, since a maximum measurable R2-star value can otherwise be reached, beyond which further increases in true iron concentration can no longer be distinguished, a technical ceiling effect that becomes clinically relevant in the most heavily iron-loaded transfusion-dependent patients.

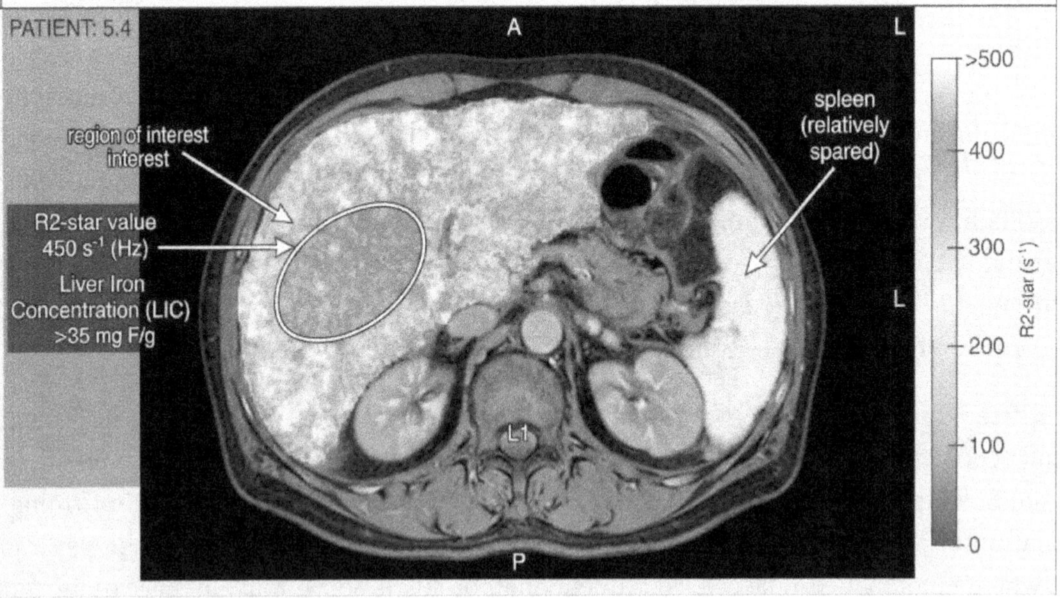

Figure 5.4 — Diagnostic Imaging: R2-Star Map of Severe Hepatic Iron Overload

Complications and Long-Term Prognosis of Diffuse Liver Disease

The long-term consequences of untreated or progressive diffuse liver disease converge on a shared final pathway regardless of underlying etiology: progressive fibrosis leading to cirrhosis, portal hypertension with its attendant risks of variceal hemorrhage and ascites, hepatic synthetic dysfunction manifesting as coagulopathy and hypoalbuminemia, and a substantially elevated risk of hepatocellular carcinoma that, in cirrhotic patients regardless of the fibrosis-causing etiology, justifies the biannual surveillance protocols detailed in the following chapter's discussion of the LI-RADS framework. Hereditary hemochromatosis carries a distinctive additional risk profile, an elevated hepatocellular carcinoma risk that can occur even in the absence of cirrhosis, thought to relate to iron's direct role in generating oxidative DNA damage through Fenton chemistry, reinforcing why iron quantification and appropriate chelation or phlebotomy therapy have prognostic significance beyond their effect on liver stiffness alone. Quantitative MRI's role in this prognostic picture extends beyond a single diagnostic snapshot: because fat fraction, elastography stiffness, and iron concentration are all reproducible, noninvasive measurements suitable for repeated longitudinal assessment, they increasingly function as surrogate endpoints for tracking disease trajectory over years of clinical follow-up, identifying patients whose fibrosis is progressing despite treatment and warrants escalated management, and confirming regression in patients responding favorably to weight loss, antiviral therapy, alcohol cessation, or iron reduction therapy, a longitudinal monitoring role that a single liver biopsy, with its attendant procedural risk and sampling variability, cannot practically fulfill.

Special Populations: Pediatric and Pregnancy Considerations

Pediatric hepatic steatosis, increasingly encountered given rising rates of childhood obesity, presents unique diagnostic considerations, since normative proton density fat fraction and elastography stiffness thresholds validated in adult populations may not directly apply to a growing liver, and pediatric-specific reference ranges and protocol adaptations, including the coil selection and sequence modifications discussed in the patient preparation chapter earlier in this book, should be used when available rather than reflexively applying adult thresholds to a pediatric examination. Distinguishing metabolic dysfunction-associated steatotic liver disease from the range of inherited pediatric metabolic and glycogen storage disorders that can also produce hepatic steatosis in childhood is a further diagnostic consideration specific to this population, generally requiring correlation with growth parameters, additional laboratory testing, and, in ambiguous cases, genetic evaluation, since the imaging appearance of steatosis alone does not reliably distinguish between these etiologically distinct pediatric conditions. Pregnancy introduces a different set of considerations, since gadolinium-based contrast administration is generally avoided when not clinically essential, as discussed in the contrast safety chapter, and since acute fatty liver of pregnancy, a rare but life-threatening condition distinct from the chronic steatotic processes emphasized throughout this chapter, requires urgent recognition and obstetric management rather than the elective, quantitative workup pathway described here; the specific protocol modifications and differential diagnostic considerations for body MRI throughout pregnancy are addressed comprehensively in a later chapter of this book.

Clinical Case Presentations

Case 1. A 48-year-old man with type 2 diabetes and a body mass index of thirty-four is referred for MRI proton density fat fraction and elastography as part of a metabolic dysfunction-associated steatotic liver disease evaluation. The fat fraction map demonstrates a value of twenty-six percent, in the severe steatosis range, with a normal R2-star value excluding iron confounding, and the elastography stiffness measures three point one kilopascals, consistent with mild to moderate fibrosis rather than advanced fibrosis or cirrhosis. The combination of severe steatosis with only mild fibrosis is specifically noted in the report as distinguishing a patient at significant risk for disease progression, given the severity of the metabolic driver, from one who has already progressed to advanced structural liver disease, information that directly informs the intensity of the lifestyle and pharmacologic intervention the referring endocrinologist subsequently pursues.

Case 2. A 61-year-old woman with a remote history of viral hepatitis C, successfully treated with antiviral therapy several years earlier, undergoes surveillance MRI with fat fraction and elastography. The elastography stiffness measures five point eight kilopascals, in the cirrhosis range, but the radiologist notes that the patient was hospitalized two weeks earlier for a heart failure exacerbation with documented volume overload, and that hepatic and inferior vena caval dilation is present on the same examination. Recognizing venous congestion as a plausible confounder given this timing, the radiologist recommends deferred repeat elastography after the patient's heart failure is optimized and volume status has normalized, rather than immediately reporting a cirrhosis stage, and a repeat examination six weeks later, after cardiac optimization, demonstrates a stiffness of three point six kilopascals, consistent with moderate rather than cirrhotic fibrosis, confirming that the initial elevated value substantially reflected congestion rather than true fibrosis stage.

Case 3. A 39-year-old man of Northern European ancestry with a family history of hemochromatosis and mildly elevated ferritin undergoes MRI for hepatic iron quantification. The R2-star map demonstrates markedly elevated hepatic iron concentration with a relatively spared spleen and pancreas, a distribution pattern consistent with primary hereditary iron overload rather than a transfusion-related secondary process, correlating with the patient's clinical history and supporting confirmatory HFE genetic testing. The quantified liver iron concentration is used directly by the patient's hematologist to establish a baseline for monitoring the response to therapeutic phlebotomy, illustrating how quantitative MRI iron assessment functions not only as a diagnostic tool but as a longitudinal monitoring biomarker throughout treatment.

Case 4. A 55-year-old woman with biopsy-proven metabolic dysfunction-associated steatohepatitis and stage F2 fibrosis two years earlier returns for interval MRI to assess treatment response following a structured weight loss program and initiation of a glucagon-like peptide-1 receptor agonist. The current examination demonstrates a proton density fat fraction of nine percent, down from a baseline of twenty-four percent documented at the time of her original diagnosis, and an elastography stiffness of two point six kilopascals, near the upper limit of normal and substantially improved from her prior stiffness of three point eight kilopascals. The report explicitly compares both quantitative values against the patient's own prior examination rather than presenting them only as isolated absolute measurements, allowing the referring hepatologist to document objective, biopsy-free evidence of both steatosis regression and fibrosis improvement in response to treatment, a comparison that meaningfully supports continuing the current management approach rather than escalating to more invasive intervention.

THE SIGNAL-TO-CATEGORY DECISION SYSTEM — Diffuse Liver Disease Quantification Arc

The Signal Pattern: This chapter's two patterns, iron-confounded fat quantification and inflammation- or congestion-confounded elastography, both involve a quantitative MRI biomarker whose numeric value can be distorted by a second, coexisting physiologic process.

Category Signature: A fat fraction or stiffness value is categorized as reliable only when the specific confounder relevant to that measurement, iron for fat fraction, acute inflammation or congestion for stiffness, has been explicitly excluded using the corresponding corroborating map or clinical correlation.

The Decision: Reliable values are used directly for grading, staging, and longitudinal monitoring; confounded values prompt either correction using corroborating data already acquired in the same examination or deferral and repeat measurement once the confounding process has resolved.

Trap Logic: Both patterns share the same trap: interpreting a single quantitative number in isolation without reviewing the corroborating map or clinical context that would reveal a confounder, a mistake made easier by how confident and precise a single numeric output can appear even when it is quietly wrong.

Pattern Anchor: Never report a quantitative fat fraction or elastography stiffness value without checking its specific corresponding confounder, R2-star for fat, clinical and venous congestion status for stiffness.

Summary and Key Concepts

Hepatic steatosis results from hepatocyte triglyceride accumulation exceeding export and oxidative capacity, most commonly driven by insulin resistance in metabolic dysfunction-associated steatotic liver disease, and is graded quantitatively by proton density fat fraction.

Confounder-corrected proton density fat fraction accounts for fat's multi-peak spectral complexity, T1 bias, and T2-star decay, and must always be interpreted alongside the R2-star map to exclude iron confounding.

Progressive hepatic fibrosis reflects hepatic stellate cell activation and collagen deposition, culminating in cirrhosis, defined by diffuse fibrosis with regenerative nodules and altered vascular architecture producing portal hypertension.

MR elastography directly measures hepatic shear stiffness, which increases with fibrosis stage, providing a noninvasive, reproducible alternative to biopsy for fibrosis staging and longitudinal monitoring.

Elastography stiffness can be falsely elevated by acute hepatic inflammation or hepatic venous congestion, and elevated values in these clinical contexts should prompt deferral or clinical correlation rather than immediate fibrosis staging.

Hereditary hemochromatosis produces predominantly hepatocellular iron deposition, while transfusion-related secondary iron overload initially deposits in the reticuloendothelial system, a distinction reflected in differing splenic and pancreatic involvement on imaging.

R2-star and T2-star mapping quantify hepatic iron concentration noninvasively, though very severe iron overload can exceed the measurable ceiling of standard sequences, requiring shorter minimum echo times in heavily iron-loaded patients.

CHAPTER 6: FOCAL LIVER LESIONS AND THE LI-RADS FRAMEWORK

Learning Objectives

1. Characterize the classic MRI appearance of common benign focal liver lesions, including simple cysts, hemangiomas, and focal nodular hyperplasia, and distinguish them from malignant mimics.
2. Classify hepatocellular adenoma subtypes and relate subtype to malignant transformation and hemorrhage risk.
3. Apply the LI-RADS major and ancillary imaging features to characterize a focal observation in a patient at risk for hepatocellular carcinoma.
4. Assign an appropriate LI-RADS category based on major feature combination and explain the corresponding management implication of each category.
5. Recognize the imaging pattern of hepatic metastatic disease and distinguish it from primary hepatocellular carcinoma and benign mimics.

Clinical Overview

Few tasks in body MRI carry as much immediate clinical consequence as characterizing a focal hepatic observation, since the differential spans entirely benign, no-action lesions at one end to hepatocellular carcinoma requiring urgent oncologic management at the other, with a wide range of intermediate and indeterminate possibilities between them. This chapter builds outward from the classic benign lesions every reader must recognize confidently and without hesitation, through the LI-RADS framework that has standardized hepatocellular carcinoma characterization across the field, to hepatic metastatic disease, the most common malignant focal liver process encountered in general practice.

The LI-RADS framework, introduced by the American College of Radiology specifically for use in patients at risk for hepatocellular carcinoma, is not a generic lesion characterization system applicable to every patient; it is a purpose-built categorization scheme whose major features and category thresholds were validated specifically in the cirrhotic and chronic hepatitis B population, and applying it outside that intended population, discussed further below, is one of the most consequential category errors a reader can make. Two instances of the Signal-to-Category Decision System are applied in this chapter, to hemangioma-versus-hypervascular-malignancy discrimination and to LI-RADS category assignment itself, extending the pattern-recognition framework introduced earlier in this book to what is arguably its highest-stakes application.

Benign Focal Liver Lesions: Cysts, Hemangiomas, and Focal Nodular Hyperplasia

Simple Hepatic Cysts

Simple hepatic cysts, among the most common incidental focal liver findings encountered in clinical practice, demonstrate a uniform, unambiguous MRI signature: markedly hyperintense signal on T2-weighted sequences, comparable to or exceeding cerebrospinal fluid, homogeneous low signal on T1-weighted sequences, sharply defined thin or imperceptible walls without internal septation or nodularity, and, critically, absence of any enhancement following contrast administration, a feature that definitively excludes the cystic or necrotic malignant lesions that can otherwise mimic a simple cyst's fluid signal characteristics on precontrast sequences alone. When a lesion demonstrates every one of these features, no further characterization or follow-up is required, and this represents one of the clearest examples in body MRI of a finding that can be dismissed with complete diagnostic confidence based on imaging alone, without biopsy or interval surveillance.

Peribiliary cysts, a distinct variant arising from obstructed peribiliary glands rather than from the biliary epithelium itself, characteristically cluster along the portal triads in a linear, tram-track-like distribution rather than the more randomly scattered distribution typical of simple hepatic cysts, and are encountered most often in patients with advanced cirrhosis or chronic biliary disease; recognizing their distinctive periportal location prevents them from being mistaken for a dilated, obstructed biliary system, particularly on sequences or in patients where the two entities might otherwise be conflated at first glance, since the clinical management of asymptomatic peribiliary cysts, essentially observation only, differs substantially from the workup that would be triggered by a concern for true biliary obstruction.

Hepatic Abscess and Infectious Mimics

Pyogenic hepatic abscess presents a pattern distinct from both simple and complicated cysts, typically demonstrating a thick, irregular, enhancing rim surrounding a central non-enhancing collection, often with surrounding parenchymal edema manifesting as ill-defined perilesional T2 hyperintensity and, characteristically, restricted diffusion within the central collection itself, reflecting the viscous, cellular content of frank pus, a feature that helps distinguish abscess from the non-restricting fluid of a simple or complicated cyst. Multiloculated or cluster-type abscesses, in which several smaller, confluent collections coalesce, are a recognized morphologic variant and should not be mistaken for a cystic neoplasm, particularly given the clinical urgency of correctly identifying an abscess given the need for prompt drainage and antimicrobial therapy. Amebic abscess, more common in patients with relevant travel or exposure history, shares substantial imaging overlap with pyogenic abscess but is more often solitary and peripherally located, and definitive distinction between pyogenic and amebic etiology ultimately depends on serologic testing and clinical context rather than imaging appearance alone, reinforcing that a confidently diagnosed abscess pattern should prompt urgent clinical correlation and, where appropriate, sampling, rather than an attempt to determine microbiologic etiology from imaging features in isolation.

Complicated Cysts and Biliary Hamartomas

Complicated cysts, containing internal hemorrhage, proteinaceous debris, or infection, deviate from the simple cyst pattern by demonstrating heterogeneous or elevated T1 signal and variable, sometimes markedly reduced, T2 signal, and the absence of any enhancing solid component remains the key discriminator confirming a complicated but still benign process rather than a cystic or necrotic neoplasm; enhancement of a thin, smooth wall alone, reflecting normal surrounding compressed hepatic parenchyma rather than a true neoplastic capsule, is an accepted feature of a complicated but benign cyst and should not by itself trigger malignancy concern. Biliary hamartomas, also called von Meyenburg complexes, present a related but distinct pattern: numerous, typically subcentimeter, T2-hyperintense foci scattered throughout the liver without mass effect or enhancement, representing small malformative bile duct clusters of no clinical significance in isolation, though their innumerable, scattered appearance can superficially suggest metastatic disease to an unfamiliar reader, a distinction usually resolved by their uniform small size, lack of any enhancing component, and, when available, comparison with prior imaging demonstrating long-term stability.

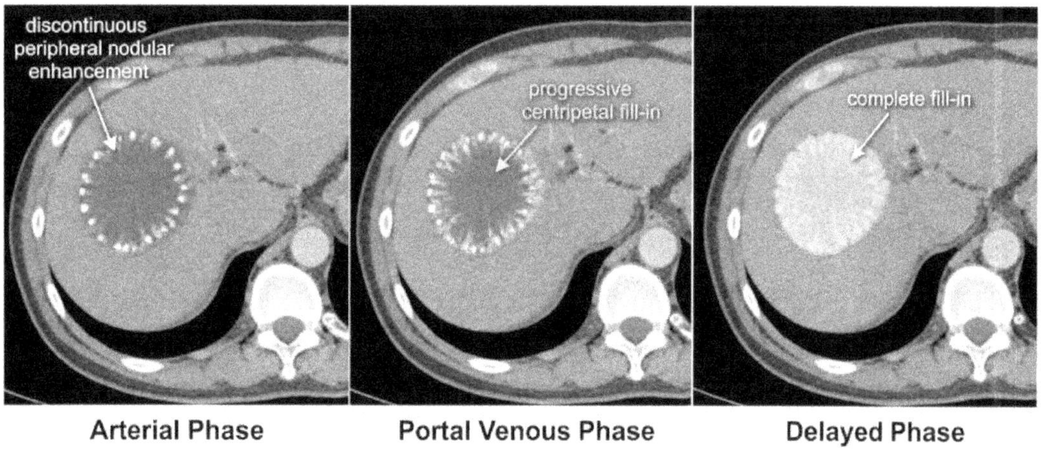

Figure 6.1: Classic Peripheral Nodular Enhancement Pattern of Hepatic **Hemangioma**

Hepatic Hemangioma

Hepatic hemangioma, the most common benign solid hepatic neoplasm, is composed of blood-filled vascular channels lined by endothelium, and its MRI appearance directly reflects this vascular architecture: markedly T2-hyperintense signal, though characteristically somewhat less intense than a simple cyst, and a highly distinctive enhancement pattern of discontinuous, peripheral, nodular enhancement on early postcontrast imaging that progressively fills in toward the lesion's center on delayed phase imaging, ultimately achieving uniform or near-uniform enhancement matching or exceeding blood pool signal, a pattern that reflects progressive contrast filling of the lesion's vascular channels over time rather than tumor-associated neovascularity. Small hemangiomas, particularly those below one to one and a half centimeters, can occasionally demonstrate rapid, uniform enhancement on arterial phase imaging without the classic discontinuous nodular pattern, a variant sometimes called a flash-filling hemangioma, which can superficially resemble a hypervascular malignancy on arterial phase imaging alone and requires the same-lesion comparison across all dynamic phases, not the arterial phase in isolation, to correctly identify the sustained, blood pool-matching enhancement on delayed imaging that confirms the benign diagnosis.

THE SIGNAL-TO-CATEGORY DECISION SYSTEM — Flash-Filling Hemangioma Mimicking a Hypervascular Malignancy

---

The Signal Pattern: A small hepatic lesion demonstrates uniform, intense arterial phase hyperenhancement without the classic discontinuous peripheral nodular pattern typically associated with hemangioma.

Category Signature: A lesion that remains uniformly, intensely enhancing and matches or exceeds blood pool signal on portal venous and delayed phase imaging, without washout, is categorized as a flash-filling hemangioma; a lesion that shows washout relative to background liver on delayed imaging is categorized as a potential hypervascular malignancy requiring further characterization.

The Decision: A confirmed flash-filling hemangioma, sustained and matched to blood pool across all postcontrast phases, requires no further workup; any degree of washout, even if only subtle relative hypointensity on delayed phase imaging, should prompt evaluation under the LI-RADS framework detailed later in this chapter or, in a non-cirrhotic patient outside the LI-RADS intended population, consideration of metastatic disease or another primary hepatic malignancy.

Trap Logic: The arterial phase alone is never sufficient to diagnose a flash-filling hemangioma, since intense arterial enhancement is shared by hemangioma and truly hypervascular malignancy alike; the discriminating step is always tracking the lesion's signal intensity relative to blood pool and background liver across every subsequent postcontrast phase, since sustained, blood pool-matching enhancement without washout is what separates the two, not the arterial phase appearance.

Pattern Anchor: A small, intensely arterial-enhancing lesion is only confirmed benign once it is shown to remain matched to blood pool, without washout, through the delayed phase; never diagnose a flash-filling hemangioma from the arterial phase alone.

Focal Nodular Hyperplasia

Focal nodular hyperplasia, a benign hyperplastic response of hepatocytes to a congenital or acquired arterial malformation rather than a true neoplasm, characteristically demonstrates near-isointensity to background liver on both T1- and T2-weighted precontrast sequences, reflecting its composition of essentially normal hepatocytes, along with a central scar in larger lesions that is T2-hyperintense, reflecting its myxoid stromal and vascular composition, and typically demonstrates delayed enhancement distinct from the surrounding lesion. On dynamic contrast imaging, focal nodular hyperplasia shows intense, uniform arterial phase hyperenhancement reflecting its predominantly arterial blood supply, followed by near-isointensity to background liver on portal venous and delayed phases, without true washout, a pattern that, together with the central scar when present, is highly specific for the diagnosis. On hepatobiliary phase imaging, obtained after administration of a hepatobiliary-specific contrast agent as discussed in the earlier chapter on contrast agents, focal nodular hyperplasia characteristically retains contrast and appears iso- to hyperintense relative to background liver, a distinctive and highly specific finding that reflects the presence of functioning, if architecturally disorganized, hepatocytes and biliary canaliculi within the lesion, in direct contrast to the hepatocellular adenoma discussed next, which typically appears hypointense on the hepatobiliary phase due to its diminished or absent normal biliary excretory function.

Hepatocellular Adenoma: Subtypes and Risk Stratification

Molecular Subtypes and Their Distinguishing Features

Hepatocellular adenoma, a true benign hepatocellular neoplasm strongly associated with oral contraceptive use, anabolic steroid use, and metabolic syndrome, is now recognized to comprise several molecularly distinct subtypes with meaningfully different imaging appearances and, more importantly, different malignant transformation and hemorrhage risk. The hepatocyte nuclear factor 1-alpha-inactivated subtype characteristically demonstrates diffuse, homogeneous intralesional fat, evident as signal loss on opposed-phase relative to in-phase imaging in a pattern distinct from the focal, boundary-limited chemical shift artifact discussed in the first chapter of this book, and carries a comparatively low risk of malignant transformation. The inflammatory subtype, the most common subtype overall, demonstrates a characteristic combination of T2 hyperintensity, often most pronounced peripherally, described as an atoll sign, along with persistent enhancement into the delayed phase reflecting sinusoidal dilation and inflammatory change, and carries an intermediate risk of both hemorrhage and, to a lesser degree, malignant transformation. The beta-catenin-activated subtype, less common but of particular concern, lacks a specific, reliable imaging signature distinguishing it from other subtypes yet carries the highest risk of malignant transformation among all adenoma subtypes, which is an important limitation to acknowledge explicitly in any report characterizing a probable adenoma, since imaging subtype prediction, while clinically useful, cannot fully substitute for the risk stratification that pathologic subtyping after biopsy or resection provides.

Hemorrhage, the most common acute complication prompting emergent presentation in a patient with an unrecognized hepatocellular adenoma, produces a recognizable, if variable, MRI pattern depending on the age of the blood products present: acute hemorrhage typically demonstrates heterogeneous, often T1-hyperintense signal reflecting methemoglobin formation within days of the bleeding episode, with fluid-fluid levels representing layering of blood products of differing density a frequently encountered and highly suggestive finding, and surrounding perilesional or, in more severe cases, perihepatic or intraperitoneal hemorrhage when the bleeding has extended beyond the lesion's capsule. Because active or recent hemorrhage substantially alters the lesion's baseline signal characteristics and can obscure the specific subtyping features described above, a lesion imaged in the acute post-hemorrhagic period is often better characterized on a follow-up examination performed after the hemorrhage has resolved and evolved, at which point the underlying adenoma's true subtype-specific features become more reliably assessable, an important practical point when counseling a patient or referring clinician about the timing and interpretation of follow-up imaging after an acute hemorrhagic presentation.

Management Implications of Adenoma Size and Subtype

Management of a confirmed or probable hepatocellular adenoma is stratified primarily by size and, where determinable, molecular subtype, with lesions smaller than five centimeters in a patient without concerning subtype features generally managed with cessation of any implicated hormonal exposure and imaging surveillance, reflecting the relatively low absolute risk of clinically significant hemorrhage or malignant transformation below this threshold, while lesions exceeding five centimeters, those demonstrating interval growth, those in male patients, in whom adenoma is less common overall but carries a disproportionately higher malignant transformation risk when it does occur, and those with beta-catenin-activated subtype features or definitively increased size on serial imaging are generally considered for resection given the cumulative risk these factors confer. This size- and subtype-based risk stratification underscores why precise, reproducible lesion measurement and subtype characterization, including explicit statement of whether the adenoma pattern is more consistent with the hepatocyte nuclear factor 1-alpha-inactivated, inflammatory, or an indeterminate subtype, adds substantial clinical value beyond simply identifying that an adenoma is present, since this information directly shapes the surgical referral threshold applied by the managing hepatobiliary team.

The LI-RADS Framework: Major and Ancillary Imaging Features

The LI-RADS Major Features

The LI-RADS framework organizes hepatocellular carcinoma risk assessment around a small set of major imaging features, each individually well validated and, in combination, forming the basis of category assignment. Nonrim arterial phase hyperenhancement describes enhancement of the observation exceeding that of background liver on arterial phase imaging, distributed relatively uniformly across the lesion rather than confined to a thin peripheral rim, the latter pattern instead favoring a different diagnosis discussed later in this chapter. Nonperipheral washout describes relative hypointensity of the observation compared to background liver on portal venous or delayed phase imaging, again distributed centrally within the lesion rather than only at its periphery, reflecting the more rapid contrast egress characteristic of hepatocellular carcinoma's abnormal, capillarized sinusoidal architecture relative to surrounding cirrhotic parenchyma. Enhancing capsule describes a smooth, uniformly enhancing rim, typically most conspicuous on portal venous or delayed phase imaging, corresponding histologically to a true fibrous pseudocapsule that forms as hepatocellular carcinoma compresses and remodels adjacent parenchyma, a feature that in this specific hepatocellular carcinoma-risk context favors malignancy, in contrast to the frequently encountered nonspecific rim enhancement of a benign complicated cyst discussed earlier in this chapter, which occurs in a fundamentally different lesion population and must not be conflated with the LI-RADS capsule feature. Threshold growth, an increase in lesion size meeting a defined magnitude within a defined time interval on serial imaging, is the fourth major feature and is unique among the four in requiring comparison imaging rather than being assessable from a single examination.

Ancillary Features That Favor or Disfavor Malignancy

Beyond the major features, LI-RADS incorporates a defined set of ancillary features that, while not sufficient alone to establish a definitive category, can adjust category assignment within defined limits when major features alone leave genuine ambiguity. Features favoring malignancy include mild-moderate T2 hyperintensity, restricted diffusion, and corona enhancement, a thin zone of enhancement surrounding the observation on late arterial or early portal venous phase imaging reflecting compressed peritumoral sinusoids, while features favoring a benign observation include marked T2 hyperintensity, more typical of a hemangioma or cyst as detailed earlier in this chapter, undistorted vessels passing through the observation without displacement, and stability over an extended surveillance interval. The hepatobiliary phase, when a hepatobiliary-specific contrast agent is used, contributes its own ancillary information: hepatocellular carcinoma typically appears hypointense on the hepatobiliary phase due to loss of normal hepatocyte transporter function, though a minority of well-differentiated hepatocellular carcinomas can retain iso- or hyperintense hepatobiliary phase signal, an important exception to keep in mind since an isointense hepatobiliary phase appearance alone should not be used to exclude malignancy in an otherwise concerning observation.

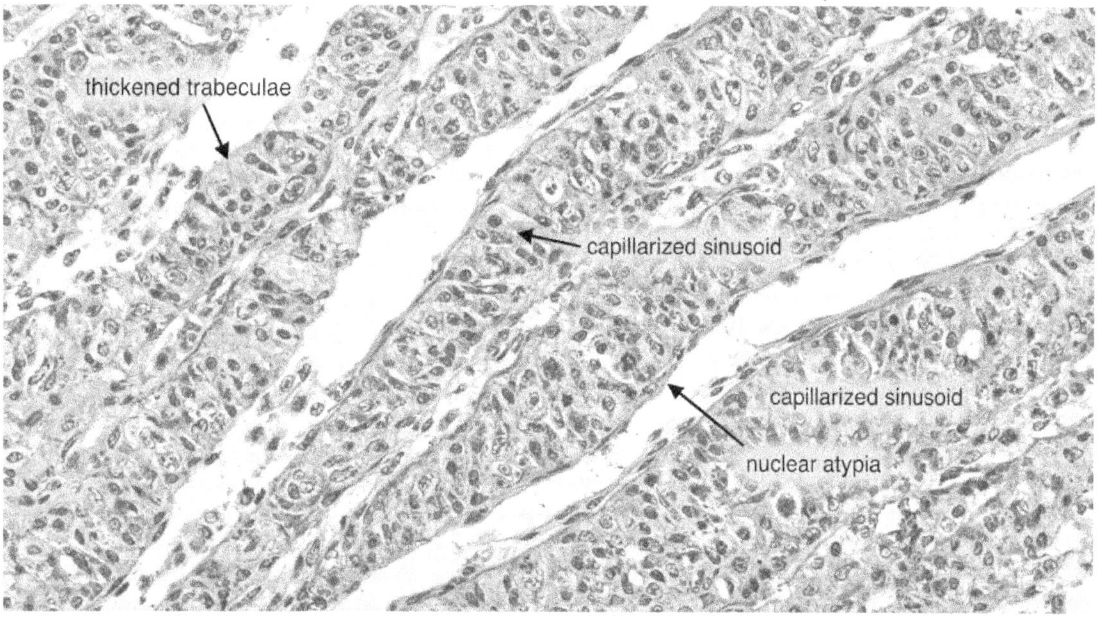

LI-RADS Category Assignment and Management Implications

The LI-RADS Category System

LI-RADS categories range from LR-1, definitely benign, through LR-2, probably benign, LR-3, intermediate probability of malignancy, LR-4, probably hepatocellular carcinoma, LR-5, definitely hepatocellular carcinoma, LR-M, probably or definitely malignant but not specific for hepatocellular carcinoma, and LR-TIV, definite tumor in vein, with category assignment determined by a defined algorithm combining observation size with the specific combination of major features present. An observation demonstrating nonrim arterial phase hyperenhancement together with either nonperipheral washout or enhancing capsule, at a size meeting the algorithm's defined threshold, achieves LR-5 categorization, treated clinically as definitive for hepatocellular carcinoma without requiring biopsy confirmation before treatment planning in most practice settings, a remarkable degree of diagnostic confidence that reflects the extensive validation underlying the LR-5 category specifically. LR-4 observations demonstrate a similar but less complete or less robust combination of major features, typically warranting biopsy or short-interval follow-up imaging rather than immediate treatment, while LR-3 observations lack sufficient major features to favor malignancy strongly but cannot be dismissed as definitely benign, generally warranting continued surveillance at a defined interval rather than immediate intervention.

Two additional categories complete the system and address specific technical or vascular scenarios not captured by the standard feature-based algorithm. LR-NC designates an observation that cannot be categorized because the examination is technically inadequate, most often due to one of the artifact patterns discussed in the preceding chapter degrading a phase critical to feature assessment, and its assignment is itself an important quality signal prompting a repeat, technically adequate examination rather than a forced categorization from suboptimal images. LR-TIV, definite tumor in vein, is assigned when unambiguous enhancing soft tissue is identified expanding the lumen of the portal or hepatic venous system, a finding with major treatment and prognostic implications since venous invasion generally excludes curative resection or transplantation and is managed instead with systemic or locoregional therapy, and distinguishing true tumor thrombus, which enhances and often demonstrates restricted diffusion similar to the parent tumor, from bland, nonenhancing thrombus, which carries no comparable prognostic weight, is a distinction of substantial clinical consequence resting on the same enhancement-based reasoning applied throughout this chapter.

LR-M and the Importance of Population Context

The LR-M category deserves particular emphasis because it captures a clinically crucial distinction that the size- and feature-based LR-1 through LR-5 algorithm alone does not: an observation demonstrating rim rather than nonrim arterial phase hyperenhancement, peripheral rather than nonperipheral washout, marked diffusion restriction, or other atypical features is categorized LR-M specifically because these features suggest a malignancy other than typical hepatocellular carcinoma, most often intrahepatic cholangiocarcinoma or a combined hepatocellular-cholangiocarcinoma tumor, which is managed differently and carries a different prognosis than typical hepatocellular carcinoma, making the LR-M distinction directly actionable rather than a mere technical subclassification. It bears repeated emphasis that the entire LI-RADS algorithm, including every category described here, is validated specifically for use in patients with cirrhosis, chronic hepatitis B infection, or a current or prior hepatocellular carcinoma, and applying LI-RADS categorization to a focal liver observation in a patient outside this specific risk population, a young patient with no liver disease risk factors, for instance, is a category error that can produce a misleading categorical label; in such patients, the differential and appropriate framework for lesion characterization instead follows the benign lesion and metastatic disease patterns discussed elsewhere in this chapter, not the LI-RADS algorithm.

Applying LI-RADS to Treatment Response Assessment

Beyond initial diagnosis, a parallel LI-RADS treatment response framework applies specifically to hepatocellular carcinoma lesions that have undergone locoregional therapy, such as transarterial chemoembolization or thermal ablation, using a distinct set of categories, viable, equivocal, and nonviable, that assess residual tumor activity rather than initial diagnostic probability. Viable tumor after treatment characteristically retains the same nonrim arterial phase hyperenhancement and washout pattern used in initial diagnosis, now interpreted specifically within or along the margin of the treated lesion bed rather than as a new, previously uncharacterized observation, while a nonviable, successfully treated lesion demonstrates absence of any enhancing tissue within the treatment zone, though distinguishing this from the expected postprocedural rim enhancement of benign granulation tissue and reactive change, particularly in the early postablation period, requires familiarity with the specific expected time course of typical treatment response versus atypical, concerning enhancement patterns. Correctly applying this treatment-response framework, rather than reflexively reapplying the initial diagnostic LI-RADS category system to a post-treatment lesion, is essential for accurately guiding the decision between continued surveillance and additional locoregional or systemic therapy, and conflating the two frameworks is a recognized source of miscommunication between radiology and the treating oncologic team.

THE SIGNAL-TO-CATEGORY DECISION SYSTEM — LI-RADS Category Assignment and the Pseudocapsule Trap

---

The Signal Pattern: A hepatic observation in a cirrhotic patient demonstrates nonrim arterial phase hyperenhancement together with a smooth, enhancing peripheral rim most conspicuous on delayed imaging.

Category Signature: A smooth, complete, uniformly enhancing rim in this specific at-risk population is categorized as an enhancing capsule, a major feature favoring LR-5 when combined with arterial phase hyperenhancement; an incomplete, irregular, or nodular rim, or rim enhancement occurring earlier, on the arterial phase itself, rather than on delayed imaging, is categorized differently and should raise consideration of LR-M or an alternative diagnosis rather than being assumed to represent a true capsule.

The Decision: A confirmed enhancing capsule combined with arterial phase hyperenhancement, at appropriate size, supports LR-5 categorization and definitive hepatocellular carcinoma management without biopsy; an atypical, incomplete, or early-arterial rim pattern should prompt LR-M consideration or additional characterization rather than default LR-5 assignment.

Trap Logic: The most consequential error is applying the enhancing capsule feature outside its validated context or without confirming its specific timing and completeness; a thin, smooth rim of transient perilesional enhancement on arterial phase imaging alone, a corona-type ancillary feature rather than a true delayed capsule, is sometimes mistaken for the capsule major feature, and confusing the two can lead to inappropriate category assignment in either direction.

Pattern Anchor: A true LI-RADS capsule is a smooth, complete rim best seen on delayed rather than arterial phase imaging in a patient within the validated risk population; confirm timing, completeness, and population before applying this major feature.

Figure 6.3: LR-5 Observation Demonstrating Arterial Hyperenhancement, Washout, and Capsule

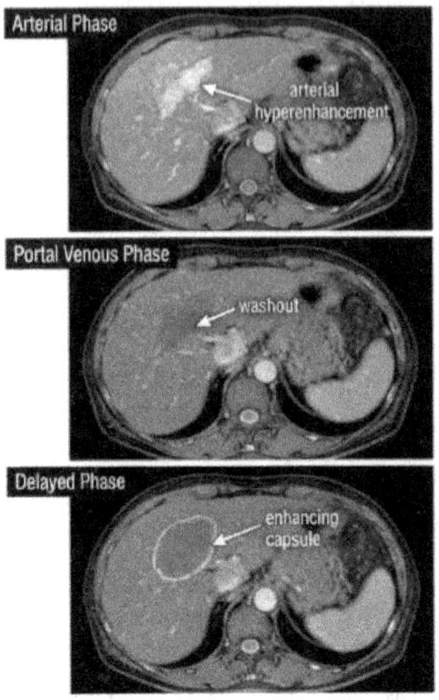

Figure 6.3 — Diagnostic Imaging: LI-RADS 5 Hepatic Observation

Hepatic Metastases and Other Malignant Focal Lesions

Imaging Patterns of Hepatic Metastatic Disease

Hepatic metastases are, in aggregate, the most common malignant hepatic lesions encountered in general clinical practice, far outnumbering primary hepatocellular carcinoma in a non-cirrhotic population, and their imaging appearance varies substantially with the primary tumor type, though several patterns recur commonly enough to warrant specific recognition. Hypovascular metastases, characteristic of colorectal, lung, and most gastric and pancreatic primary tumors, demonstrate relatively low signal on arterial and portal venous phase imaging relative to background liver, often with a thin rim of peripheral enhancement, and are typically best detected on portal venous phase imaging, when the contrast between maximally enhancing background parenchyma and the relatively hypoenhancing metastasis is greatest, reinforcing the portal venous phase's importance as the primary detection phase emphasized in the protocol design chapter earlier in this book. Hypervascular metastases, characteristic of neuroendocrine tumors, renal cell carcinoma, thyroid carcinoma, and melanoma, instead demonstrate arterial phase hyperenhancement that can superficially resemble a benign hemangioma or, in an at-risk patient, hepatocellular carcinoma, distinguished primarily by the presence of multiple lesions, a known extrahepatic primary malignancy, and, when present, washout patterns or restricted diffusion inconsistent with the specific benign patterns detailed earlier in this chapter.

Distinguishing Metastatic Disease From Its Principal Mimics

The single most useful discriminating principle when hepatic metastatic disease is suspected is multiplicity and clinical context: multiple lesions of similar imaging appearance in a patient with a known primary malignancy overwhelmingly favor metastatic disease over a coincidental benign process, whereas a solitary lesion in a patient without a known malignancy warrants more careful consideration of the benign entities detailed earlier in this chapter before metastatic disease is assumed. Diffusion-weighted imaging is particularly valuable in this differential, since most hepatic metastases demonstrate restricted diffusion reflecting their high cellular density, a feature shared with hepatocellular carcinoma but not with hemangioma, simple cyst, or the hepatobiliary-phase-retaining focal nodular hyperplasia, making diffusion-weighted imaging a useful adjunct across nearly every scenario addressed in this chapter, and the hepatobiliary phase, when used, is similarly valuable since virtually all metastatic lesions, like hepatocellular carcinoma, appear hypointense due to the complete absence of functioning hepatocyte transporter activity within metastatic tissue, though this hepatobiliary phase hypointensity is nonspecific and does not by itself distinguish metastatic disease from hepatocellular carcinoma, a distinction that instead relies on the specific enhancement pattern, clinical history, and multiplicity considerations detailed throughout this section.

Metastatic lesions that have responded to systemic chemotherapy present their own interpretive nuance: a treated lesion may decrease in size, develop internal cystic or necrotic change, or, in the specific case of colorectal metastases treated with certain chemotherapy regimens, transform into a predominantly cystic-appearing lesion that can be mistaken for a new benign cyst if the patient's treatment history is not available at the time of interpretation, underscoring why reviewing prior oncologic treatment history is as essential to accurate hepatic lesion interpretation as the imaging findings themselves. Conversely, lesions demonstrating new or increasing size, new restricted diffusion, or new enhancement components after a period of treatment-related stability or regression should be flagged as possible disease progression, and correlating the current examination directly against the most recent prior study, rather than assessing the current study in isolation, is essential for reliably detecting this kind of interval change, particularly for small lesions near the threshold of detectability where subtle growth is easy to overlook without direct side-by-side comparison.

Special Populations and Incidental Lesion Management

Incidentally discovered hepatic lesions in patients without a known malignancy or cirrhosis risk factor, an exceedingly common scenario given the frequency of abdominal imaging performed for unrelated indications, should be managed according to established incidental lesion management guidelines that stratify follow-up recommendations by lesion size, imaging characteristics, and patient risk factors, rather than by reflexive application of either the LI-RADS or the oncologic surveillance frameworks detailed above, both of which presume a specific at-risk population that most patients with a truly incidental finding do not belong to. In pregnant patients, discussed in greater detail in a later chapter of this book, hepatic hemangioma and focal nodular hyperplasia both remain the most common benign incidental findings, and their characteristic appearance, together with avoidance of gadolinium-based contrast when not essential as discussed in the contrast safety chapter, generally allows confident, contrast-sparing or contrast-deferred characterization using precontrast T1 and T2 signal characteristics alone, reserving contrast-enhanced characterization for genuinely indeterminate lesions where the diagnostic benefit outweighs the preference to avoid contrast during pregnancy.

Intrahepatic Cholangiocarcinoma and Other Rare Primary Malignancies

Intrahepatic cholangiocarcinoma, the primary malignancy most often responsible for the LR-M categorization discussed earlier in this chapter, arises from the intrahepatic bile duct epithelium and characteristically demonstrates a mass-forming pattern with progressive, delayed enhancement reflecting its dense fibrous stroma, in contrast to the washout pattern typical of hepatocellular carcinoma, along with capsular retraction of the overlying liver surface, upstream biliary ductal dilation when the tumor obstructs an adjacent duct, and, frequently, satellite nodules surrounding the dominant mass, none of which are typical features of hepatocellular carcinoma. Because intrahepatic cholangiocarcinoma is managed with a fundamentally different surgical and systemic treatment approach than hepatocellular carcinoma, and because it arises with some increased frequency in the same cirrhotic population at risk for hepatocellular carcinoma, correctly recognizing this progressive, delayed-enhancing, capsule-retracting pattern rather than defaulting to a hepatocellular carcinoma-pattern interpretation is one of the most clinically consequential distinctions addressed in this chapter, and is precisely the distinction the LR-M category was designed to flag. Hepatic angiosarcoma, a rare but aggressive malignant vascular neoplasm, and combined hepatocellular-cholangiocarcinoma tumors, which display overlapping imaging features of both parent lesion types, represent further, less common entities within the LR-M category, underscoring that LR-M is intentionally a heterogeneous category capturing several distinct malignant entities united by their atypical, non-hepatocellular-carcinoma-pattern imaging appearance rather than a single specific diagnosis.

Figure 6.4 — Percutaneous Image-Guided Biopsy Technique for an Indeterminate Hepatic Lesion

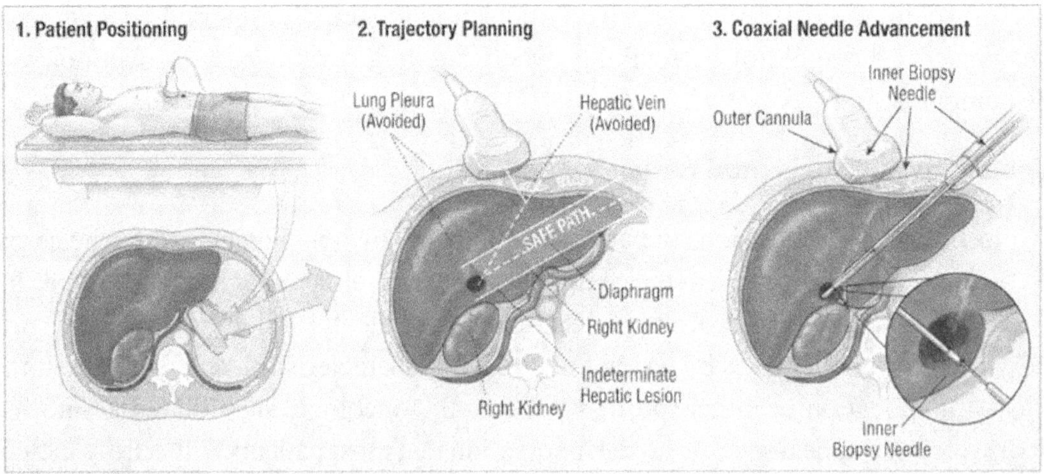

1. Patient Positioning — Patient positioned for image-guided access to the liver lesion, utilizing ultrasound.
2. Trajectory Planning — Planning needle path to reach the hepatic lesion while avoiding critical structures (pleura, vessels).
3. Coaxial Needle Advancement — Advancement of the coaxial introducer system under image guidance for core biopsy sample acquisition.

Clinical Case Presentations

Case 1. A 44-year-old woman with no liver disease risk factors undergoes MRI for evaluation of a hepatic lesion identified incidentally on ultrasound. The lesion demonstrates near-isointensity to background liver on precontrast sequences, intense uniform arterial phase enhancement, near-isointensity on portal venous and delayed phases without washout, and a central T2-hyperintense scar. On hepatobiliary phase imaging obtained as part of the protocol, the lesion is mildly hyperintense relative to background liver. This complete constellation of findings, including the diagnostic hepatobiliary phase retention, allows the radiologist to confidently characterize the lesion as focal nodular hyperplasia without biopsy, and the report explicitly notes that no further imaging follow-up is required given the specificity of this combined finding set.

Case 2. A 58-year-old man with hepatitis B-related cirrhosis undergoes surveillance MRI. A 2.2-centimeter observation in segment 7 demonstrates nonrim arterial phase hyperenhancement and nonperipheral washout on the portal venous phase, but the delayed phase rim enhancement is subtle, irregular, and better appreciated on the arterial than the delayed phase, raising the radiologist's suspicion that this represents corona enhancement rather than a true capsule. Applying the category assignment framework carefully, the radiologist categorizes the observation as LR-4 rather than LR-5, given the atypical capsule-like feature, and recommends multidisciplinary tumor board discussion and probable biopsy rather than proceeding directly to LR-5-driven treatment planning, illustrating the clinical consequence of correctly distinguishing a true capsule from corona enhancement rather than defaulting to the more definitive category.

Case 3. A 62-year-old woman with a history of colorectal cancer treated three years earlier undergoes surveillance MRI, which demonstrates five new hepatic lesions ranging from 0.8 to 2.1 centimeters, each showing relatively hypovascular enhancement on all dynamic phases with thin peripheral rim enhancement, best conspicuous on the portal venous phase, and restricted diffusion on high b-value and apparent diffusion coefficient imaging. Given the multiplicity, the patient's oncologic history, and the characteristic hypovascular pattern with restricted diffusion, the radiologist confidently characterizes these as metastatic disease without requiring biopsy of every lesion, recommending biopsy of a single representative lesion only if tissue confirmation is specifically needed for treatment planning purposes, and the report is structured to clearly convey the number, size, and distribution of lesions in a format directly usable for the patient's oncologic staging and treatment planning discussion.

Case 4. A 51-year-old woman with hepatitis B-related cirrhosis returns for follow-up MRI eight weeks after transarterial chemoembolization of a previously confirmed LR-5 observation in segment 6. The treatment zone demonstrates a large area of expected nonenhancing embolized tumor with peripheral rim enhancement, and the radiologist, applying the LI-RADS treatment response framework rather than the initial diagnostic algorithm, notes a small, 8-millimeter focus of nodular, nonrim arterial phase hyperenhancement with washout along the posterior margin of the treatment zone, distinct from the expected thin, smooth rim enhancement pattern of benign post-treatment change. This focus is categorized as viable residual tumor under the treatment response framework, and the report explicitly distinguishes this specific, actionable finding from the surrounding expected nonviable treatment bed, prompting the interventional radiology team to plan a targeted repeat treatment to the residual focus rather than assuming complete treatment response based on the overall appearance of the treatment zone.

THE SIGNAL-TO-CATEGORY DECISION SYSTEM — Focal Liver Lesion Characterization Arc

---

The Signal Pattern: This chapter's patterns span the full spectrum of focal liver lesion characterization, from the flash-filling hemangioma that mimics malignancy to the pseudocapsule that can mislead LI-RADS category assignment.

Category Signature: Benign lesions are categorized by their complete, specific imaging signature across every relevant phase and sequence, never by a single feature in isolation; LI-RADS categories are assigned only within the validated at-risk population, using precisely defined major features whose timing and completeness must be confirmed rather than assumed.

The Decision: A complete, specific benign signature ends the workup without biopsy; an incomplete or atypical pattern, whether in a benign lesion mimicking malignancy or a hepatocellular carcinoma mimic lacking a true capsule, triggers either LI-RADS-appropriate management or a step down to a less definitive category and further evaluation.

The Trap Logic: Every pattern in this chapter shares the same underlying trap: relying on a single phase or a single feature, an arterial phase alone, a rim of enhancement alone, without confirming its full behavior across every relevant sequence and its validity within the correct patient population.

Pattern Anchor: Never characterize a focal liver lesion from a single phase or feature; confirm the complete signature across all dynamic phases, and confirm LI-RADS applies to this specific patient, before finalizing a category.

Summary and Key Concepts

Simple hepatic cysts demonstrate uniform T2 hyperintensity, T1 hypointensity, and absent enhancement, allowing confident diagnosis without follow-up; complicated cysts and biliary hamartomas deviate from this pattern but remain benign in the absence of a true enhancing solid component.

Hemangioma demonstrates discontinuous peripheral nodular enhancement with centripetal fill-in; small flash-filling hemangiomas require confirmation of sustained, blood pool-matched enhancement across all postcontrast phases, not the arterial phase alone.

Focal nodular hyperplasia shows near-isointensity to liver precontrast, intense arterial hyperenhancement without washout, a central scar in larger lesions, and characteristic hepatobiliary phase retention distinguishing it from hepatocellular adenoma.

Hepatocellular adenoma subtypes, hepatocyte nuclear factor 1-alpha-inactivated, inflammatory, and beta-catenin-activated, carry different malignant transformation and hemorrhage risk, and management is stratified by size, subtype, and patient sex.

The LI-RADS major features, nonrim arterial phase hyperenhancement, nonperipheral washout, enhancing capsule, and threshold growth, combine algorithmically to assign categories from LR-1 through LR-5, LR-M, and LR-TIV, validated specifically in cirrhotic and chronic hepatitis B populations.

The enhancing capsule major feature must be smooth, complete, and best seen on delayed rather than arterial phase imaging to be distinguished from corona enhancement, an ancillary feature that does not carry the same category-defining weight.

Hepatic metastases are distinguished from primary hepatocellular carcinoma and benign mimics primarily by multiplicity, clinical history, hypovascular portal venous phase conspicuity for most primary tumor types, and restricted diffusion.

CHAPTER 7: BILIARY TRACT DISORDERS AND MRCP

Learning Objectives

1. Recognize the MRCP appearance of choledocholithiasis and distinguish true filling defects from common technical mimics.
2. Differentiate benign from malignant biliary strictures based on morphology, length, and associated findings.
3. Apply the Bismuth-Corlette classification to perihilar cholangiocarcinoma and relate classification to surgical planning.
4. Recognize the imaging features of congenital biliary anomalies, including choledochal cysts and Caroli disease, and their associated malignancy risk.
5. Distinguish primary sclerosing cholangitis and other inflammatory biliary conditions from malignant biliary obstruction.

Clinical Overview

Magnetic resonance cholangiopancreatography, introduced in the protocol design chapter earlier in this book, provides a noninvasive, contrast-independent window into the biliary tree that has substantially reduced the diagnostic role of endoscopic retrograde cholangiopancreatography, now reserved primarily for therapeutic rather than purely diagnostic indications. This chapter builds the clinical interpretive framework for that window: how to distinguish a true filling defect from ductal fluid signal artifact, how to characterize a stricture's morphology in a way that meaningfully narrows the differential between benign and malignant causes, and how to recognize the specific congenital and inflammatory conditions that carry their own distinct malignancy risk and management pathway.

Biliary pathology sits at a genuine diagnostic crossroads in body MRI, where a missed or mischaracterized finding can mean either an unnecessary invasive procedure for a benign process or, in the opposite direction, a delayed diagnosis of a malignancy whose curability depends heavily on early, accurate staging. Two instances of the Signal-to-Category Decision System are applied in this chapter, to distinguishing a true ductal filling defect from pneumobilia and other artifactual mimics, and to distinguishing a malignant from a benign-appearing biliary stricture.

Choledocholithiasis and Biliary Obstruction

MRCP Appearance of Ductal Calculi

Choledocholithiasis characteristically appears on heavily T2-weighted MRCP sequences as a rounded or faceted filling defect, low in signal against the surrounding bright, T2-hyperintense bile, typically outlined by a thin rim of bile creating a meniscus sign at its interface with the duct wall, a pattern most reliably appreciated on thin-section source images reviewed individually rather than on the maximum intensity projection reconstruction alone, since small or multiple calculi can be obscured by overlapping structures on the projection image even when clearly visible on the source data. Ductal dilation proximal to an obstructing calculus is a common but not universal associated finding, since a calculus can be present without producing significant proximal dilation, particularly if it is small, nonobstructing, or intermittently mobile, which is why the absence of ductal dilation should not by itself be used to exclude choledocholithiasis when a filling defect meeting the characteristic signal and morphologic criteria is otherwise identified.

Intrahepatic calculi, less common than choledocholithiasis but encountered in the setting of recurrent pyogenic cholangitis discussed later in this chapter, primary sclerosing cholangitis, or chronic biliary stasis of any cause, follow the same fundamental signal characteristics as extrahepatic calculi but require careful, segment-by-segment review of the intrahepatic ductal branches on the thin-section source images, since small intrahepatic stones are easily overlooked on the maximum intensity projection view, where they can be obscured by overlapping vascular structures or by the inherently lower conspicuity of a small filling defect within a smaller-caliber duct. Sensitivity for small calculi, whether extrahepatic or intrahepatic, is generally highest on heavily T2-weighted thin-section sequences with the shortest achievable echo time consistent with adequate T2 weighting, since calculi smaller than the section thickness are subject to the same partial volume averaging discussed in the artifact chapter, which can render a genuinely present small stone falsely inconspicuous or falsely absent on thicker-slice acquisitions.

Distinguishing True Calculi From Artifactual Filling Defects

Pneumobilia, air within the biliary tree most often resulting from a prior sphincterotomy, biliary-enteric anastomosis, or, less commonly, a spontaneous biliary-enteric fistula, produces a filling defect that can superficially resemble a calculus but is distinguished by its tendency to layer nondependently, typically anteriorly with the patient supine, in contrast to a calculus, which layers dependently under gravity, and by its characteristic susceptibility-related signal void and blooming on gradient-echo sequences, a pattern not shared by the more sharply marginated signal void of a true calculus on heavily T2-weighted sequences. Flow-related signal voids and the vascular pulsation ghosting discussed in the artifact chapter earlier in this book can occasionally be mistaken for a ductal filling defect when a vessel courses in close proximity to the biliary tree, and confirming that a suspicious filling defect is present in exactly the same location and configuration across multiple sequences and imaging planes, rather than relying on a single MRCP sequence in isolation, is the standard discriminating maneuver that resolves the great majority of ambiguous cases.

A further, more subtle mimic arises from residual T2-hyperintense signal within a partially collapsed or poorly distended duct, particularly in the setting of respiratory or bulk motion during MRCP acquisition, where inconsistent ductal caliber across the respiratory cycle can create an apparent filling defect at the transition between differently distended segments, a phenomenon conceptually analogous to the bowel distension artifact discussed in the protocol design chapter earlier in this book. This artifact is generally resolved by reviewing multiple MRCP acquisitions if available, since a true calculus persists in the same location and configuration regardless of respiratory phase or acquisition technique, while a distension-related apparent defect typically shifts or resolves on a differently timed or differently gated acquisition, reinforcing the same reproducibility-across-technical-variation principle applied throughout the artifact chapter to this specific biliary context.

Figure 7.1

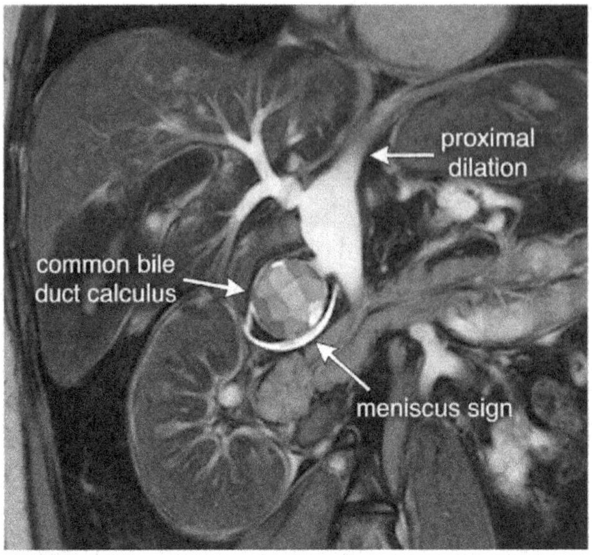

THE SIGNAL-TO-CATEGORY DECISION SYSTEM — True Ductal Calculus versus Pneumobilia

---

The Signal Pattern: A filling defect is identified within the common bile duct on MRCP, appearing as a signal void against the surrounding bright bile signal.

Category Signature: A filling defect that layers dependently, is sharply rounded or faceted, and does not demonstrate blooming on gradient-echo sequences is categorized as a true calculus; a filling defect that layers nondependently, demonstrates blooming artifact, and correlates with a known history of sphincterotomy or biliary-enteric anastomosis is categorized as pneumobilia.

The Decision: A confirmed true calculus, particularly if obstructing or symptomatic, warrants referral for endoscopic or surgical extraction; confirmed pneumobilia requires no intervention and should be explicitly distinguished in the report from a retained or recurrent calculus, particularly in a post-cholecystectomy or post-sphincterotomy patient in whom this distinction is frequently clinically relevant.

Trap Logic: Layering position alone can occasionally be ambiguous depending on patient positioning and duct orientation; the more reliable discriminating feature is the presence or absence of blooming artifact on a gradient-echo sequence, since true calculi, lacking the strong susceptibility effect of air, do not bloom to the same degree, and this comparison should be made whenever layering position alone leaves genuine uncertainty.

Pattern Anchor: When a ductal filling defect is ambiguous, check for blooming on a gradient-echo sequence and correlate with prior sphincterotomy or biliary-enteric surgical history before diagnosing a retained calculus.

Biliary Strictures: Benign and Malignant Differentiation

Morphologic Features Favoring Malignancy

A malignant biliary stricture characteristically demonstrates an abrupt, shouldered transition from normal to narrowed duct caliber, often with irregular, asymmetric margins, in contrast to the smooth, gradually tapering transition more typical of a benign process, and is frequently accompanied by an associated soft tissue mass, either subtle mural thickening and enhancement of the duct wall itself or a more overt discrete mass, that enhances progressively into the delayed phase, reflecting the fibrous stromal composition shared with the intrahepatic cholangiocarcinoma pattern discussed in the preceding chapter. Marked, asymmetric proximal ductal dilation disproportionate to the degree of luminal narrowing, and the length of the stricture itself, with longer segments of involvement generally favoring malignancy over the typically shorter, more focal narrowing of most benign strictures, are further morphologic features that, in combination rather than individually, meaningfully shift the differential toward a malignant process warranting tissue sampling and oncologic staging.

Morphologic Features Favoring a Benign Process

Benign strictures, whether related to prior surgery, chronic pancreatitis extending to involve the intrapancreatic bile duct, or an inflammatory condition such as primary sclerosing cholangitis discussed later in this chapter, more often demonstrate smooth, symmetric, gradually tapering margins without an associated soft tissue mass, and a clinical history of prior biliary surgery, recurrent pancreatitis, or a known inflammatory bowel disease association, as is frequently the case with primary sclerosing cholangitis, should be actively sought and weighted heavily in the overall assessment, since a benign clinical context substantially strengthens the case for a benign stricture even when the morphologic features alone leave some residual ambiguity. It bears emphasis that morphologic stricture characterization, while a valuable and validated diagnostic tool, does not achieve the same near-definitive diagnostic confidence that the LI-RADS LR-5 category provides for hepatocellular carcinoma, and a stricture with any concerning feature, even in a clinical context favoring a benign process, generally still warrants tissue sampling before a benign diagnosis is definitively accepted, reflecting biliary malignancy's comparatively higher diagnostic stakes and the recognized limitations of imaging-only stricture characterization.

Mirizzi Syndrome and Gallbladder-Related Biliary Obstruction

Mirizzi syndrome, extrinsic compression of the common hepatic duct by a large calculus impacted within the gallbladder neck or cystic duct, produces biliary obstruction through a mechanism distinct from the intrinsic ductal strictures discussed above, and its correct recognition matters substantially for surgical planning, since a standard laparoscopic cholecystectomy in the presence of Mirizzi syndrome carries an elevated risk of biliary injury given the distorted anatomy and dense inflammatory adhesion typically present at the site of chronic compression. On MRI, Mirizzi syndrome is suggested by the combination of a large, impacted gallbladder neck or cystic duct calculus, smooth extrinsic compression and narrowing of the adjacent common hepatic duct at that specific level, corresponding to the site of compression rather than an intrinsic ductal abnormality, and dilation of the intrahepatic ducts and common hepatic duct proximal to the compression, with a normal-caliber duct distal to it, a pattern distinguishable from an intrinsic malignant stricture by the absence of any mural thickening or enhancement of the compressed ductal segment itself, since the narrowing here reflects extrinsic mass effect from the adjacent inflamed gallbladder and impacted stone rather than a process arising within the ductal wall.

Cholangiocarcinoma and Perihilar Biliary Malignancy

Perihilar Cholangiocarcinoma and the Bismuth-Corlette Classification

Perihilar cholangiocarcinoma, also called a Klatskin tumor, arises at or near the confluence of the right and left hepatic ducts and is classified using the Bismuth-Corlette system based on the precise pattern of ductal involvement, a classification with direct surgical planning implications: type I tumors are confined to the common hepatic duct below the confluence, type II tumors involve the confluence itself without extending into either secondary intrahepatic duct, type IIIa and IIIb tumors extend into the right or left secondary intrahepatic ducts respectively, and type IV tumors involve both secondary ducts or are multicentric, with increasing type generally corresponding to increasing surgical complexity and, in the most advanced types, unresectability. Because MRCP depicts the full three-dimensional architecture of the biliary tree noninvasively, it has become the preferred noninvasive method for Bismuth-Corlette classification, and the report should explicitly state the classification type using the surgical team's expected terminology, along with a description of any vascular encasement or invasion, since the combination of biliary and vascular involvement together determines resectability more completely than either assessment alone.

Distal Cholangiocarcinoma and Ampullary Malignancy

Distal cholangiocarcinoma, arising in the intrapancreatic portion of the common bile duct, and ampullary carcinoma, arising at the ampulla of Vater, both present with progressive biliary obstruction but carry distinct anatomic and surgical considerations from perihilar disease, since both are potentially addressed by pancreaticoduodenectomy when resectable, a fundamentally different operation from the hepatic resection required for perihilar disease. Ampullary carcinoma in particular can be subtle on cross-sectional imaging, sometimes presenting as only mild, nonspecific ampullary thickening or asymmetric enhancement without an obvious discrete mass, and the combination of both common bile duct and pancreatic duct dilation, the so-called double duct sign, in the absence of an obvious pancreatic head mass, should specifically raise suspicion for an ampullary or distal common bile duct process and prompt dedicated ampullary imaging and endoscopic evaluation, since this specific combined dilation pattern is a well-recognized indirect sign of ampullary pathology even when the primary lesion itself is not clearly visualized.

Ampullary adenoma, a benign precursor lesion related to ampullary carcinoma through an adenoma-carcinoma progression sequence analogous to colonic polyp progression, presents a diagnostic and management challenge distinct from an already-invasive ampullary carcinoma, since an adenoma may be amenable to endoscopic papillectomy rather than requiring pancreaticoduodenectomy, making the distinction between adenoma and early invasive carcinoma clinically significant despite their potential imaging overlap. MRI features that raise concern for invasive transformation within an ampullary lesion include a size generally exceeding one to one and a half centimeters, irregular rather than smooth margins, evidence of extension beyond the ampullary complex into the adjacent duodenal wall or pancreatic parenchyma, and associated lymphadenopathy, none of which are expected findings in a purely benign adenoma, and endoscopic ultrasound with biopsy, rather than MRI alone, typically provides the definitive tissue diagnosis and local staging precision needed to confidently select between papillectomy and formal surgical resection.

Figure 7.2: Bismuth-Corlette Classification of Perihilar Cholangiocarcinoma

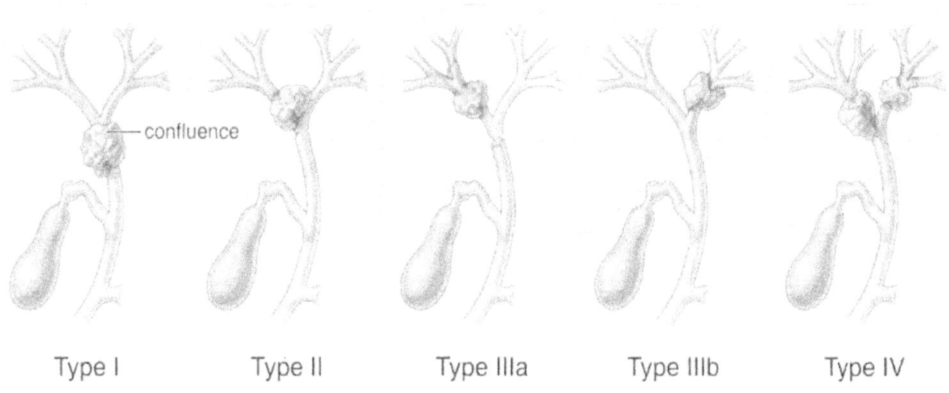

Staging Considerations for Malignant Biliary Obstruction

Beyond the Bismuth-Corlette classification's specific application to perihilar disease, comprehensive staging of any biliary malignancy identified on MRI requires systematic assessment of several additional factors that together determine resectability and guide the multidisciplinary treatment planning discussion. Vascular involvement, specifically encasement, narrowing, or occlusion of the portal vein or hepatic artery and their major branches, is assessed on the same dynamic contrast-enhanced sequences used for parenchymal lesion characterization and is generally described using a defined degree-of-circumferential-contact threshold, since partial contact without frank encasement carries different surgical implications than circumferential involvement. Regional lymphadenopathy, hepatic parenchymal metastatic disease, which should prompt the same careful whole-liver review applied throughout the preceding chapter, and peritoneal or distant metastatic spread must all be systematically assessed and reported, since the presence of any of these findings can shift a patient from a potentially curative surgical pathway to a palliative systemic therapy pathway, making the completeness of this staging assessment as clinically con sequential as the primary tumor characterization itself.

THE SIGNAL-TO-CATEGORY DECISION SYSTEM — Malignant Stricture versus Post-Inflammatory Benign Stricture

---

The Signal Pattern: A focal biliary stricture is identified with proximal ductal dilation, and the referring history includes either a remote biliary surgery, chronic pancreatitis, or no clear prior biliary history at all.

Category Signature: A short, smooth, symmetrically tapering stricture without an associated enhancing mass, occurring at a site anatomically consistent with prior surgery or chronic pancreatitis, is categorized as probably benign; a longer, irregular, shouldered stricture with associated progressive delayed enhancement or a discrete mass is categorized as probably malignant.

The Decision: A probably benign stricture with a clearly corroborating surgical or inflammatory history can reasonably be managed with surveillance imaging in appropriate clinical contexts; any stricture with a concerning morphologic feature, or one without a clear benign explanation, should proceed to endoscopic tissue sampling regardless of how reassuring the remainder of the imaging appears, given the comparatively high diagnostic stakes of missed biliary malignancy.

Trap Logic: A postsurgical anastomotic stricture can occasionally appear more irregular than a typical benign stricture due to postsurgical scarring and altered anatomy, risking an incorrect malignant categorization; conversely, a well-differentiated, densely fibrotic cholangiocarcinoma can occasionally present with a deceptively smooth, short-segment appearance, risking under-characterization. The discriminating step in genuinely ambiguous cases is not morphology alone but the presence or absence of an associated enhancing soft tissue component, which remains the single most specific discriminator between the two.

Pattern Anchor: When stricture morphology and clinical history are discordant or ambiguous, base the categorization primarily on the presence or absence of an associated enhancing soft tissue component, and proceed to tissue sampling when genuine uncertainty remains.

Congenital Biliary Anomalies and Cystic Disease

Choledochal Cysts and the Todani Classification

Choledochal cysts, congenital dilations of the biliary tree classified by the Todani system into five types based on the location and pattern of dilation, most commonly present as type I, fusiform or cystic dilation of the extrahepatic common bile duct, though the classification also encompasses diverticular, choledochocele, and combined intrahepatic and extrahepatic dilation patterns. Beyond their direct anatomic effect, choledochal cysts carry a substantially elevated lifetime risk of biliary malignancy, thought to relate to chronic biliary stasis, recurrent inflammation, and, in many cases, an anomalous pancreaticobiliary ductal union allowing reflux of pancreatic enzymes into the biliary tree, and this elevated malignancy risk is the primary reason surgical excision, rather than observation alone, is generally recommended for a confirmed choledochal cyst in a surgical candidate, making accurate MRCP-based classification directly relevant to operative planning rather than a purely descriptive exercise.

Type IV choledochal cysts, involving both extrahepatic and intrahepatic ductal dilation, and type V, which corresponds to Caroli disease and is discussed separately below given its distinct clinical associations, carry the most extensive surgical planning implications since intrahepatic involvement may require partial hepatectomy in addition to extrahepatic cyst excision and biliary-enteric reconstruction, whereas type I and type II cysts, confined to the extrahepatic duct, are more often addressed by extrahepatic excision alone. Type III cysts, or choledochoceles, involving cystic dilation of the intraduodenal portion of the distal common bile duct, are anatomically and often clinically distinct from the other types, sometimes identified incidentally and managed endoscopically rather than surgically given their location and generally lower associated malignancy risk relative to the more proximal cyst types, illustrating why accurate Todani subtyping, rather than a generic description of biliary cystic dilation, meaningfully changes the anticipated management pathway discussed with the surgical or gastroenterology team.

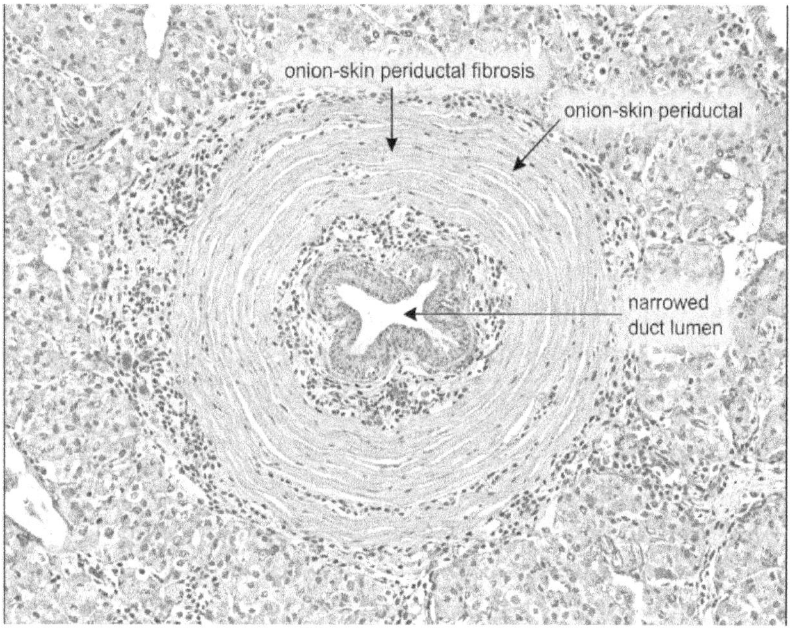

Caroli Disease and Fibropolycystic Liver Disease

Caroli disease, characterized by segmental, saccular dilation of the intrahepatic bile ducts, is distinguished on MRCP by its multifocal, communicating cystic-appearing intrahepatic ductal dilations, often containing the pathognomonic central dot sign, a small, enhancing focus of portal venous radicle surrounded by the dilated duct, reflecting the fibrovascular bundle around which the ductal dilation forms. When Caroli disease occurs in combination with congenital hepatic fibrosis, a condition frequently associated with autosomal recessive polycystic kidney disease, the resulting entity, Caroli syndrome, carries both the biliary malignancy risk discussed above and the portal hypertension risk conferred by the accompanying congenital hepatic fibrosis, and recognizing the combination on a single MRI examination, biliary ductal dilation with the central dot sign alongside renal cystic disease, allows a unifying diagnosis to be offered rather than reporting each finding as an isolated, unrelated observation.

Patients with Caroli disease or Caroli syndrome require long-term surveillance given their compound risk profile: recurrent cholangitis related to bile stasis within the dilated, poorly draining ductal segments, intrahepatic calculus formation within these same stagnant segments, and the cholangiocarcinoma risk shared with the other congenital biliary anomalies discussed in this section, generally cited as substantially elevated above the general population risk, though precise quantification varies across the limited available natural history data given the condition's rarity. Distinguishing Caroli disease from other causes of multifocal intrahepatic ductal dilation, particularly advanced primary sclerosing cholangitis, rests primarily on the central dot sign described above, which is not a feature of primary sclerosing cholangitis, together with the characteristic saccular, rather than beaded and stricturing, morphology of the ductal dilation itself, and correlating any new symptom, particularly worsening jaundice or a new dominant area of ductal narrowing, with the possibility of superimposed cholangiocarcinoma is an essential component of long-term Caroli disease management given this population's elevated baseline risk.

Inflammatory and Infectious Biliary Disease

Primary Sclerosing Cholangitis

Primary sclerosing cholangitis, a chronic, immune-mediated inflammatory condition strongly associated with inflammatory bowel disease, particularly ulcerative colitis, produces a characteristic multifocal pattern of short, annular strictures alternating with normal or mildly dilated ductal segments, producing the classic beaded appearance on MRCP that, when present in its full, multifocal form, is highly suggestive of the diagnosis and can often be recognized with substantial confidence on imaging alone in the correct clinical context. Because primary sclerosing cholangitis carries a substantially elevated risk of cholangiocarcinoma, developing in a meaningful minority of affected patients over the course of their disease, any dominant stricture, meaning one that is disproportionately more severe or that demonstrates progressive worsening compared to the patient's overall pattern of disease, should be evaluated with the same heightened suspicion for malignancy applied to any other biliary stricture discussed in this chapter, since distinguishing a dominant benign stricture from superimposed cholangiocarcinoma in a patient with known primary sclerosing cholangitis is one of the most diagnostically challenging scenarios in biliary imaging, given that the patient's baseline disease already produces multiple strictures against which a new malignant stricture must be distinguished.

IgG4-Related Sclerosing Cholangitis as a Treatable Mimic

IgG4-related sclerosing cholangitis, part of the broader spectrum of IgG4-related systemic fibroinflammatory disease, produces biliary strictures that can closely mimic both primary sclerosing cholangitis and, in some presentations, malignant biliary obstruction, but carries a fundamentally different and far more favorable prognosis, since it characteristically responds rapidly and substantially to corticosteroid therapy, making its correct recognition one of the more clinically rewarding distinctions addressed in this chapter. Features favoring IgG4-related disease over primary sclerosing cholangitis or malignancy include smooth, often long-segment biliary wall thickening rather than the short, annular, beaded pattern of primary sclerosing cholangitis, frequent coexistence with autoimmune pancreatitis, addressed in the following chapter, producing a distinctive combination of pancreatic and biliary involvement, and elevated serum IgG4 levels, though this last feature requires laboratory correlation beyond the imaging examination itself. When a stricture pattern raises genuine consideration for IgG4-related disease, particularly in a patient with coexisting pancreatic findings suggestive of autoimmune pancreatitis, explicitly raising this possibility in the report, alongside the malignant and primary sclerosing cholangitis differential, can meaningfully accelerate the correct diagnosis and appropriate steroid trial rather than proceeding directly to more invasive tissue sampling that a straightforward steroid response could have obviated.

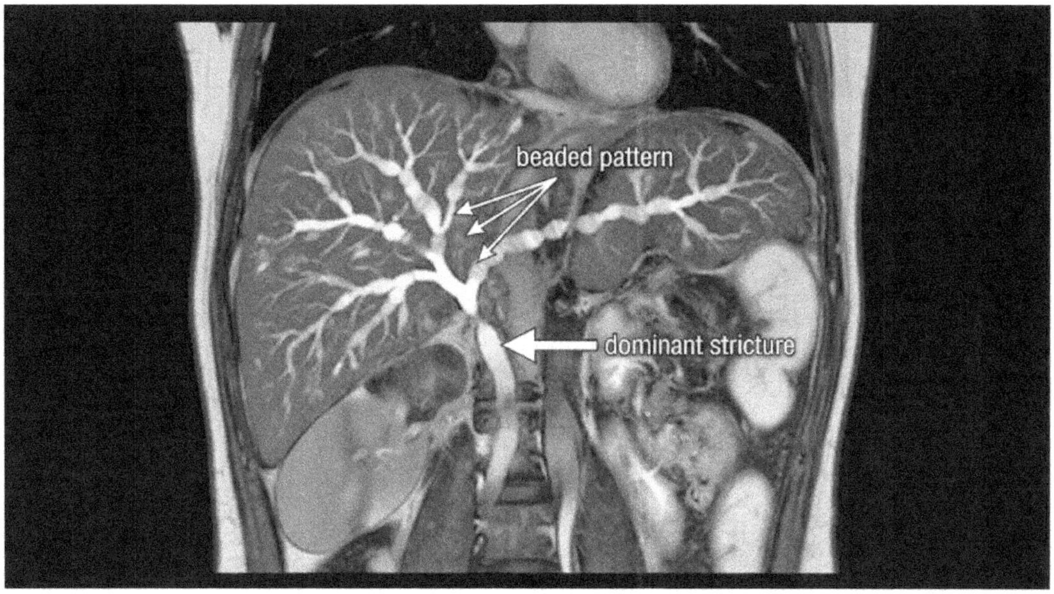

Figure 7.4 — Diagnostic Imaging: Primary Sclerosing Cholangitis with a Dominant Stricture

Acute Cholangitis and Recurrent Pyogenic Cholangitis

Acute cholangitis, most often precipitated by choledocholithiasis or a malignant or benign stricture producing bacterial superinfection of obstructed bile, is characterized on MRI by biliary ductal dilation with associated periductal edema and enhancement, hepatic parenchymal changes including transient, wedge-shaped or geographic areas of increased arterial phase enhancement reflecting localized inflammatory hyperemia, and, in progressive cases, evolution toward hepatic abscess formation as described in the preceding chapter, a clinical scenario requiring urgent recognition and biliary decompression rather than elective further imaging workup. Recurrent pyogenic cholangitis, endemic in parts of Southeast Asia but increasingly recognized elsewhere, produces a distinctive pattern of intrahepatic pigment stone formation, often predominantly involving the left hepatic lobe, together with associated ductal dilation and stricture from repeated inflammatory episodes, and carries its own long-term risk of secondary biliary cirrhosis and cholangiocarcinoma, making accurate recognition of this less commonly encountered but distinctive entity relevant to appropriately counseling and following affected patients over the long term.

Recurrent episodes of intrahepatic pigment stone formation and infection in recurrent pyogenic cholangitis progressively produce segmental atrophy of the most severely and repeatedly affected hepatic segments, most often the left lateral segment, together with compensatory hypertrophy of relatively spared segments, a pattern of asymmetric segmental volume redistribution that, while superficially similar to the cirrhotic volume redistribution discussed in the preceding chapter, reflects a fundamentally different underlying process, chronic segmental biliary obstruction and infection rather than diffuse parenchymal fibrosis, and this distinction matters because the affected, atrophic segment in recurrent pyogenic cholangitis is sometimes addressed surgically with segmental hepatectomy when recurrent symptomatic infection cannot be adequately controlled by endoscopic or percutaneous stone clearance alone, a targeted surgical option not applicable to the diffuse fibrotic process of cirrhosis.

Postoperative Biliary Complications

Bile leak, most commonly encountered after cholecystectomy or hepatic resection, presents on MRI as a discrete perihepatic or subhepatic fluid collection, sometimes difficult to distinguish from a simple postoperative seroma on conventional T2-weighted sequences alone, and hepatobiliary-specific contrast agents, introduced in the earlier chapter on contrast agents, offer a specific diagnostic solution: active extravasation of hepatobiliary-phase-excreted contrast into the collection directly confirms a bile leak and its precise site of origin, information not reliably obtainable from conventional MRCP or standard extracellular contrast imaging alone. This application, sometimes termed functional or contrast-enhanced MRCP, is particularly valuable in the postoperative patient with an equivocal or borderline finding on conventional imaging, since definitively confirming or excluding an active leak directly determines whether the patient proceeds to endoscopic biliary stenting or is managed with observation and percutaneous drainage of a sterile postoperative collection alone.

Anastomotic strictures following biliary-enteric surgery, whether performed for a choledochal cyst, prior malignancy, or benign reconstructive indication, present a specific variant of the benign stricture pattern discussed earlier in this chapter, typically occurring at the surgical anastomosis itself and demonstrating smooth, symmetric narrowing without an associated mass, though the altered postsurgical anatomy can make this distinction more challenging than in a native, unoperated biliary tree, and correlating stricture location precisely against the known surgical anatomy, ideally with reference to the original operative report when available, is essential to confidently distinguishing an expected anastomotic narrowing from a new, superimposed process requiring further evaluation.

Clinical Case Presentations

Case 1. A 34-year-old woman with acute right upper quadrant pain and mildly elevated liver enzymes undergoes MRCP, which demonstrates a rounded filling defect in the distal common bile duct with a clear meniscus sign and mild proximal ductal dilation, layering dependently on the axial source images and without blooming on the corresponding gradient-echo sequence. The radiologist confidently characterizes this as a retained common bile duct calculus rather than pneumobilia, noting the absence of any prior sphincterotomy or biliary-enteric surgical history, and the patient proceeds directly to endoscopic retrograde cholangiopancreatography for stone extraction based on the MRCP findings, avoiding a purely diagnostic endoscopic procedure.

Case 2. A 68-year-old man with painless jaundice undergoes MRCP demonstrating a short, abrupt stricture at the confluence of the right and left hepatic ducts with extension into the right secondary intrahepatic ducts but sparing of the left secondary ducts, together with an associated enhancing soft tissue component. The radiologist classifies this as Bismuth-Corlette type IIIa perihilar cholangiocarcinoma, explicitly documenting the pattern of secondary ductal involvement and assessing for portal venous encasement, which is not identified, and this specific classification directly informs the hepatobiliary surgical team's decision to proceed with a right hepatectomy and biliary reconstruction, illustrating the direct surgical relevance of precise Bismuth-Corlette subclassification beyond a general description of a hilar mass.

Case 3. A 41-year-old man with longstanding ulcerative colitis and known primary sclerosing cholangitis undergoes surveillance MRCP, which demonstrates the patient's established beaded intrahepatic ductal pattern, stable compared to prior examinations, but a new, more severe stricture in the common hepatic duct not present on the examination from eighteen months earlier, associated with new focal wall thickening and enhancement. Recognizing this as a new dominant stricture with a concerning associated soft tissue finding, distinct from the patient's chronic, stable baseline disease pattern, the radiologist recommends prompt endoscopic evaluation with brushing and biopsy to exclude superimposed cholangiocarcinoma, explicitly distinguishing this new, actionable finding from the patient's otherwise unchanged chronic disease in the comparison-based report.

Case 4. A 57-year-old woman develops a fever and right upper quadrant pain five days after laparoscopic cholecystectomy, and MRI with a hepatobiliary-specific contrast agent is obtained given equivocal findings on an initial ultrasound. Conventional T2-weighted images demonstrate a moderate-sized perihepatic fluid collection adjacent to the surgical bed, and the hepatobiliary phase images, obtained approximately twenty minutes after contrast administration, demonstrate a discrete focus of excreted contrast extending from the region of the cystic duct stump directly into the fluid collection, confirming active bile leak with the precise site of origin identified. This specific finding, distinguishing a bile leak from a sterile postoperative seroma that would show no such contrast extravasation, directly informs the surgical team's decision to proceed with endoscopic biliary stenting to divert bile flow away from the leak site, and the report explicitly documents both the leak's confirmation and its precise anatomic origin to guide the endoscopic procedure.

THE SIGNAL-TO-CATEGORY DECISION SYSTEM — Biliary Tract Characterization Arc

The Signal Pattern: This chapter's patterns span from the simplest biliary finding, a ductal filling defect, to the most consequential, a stricture that must be correctly triaged between benign and malignant causes.

Category Signature: Filling defects are categorized as calculus or artifact based on layering behavior and susceptibility blooming; strictures are categorized as probably benign or probably malignant based on morphology, length, and the presence or absence of an associated enhancing soft tissue component, always interpreted alongside clinical and surgical history.

The Decision: Confirmed calculi proceed to extraction; confirmed artifact requires no action. Probably malignant strictures proceed to tissue sampling and staging regardless of a reassuring clinical history; probably benign strictures with clear corroborating history may be managed with surveillance, always with a lower threshold for sampling than the comparatively more definitive LI-RADS framework of the preceding chapter allows.

The Trap Logic: Every pattern in this chapter is most dangerous when clinical context and imaging morphology point in different directions, a reassuring history alongside a concerning stricture, or an alarming morphology explained by a known benign process; the discriminating anchor in every such conflict is the presence or absence of an associated enhancing soft tissue component.

Pattern Anchor: When benign clinical history and concerning imaging morphology conflict for a biliary stricture, default to tissue sampling rather than reassurance; biliary malignancy's diagnostic stakes do not permit the same imaging-only confidence available in hepatocellular carcinoma.

Summary and Key Concepts

True ductal calculi layer dependently and do not bloom on gradient-echo sequences; pneumobilia layers nondependently and blooms, and the distinction should always be confirmed before diagnosing a retained stone.

Malignant biliary strictures are typically longer, irregular, and shouldered with an associated enhancing soft tissue component; benign strictures are typically shorter, smooth, and symmetric, but any concerning feature warrants tissue sampling.

The Bismuth-Corlette classification of perihilar cholangiocarcinoma, based on the specific pattern of ductal confluence and secondary duct involvement, directly determines surgical resectability and approach.

The double duct sign, combined common bile duct and pancreatic duct dilation without an obvious pancreatic head mass, should raise suspicion for ampullary or distal common bile duct malignancy.

Choledochal cysts carry a substantial lifetime malignancy risk warranting surgical excision, and Caroli disease demonstrates the pathognomonic central dot sign within multifocal intrahepatic ductal dilations.

Primary sclerosing cholangitis produces a characteristic beaded ductal pattern, and any new dominant stricture in this population warrants evaluation for superimposed cholangiocarcinoma rather than assumption of stable chronic disease.

Acute cholangitis demonstrates ductal dilation with periductal enhancement and transient geographic hepatic hyperemia, and can progress to abscess formation if biliary decompression is delayed.

CHAPTER 8: PANCREATIC DISORDERS AND PANCREATIC NEOPLASMS

Learning Objectives

1. Recognize the MRI findings of acute and chronic pancreatitis and their major local complications.
2. Classify pancreatic cystic lesions and apply worrisome feature and high-risk stigmata criteria to guide surveillance versus surgical referral.
3. Recognize the imaging features of autoimmune pancreatitis and distinguish it from pancreatic adenocarcinoma.
4. Characterize pancreatic ductal adenocarcinoma, assess vascular involvement relevant to resectability, and distinguish it from mass-forming pancreatitis.
5. Recognize the imaging appearance of pancreatic neuroendocrine tumors and relate imaging features to functional status and malignant potential.

Clinical Overview

The pancreas presents a distinctive interpretive challenge in body MRI: its retroperitoneal location, small caliber ducts, and proximity to major vasculature demand the protocol-specific attention discussed in the second chapter of this book, while its disease spectrum, from acute inflammatory processes through a wide range of cystic lesions with markedly different malignant potential to adenocarcinoma, one of the most lethal solid malignancies in oncology, demands equally careful diagnostic discipline. Few chapters in this book carry higher clinical stakes than correctly triaging a pancreatic cystic lesion between reassuring surveillance and surgical referral, or correctly distinguishing a mass-forming inflammatory process from adenocarcinoma before an unnecessary or, conversely, a delayed operation results.

This chapter moves from acute and chronic pancreatitis, through the cystic lesion spectrum where risk stratification carries the most immediate clinical consequence, to autoimmune pancreatitis as a specifically treatable adenocarcinoma mimic, to adenocarcinoma itself and its vascular staging, and finally to pancreatic neuroendocrine tumors. Two instances of the Signal-to-Category Decision System are applied here, to intraductal papillary mucinous neoplasm risk stratification and to distinguishing pancreatic adenocarcinoma from its most consequential inflammatory mimic.

Acute and Chronic Pancreatitis

Acute Pancreatitis and the Revised Atlanta Classification

Acute pancreatitis on MRI demonstrates pancreatic parenchymal enlargement with ill-defined margins, peripancreatic fat stranding manifesting as T2-hyperintense, poorly marginated signal in the normally low-signal peripancreatic fat, and, in more severe cases, peripancreatic fluid collections whose classification follows the revised Atlanta classification based on their contents and time course: acute peripancreatic fluid collections, occurring within four weeks of onset and lacking a defined wall, evolve into pseudocysts, well-defined, encapsulated fluid collections without solid debris, if they persist beyond four weeks, while acute necrotic collections, containing variable amounts of solid necrotic debris admixed with fluid, evolve into walled-off necrosis once a mature, defined wall forms. MRI's superior soft tissue contrast relative to CT, the modality more commonly used for initial acute pancreatitis assessment given its wider availability and faster acquisition, provides particular value in distinguishing a purely fluid pseudocyst from walled-off necrosis containing solid debris, a distinction with direct management implications since walled-off necrosis containing solid debris generally requires a different drainage approach, often involving a larger-caliber access or endoscopic necrosectomy, than the straightforward percutaneous or endoscopic drainage typically sufficient for a simple pseudocyst.

Chronic Pancreatitis and Its Imaging Signature

Chronic pancreatitis produces a distinct pattern reflecting cumulative, irreversible glandular injury: parenchymal atrophy, an irregular, dilated main pancreatic duct with alternating strictures and dilations producing a beaded appearance conceptually similar to the biliary beading of primary sclerosing cholangitis discussed in the preceding chapter, and, characteristically, intraductal and parenchymal calcifications, which, while more conspicuous on CT given their calcific composition, appear as signal voids on MRI sequences and are an important corroborating feature when present. Because chronic pancreatitis produces both diffuse gland signal change, typically decreased T1 signal reflecting loss of the normal, physiologically high T1 signal intensity of healthy pancreatic parenchyma related to its acinar protein content, and, in a meaningful subset of patients, a focal inflammatory mass that can be genuinely difficult to distinguish from adenocarcinoma on morphology alone, chronic pancreatitis represents one of the more diagnostically challenging contexts in this chapter, addressed further in the discussion of mass-forming pancreatitis later in this chapter.

Epidemiology and Etiology of Acute and Chronic Pancreatitis

Gallstone disease and alcohol use together account for the substantial majority of acute pancreatitis cases in most populations, with gallstones the more common cause overall and alcohol a leading cause particularly among cases presenting with recurrent or chronic disease; hypertriglyceridemia, generally when serum triglyceride levels exceed one thousand milligrams per deciliter, and post-endoscopic retrograde cholangiopancreatography pancreatitis together account for most of the remaining cases with an identifiable cause, while a meaningful minority remain idiopathic despite thorough evaluation. Chronic pancreatitis shares alcohol as a dominant etiology in adults, generally requiring sustained heavy consumption over years before clinically apparent glandular injury develops, though genetic and hereditary forms, including mutations in the cationic trypsinogen gene, the pancreatic secretory trypsin inhibitor gene, and cystic fibrosis transmembrane conductance regulator mutations, are increasingly recognized causes particularly in patients presenting at a younger age or without a substantial alcohol history, and their identification carries genetic counseling implications for affected families given the hereditary transmission pattern of the causative mutations. Obstructive chronic pancreatitis, arising downstream of a fixed ductal obstruction such as a stricture, an intraductal papillary mucinous neoplasm, or a prior traumatic injury, produces a similar imaging pattern to the more common toxic-metabolic forms but is distinguished by its localization distal to the obstructing lesion and its potential reversibility if the underlying obstruction is addressed before irreversible glandular fibrosis becomes established.

Local Complications and Vascular Sequelae of Pancreatitis

Vascular complications of pancreatitis carry disproportionate clinical significance relative to their incidence and are a specific area where MRI, particularly when combined with magnetic resonance angiography sequences, contributes materially beyond simple fluid collection characterization. Splenic vein thrombosis, arising from the vein's direct anatomic course along the posterior pancreatic body and tail where it is vulnerable to compression or direct inflammatory involvement, can produce left-sided or sinistral portal hypertension with gastric varices in the absence of generalized portal hypertension or liver disease, a specific pattern that should prompt a deliberate search for splenic vein thrombosis when gastric varices are identified without other stigmata of cirrhosis. Pseudoaneurysm formation, most often involving the splenic artery given its close anatomic relationship to the pancreatic tail and body, represents a potentially catastrophic complication arising from vascular wall injury by adjacent inflammatory or enzymatic pancreatic tissue, and its recognition on MRI as a rounded, avidly enhancing structure contiguous with a named artery, distinct from a simple fluid collection, should prompt urgent vascular consultation given the substantial hemorrhage risk if the pseudoaneurysm ruptures, particularly into an adjacent pseudocyst or the peritoneal cavity. Disconnected pancreatic duct syndrome, in which necrosis or severe inflammation causes a discontinuity in the main pancreatic duct such that the upstream, viable pancreatic segment no longer communicates with the downstream duct and duodenum, produces persistent or recurrent fluid collections despite adequate drainage of the initially identified collection, and its recognition, most reliably established with MRCP demonstrating the ductal discontinuity, is essential to selecting a definitive treatment strategy rather than pursuing repeated, ultimately unsuccessful percutaneous drainage of a persistently refilling collection.

Complication	Key Imaging Feature	Clinical Significance
Pseudocyst	Well-defined, encapsulated fluid collection without solid debris, maturing beyond four weeks	Generally amenable to percutaneous or endoscopic drainage if symptomatic or enlarging
Walled-off necrosis	Encapsulated collection containing solid necrotic debris admixed with fluid	Often requires larger-caliber or endoscopic necrosectomy drainage approach
Splenic vein thrombosis	Non-opacified splenic vein with collateral gastric varices	Produces sinistral portal hypertension without generalized liver disease
Pseudoaneurysm	Rounded, avidly enhancing structure contiguous with a named artery	Substantial hemorrhage risk; requires urgent vascular consultation

Disconnected duct syndrome	Ductal discontinuity on MRCP with persistent upstream collection	Predicts failure of simple percutaneous drainage; guides definitive therapy

Pancreatic Cystic Lesions: Classification and Risk Stratification

Intraductal Papillary Mucinous Neoplasm: Main Duct, Branch Duct, and Mixed Type

Intraductal papillary mucinous neoplasm, the most commonly encountered pancreatic cystic neoplasm in current clinical practice given its frequent incidental discovery, is classified by its relationship to the pancreatic ductal system: main duct type, involving diffuse or segmental dilation of the main pancreatic duct itself, branch duct type, involving one or more side-branch cysts communicating with, but not primarily dilating, the main duct, and mixed type, demonstrating features of both. This distinction carries substantial prognostic weight, since main duct and mixed type intraductal papillary mucinous neoplasm carry a considerably higher risk of harboring high-grade dysplasia or invasive carcinoma at the time of diagnosis than branch duct type alone, which is why main duct involvement itself, discussed further below as a high-risk stigma, generally shifts management toward surgical resection rather than surveillance regardless of the specific cyst's other characteristics.

Figure 8.1 — Diagnostic Imaging: Branch Duct IPMN with Enhancing Mural Nodule

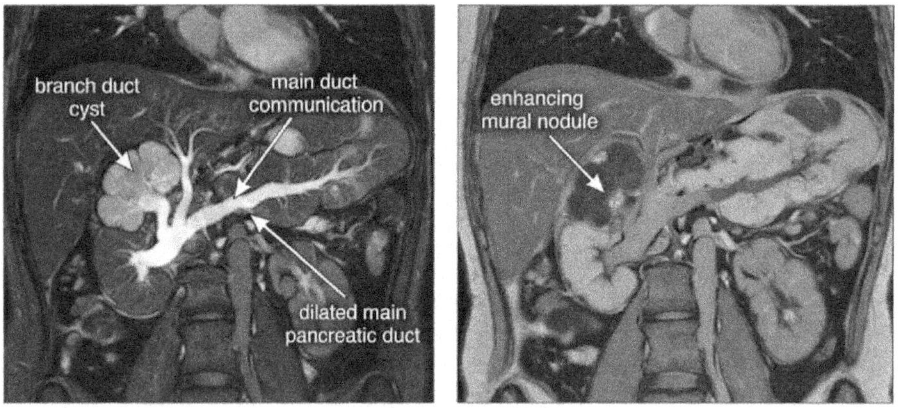

Worrisome Features and High-Risk Stigmata

Current consensus guidelines stratify intraductal papillary mucinous neoplasm management using a defined set of worrisome features and high-risk stigmata, each carrying different management implications. High-risk stigmata, findings prompting strong consideration for surgical resection essentially regardless of other factors, include an enhancing mural nodule measuring five millimeters or greater, main pancreatic duct dilation to ten millimeters or greater, and obstructive jaundice in a patient with a cystic lesion in the pancreatic head, each of these findings carrying a substantially elevated probability of underlying high-grade dysplasia or invasive malignancy. Worrisome features, findings warranting further evaluation, typically with endoscopic ultrasound and fine-needle aspiration, but not immediate resection in isolation, include cyst size of three centimeters or greater, main duct dilation between five and nine millimeters, an enhancing mural nodule smaller than five millimeters, abrupt change in duct caliber with associated distal parenchymal atrophy, and lymphadenopathy, and the presence of multiple worrisome features, or a worrisome feature that does not resolve on dedicated further evaluation, generally shifts management toward resection even in the absence of a formal high-risk stigma.

THE SIGNAL-TO-CATEGORY DECISION SYSTEM — Intraductal Papillary Mucinous Neoplasm Risk Stratification

The Signal Pattern: A pancreatic cystic lesion is identified, communicating with the main pancreatic duct on MRCP, and the reader must characterize its size, ductal involvement, and any internal enhancing component.

Category Signature: A branch duct-type cyst under three centimeters without a mural nodule, significant main duct dilation, or other worrisome feature is categorized as low-risk, appropriate for surveillance; a cyst with any high-risk stigma, an enhancing nodule five millimeters or greater, main duct dilation of ten millimeters or greater, or obstructive jaundice, is categorized as high-risk; a cyst with an intermediate feature, such as size at or above three centimeters or a smaller mural nodule, is categorized as worrisome, warranting further characterization.

The Decision: Low-risk lesions are managed with surveillance imaging at guideline-defined intervals scaled to cyst size; high-risk lesions are referred for surgical evaluation; worrisome lesions are referred for endoscopic ultrasound with fine-needle aspiration to further refine risk before a final surveillance-versus-resection decision is made.

Trap Logic: A mucin plug within the cyst or duct can mimic a true enhancing mural nodule on a single postcontrast sequence, particularly if evaluated on a single phase without careful comparison against a precontrast sequence; the discriminating step is confirming that the presumed nodule demonstrates genuine, unambiguous enhancement relative to its own precontrast signal, since a non-enhancing filling defect, however nodular in shape, represents mucin rather than a true mural nodule and does not carry the same high-risk implication.

Pattern Anchor: Never categorize a mural nodule as a high-risk stigma without confirming genuine contrast enhancement relative to a precontrast baseline; an unenhancing intraluminal filling defect is mucin, not a nodule.

Serous Cystadenoma and Mucinous Cystic Neoplasm

Serous cystadenoma, a benign cystic neoplasm with essentially negligible malignant potential, characteristically demonstrates a microcystic, honeycomb architecture composed of numerous small cysts, often with a central stellate scar and, when present, associated calcification, and does not communicate with the pancreatic ductal system, a key distinguishing feature from the intraductal papillary mucinous neoplasms discussed above; when this classic microcystic morphology is present, serous cystadenoma can generally be managed with observation alone given its minimal malignant potential, reserving intervention for the uncommon scenario of a very large lesion causing mass effect or symptoms rather than malignancy concern. Mucinous cystic neoplasm, by contrast, occurs almost exclusively in women, typically in the pancreatic body or tail, and presents as a unilocular or septated cyst with a thick, sometimes calcified wall, distinguished from a branch duct intraductal papillary mucinous neoplasm by its lack of communication with the pancreatic ductal system, and carries a meaningful malignant potential that generally warrants surgical resection in appropriately fit surgical candidates given this risk, distinct from the size- and feature-based surveillance-versus-resection algorithm applied to intraductal papillary mucinous neoplasm.

Epidemiology and Clinical Context of Pancreatic Cystic Lesions

Pancreatic cystic lesions are identified with increasing frequency as incidental findings on cross-sectional imaging performed for unrelated indications, a trend driven substantially by the growing utilization of high-resolution MRI and CT rather than by any true increase in disease incidence, and current series suggest that a meaningful proportion of the adult population, rising with advancing age, harbors at least one incidentally discovered pancreatic cyst at some point during their lifetime. This high background prevalence of predominantly low-risk lesions creates a specific interpretive tension: the overwhelming majority of incidentally discovered pancreatic cysts, particularly small branch duct intraductal papillary mucinous neoplasms without worrisome features, will never progress to clinically significant malignancy during a patient's lifetime, yet a small but clinically important minority will, and the radiologist's role in applying the worrisome feature and high-risk stigmata framework precisely, rather than either dismissing every cyst as inconsequential or referring every cyst for aggressive further evaluation, is essential to avoiding both undertreatment of the minority destined to progress and overtreatment, with its attendant surgical morbidity, of the majority that will not. Age itself factors into this calculus, since the cumulative lifetime risk of malignant transformation is necessarily higher in a younger patient with a longer remaining life expectancy over which progression could occur, a consideration that appropriately informs, without independently determining, the surveillance-versus-resection decision in borderline cases.

Feature	Serous Cystadenoma	Mucinous Cystic Neoplasm	Branch Duct IPMN
Typical demographic	Older women	Middle-aged women, almost exclusively	Either sex, older adults
Ductal communication	Absent	Absent	Present
Characteristic architecture	Microcystic, honeycomb, central scar	Unilocular or septated, thick wall	Grape-like cluster of cysts
Malignant potential	Negligible	Meaningful, generally warrants resection	Variable, risk-stratified by defined criteria

CLINICAL PEARL: When a mural nodule's enhancement is genuinely equivocal on a single postcontrast phase, direct comparison of identical window and level settings between the precontrast and postcontrast sequences, rather than visual impression on the postcontrast sequence alone, is the most reliable way to confirm true enhancement and avoid overcalling mucin as a high-risk nodule.

Autoimmune Pancreatitis

Diffuse and Focal Patterns of Autoimmune Pancreatitis

Autoimmune pancreatitis, part of the IgG4-related disease spectrum introduced in the biliary chapter's discussion of IgG4-related sclerosing cholangitis, most characteristically presents with diffuse pancreatic enlargement and a smooth, featureless, sausage-shaped contour, loss of the gland's normal lobulated architecture, and a thin, hypoenhancing peripancreatic rim or capsule-like halo that is a highly distinctive, near-pathognomonic finding when present in its classic diffuse form. A focal or mass-forming variant, involving only a portion of the gland, most often the head, presents a far greater diagnostic challenge, since it can closely mimic pancreatic adenocarcinoma both clinically, with obstructive jaundice a shared presenting feature, and on morphologic imaging, making the ancillary features discussed below, together with serum IgG4 elevation and, most definitively, the classic and dramatic response to corticosteroid therapy, essential tools for correctly identifying this specific, eminently treatable mimic rather than proceeding directly to resection for a presumed malignancy.

Type 1 Versus Type 2 Autoimmune Pancreatitis and Systemic Associations

Autoimmune pancreatitis is divided into two histologically and clinically distinct subtypes with direct relevance to interpretation and multidisciplinary management. Type 1 autoimmune pancreatitis, the IgG4-related form and the more common subtype in most populations, typically affects older men, is frequently accompanied by elevated serum IgG4 concentrations, and commonly demonstrates involvement of other organs within the IgG4-related disease spectrum, including the biliary tree as IgG4-related sclerosing cholangitis discussed in the preceding chapter, the salivary and lacrimal glands, the retroperitoneum as retroperitoneal fibrosis, and the kidneys, such that identification of one or more of these associated extrapancreatic findings on the same examination substantially strengthens confidence in the autoimmune pancreatitis diagnosis. Type 2 autoimmune pancreatitis, by contrast, typically affects a younger population without the male predominance seen in type 1, is not reliably associated with serum IgG4 elevation, and lacks the characteristic multiorgan IgG4-related disease associations, though it carries a distinctive association with inflammatory bowel disease, particularly ulcerative colitis, that should prompt consideration of this specific subtype when autoimmune pancreatitis is suspected in a patient with a known or subsequently diagnosed inflammatory bowel disease history. Both subtypes share the corticosteroid responsiveness that is among the most clinically useful confirmatory features of autoimmune pancreatitis as a category, though type 2 disease is more prone to acute presentation resembling typical acute pancreatitis than the more insidious, often painless presentation characteristic of type 1 disease.

Differential Diagnosis and Ancillary Features Distinguishing Autoimmune Pancreatitis From Adenocarcinoma

Beyond the classic diffuse sausage-shaped morphology, several ancillary imaging features help distinguish autoimmune pancreatitis from adenocarcinoma in the diagnostically more challenging focal or mass-forming presentation. A capsule-like rim, when present, is a highly specific finding essentially unique to autoimmune pancreatitis among pancreatic mass-forming processes and, when identified, should strongly favor this diagnosis over adenocarcinoma even in the focal form. Multiple strictures of the main pancreatic duct without significant proximal upstream dilation, a pattern termed skip lesions when multiple discontinuous strictures are present, favors autoimmune pancreatitis, since adenocarcinoma-related ductal obstruction typically produces a single, more abrupt stricture with more pronounced proximal ductal dilation than is characteristic of the diffusely narrowed but not markedly obstructed duct seen in autoimmune pancreatitis. Restricted diffusion is frequently present in both entities and is therefore of limited value for this specific differential, unlike its greater discriminating value elsewhere in this book, and should not be relied upon in isolation to favor one diagnosis over the other in this specific clinical context. When imaging remains genuinely ambiguous despite attention to these ancillary features, a corticosteroid trial with close interval imaging follow-up, reserved for cases where malignancy has been reasonably excluded through tissue sampling or a sufficiently low pretest probability, remains the most definitive diagnostic maneuver available, given the dramatic and rapid response autoimmune pancreatitis characteristically demonstrates.

PATIENT EDUCATION: Patients diagnosed with autoimmune pancreatitis should understand that this is a treatable inflammatory condition distinct from cancer, that corticosteroid therapy is typically highly effective, and that long-term surveillance is still recommended given a meaningful relapse rate and the described association with other organ involvement.

Solid Pancreatic Neoplasms: Adenocarcinoma and Its Mimics

Pancreatic Ductal Adenocarcinoma: Imaging Features and Detection

Pancreatic ductal adenocarcinoma characteristically presents as an ill-defined, infiltrative mass that is relatively hypointense to normal pancreatic parenchyma on T1-weighted imaging, reflecting loss of the normal gland's high T1 signal, and demonstrates relatively hypovascular enhancement on arterial and portal venous phase imaging compared to the intensely enhancing normal surrounding parenchyma, a pattern of relative hypoenhancement that, as discussed in the protocol design chapter, is often most conspicuous on the pancreatic parenchymal phase specifically timed earlier than the hepatic arterial phase for exactly this reason. Indirect secondary signs are frequently as important as direct mass visualization for small, subtle tumors that can be genuinely difficult to see directly: abrupt pancreatic duct cutoff with upstream ductal dilation, the double duct sign discussed in the preceding chapter when the tumor is located in the pancreatic head near the distal common bile duct, and focal parenchymal atrophy distal to an area of ductal obstruction, any of which should prompt a deliberate, focused search for a subtle underlying mass even when one is not immediately obvious on initial review, since missing a small, potentially resectable adenocarcinoma at this early stage carries some of the highest stakes of any diagnostic error addressed in this book.

Vascular Staging and Resectability Assessment

Resectability of pancreatic ductal adenocarcinoma depends substantially on the tumor's relationship to the major peripancreatic vasculature, assessed using the same degree-of-circumferential-contact framework introduced in the preceding chapter's discussion of biliary malignancy staging: contact with the superior mesenteric artery, celiac axis, or common hepatic artery exceeding one hundred eighty degrees of vessel circumference generally indicates unresectable disease, contact between the artery and tumor at or below this threshold, together with reconstructible venous involvement, generally defines the borderline resectable category appropriate for neoadjuvant therapy consideration, and tumors without significant arterial contact and with venous involvement, if present, amenable to reconstruction are generally considered resectable. Venous involvement of the superior mesenteric or portal vein is assessed similarly but carries a somewhat more favorable resectability threshold than arterial involvement given the greater surgical feasibility of venous resection and reconstruction, and the report should explicitly state the specific degree of contact with each relevant vessel using this standardized, degree-based framework, since a vague description of tumor proximity to vasculature, without this specific quantification, provides insufficient information for the multidisciplinary tumor board's resectability determination.

Epidemiology, Risk Factors, and Molecular Pathogenesis of Pancreatic Ductal Adenocarcinoma

Pancreatic ductal adenocarcinoma incidence has risen steadily in recent decades and current projections suggest it will become one of the leading causes of cancer mortality in coming years, a trajectory reflecting both an aging population and the disease's persistently poor prognosis relative to more treatable malignancies rather than any dramatic rise in age-adjusted incidence alone. Established risk factors include cigarette smoking, one of the most consistently identified and modifiable risk factors across epidemiologic studies, longstanding type 2 diabetes mellitus, which carries a bidirectional relationship with pancreatic cancer since new-onset diabetes in an older adult can itself represent a paraneoplastic manifestation of an occult tumor, chronic pancreatitis as discussed earlier in this chapter, obesity, and hereditary syndromes including hereditary pancreatitis, Peutz-Jeghers syndrome, and germline mutations in genes including BRCA2, BRCA1, and the mismatch repair genes associated with Lynch syndrome, the identification of which carries direct implications for genetic counseling and, in some cases, targeted systemic therapy selection. At the molecular level, pancreatic ductal adenocarcinoma is characterized by near-universal activating mutations in the KRAS oncogene together with frequent inactivating mutations in the TP53, CDKN2A, and SMAD4 tumor suppressor genes, a mutational profile that underlies the tumor's characteristic desmoplastic stromal response and contributes to its relative resistance to many systemic therapies effective against other solid tumors, an area of active therapeutic research beyond the scope of this chapter's imaging focus.

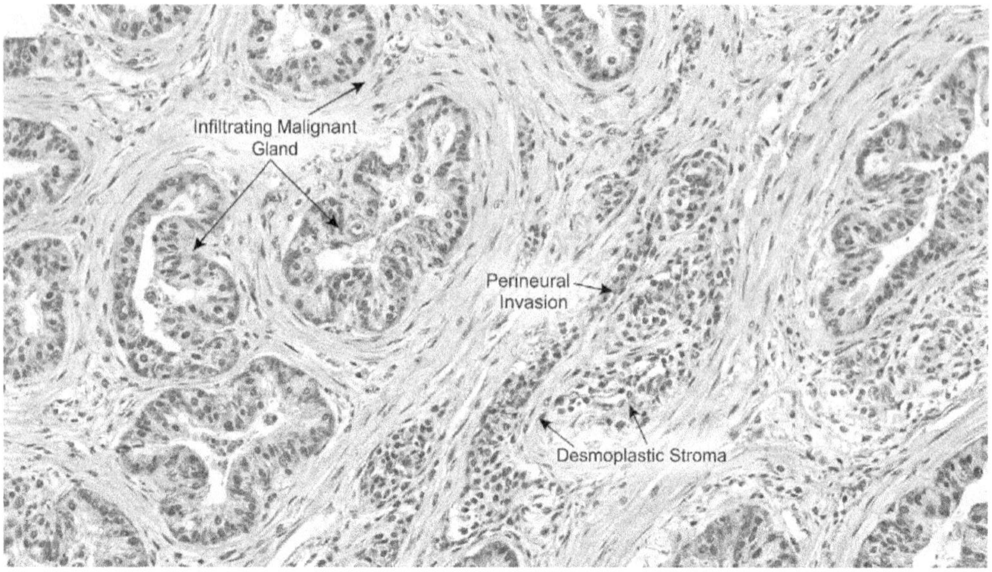

THE SIGNAL-TO-CATEGORY DECISION SYSTEM — Adenocarcinoma versus Mass-Forming Pancreatitis

---

The Signal Pattern: A focal pancreatic mass is identified, hypovascular relative to background parenchyma, with associated upstream ductal dilation, in a patient with a history that could support either malignancy or chronic pancreatitis.

Category Signature: A mass with ill-defined, infiltrative margins, duct-penetrating rather than duct-displacing morphology, in which the pancreatic duct appears to pass directly through and be obliterated by the mass rather than being smoothly displaced around it, and progressive, rather than diminishing, size on interval imaging is categorized as favoring adenocarcinoma; a mass with more defined margins, a visible duct penetrating and continuing through the mass without obliteration, the so-called duct-penetrating sign, and stability or improvement on treatment or interval imaging is categorized as favoring mass-forming pancreatitis.

The Decision: A mass favoring adenocarcinoma proceeds to tissue sampling, typically endoscopic ultrasound-guided fine-needle aspiration or biopsy, and full staging; a mass favoring pancreatitis, particularly one demonstrating the duct-penetrating sign, may be managed with a trial of medical therapy and close interval imaging follow-up, though genuine diagnostic uncertainty in either direction should still prompt tissue sampling given the consequences of a missed malignancy.

The Trap Logic: Chronic pancreatitis and adenocarcinoma frequently coexist in the same gland, since chronic inflammation is itself a risk factor for malignant transformation, and a mass arising within a background of chronic pancreatitis can be obscured by the surrounding inflammatory change, both radiologically and, at times, even on core biopsy if the sampled tissue happens to capture inflammatory rather than malignant tissue; the discriminating step in persistently ambiguous cases is a low threshold for repeat sampling, additional imaging with diffusion-weighted or hepatobiliary-phase-equivalent pancreatic-specific sequences, or multidisciplinary discussion rather than accepting a single reassuring biopsy result as definitively excluding malignancy in a highly suspicious mass.

Pattern Anchor: The duct-penetrating sign, a duct passing through rather than being obliterated by a mass, favors pancreatitis; duct-penetrating morphology should not be treated as absolutely excluding malignancy when other features remain highly suspicious, and low-threshold repeat sampling remains appropriate in genuinely discordant cases.

Complications, Prognosis, and Special Populations Considerations

Prognosis in pancreatic ductal adenocarcinoma remains guarded even following complete surgical resection, with recurrence, most often at distant sites including the liver and peritoneum, common within the first two years following an ostensibly curative operation, underscoring the importance of the accurate preoperative staging discussed throughout this chapter in appropriately selecting patients most likely to benefit from resection rather than proceeding to an operation unlikely to achieve durable disease control. Common complications following pancreaticoduodenectomy, the surgical procedure for resectable pancreatic head tumors, include postoperative pancreatic fistula, arising from leakage at the pancreaticojejunal anastomosis and best characterized on postoperative imaging as a peripancreatic fluid collection with associated elevated drain amylase, delayed gastric emptying, and, less commonly, postpancreatectomy hemorrhage, a potentially life-threatening complication that may require urgent angiographic or surgical intervention. Special population considerations include the pregnant patient, in whom MRI without gadolinium contrast remains the preferred modality for pancreatic evaluation when imaging is required, and the older adult with substantial medical comorbidity, in whom the decision to pursue an operation as extensive as pancreaticoduodenectomy requires careful multidisciplinary assessment of physiologic reserve independent of tumor resectability alone, since perioperative mortality following this procedure, while substantially improved at high-volume centers, remains meaningfully higher than for most other gastrointestinal operations discussed elsewhere in this book, a consideration the radiologist's report can support by clearly documenting the full extent of disease relevant to this risk-benefit discussion.

CAUTION: A vague resectability description such as tumor abuts the superior mesenteric artery, without the specific degree of circumferential contact this chapter's framework requires, provides insufficient information for multidisciplinary tumor board planning and should be avoided in favor of an explicit degree-based assessment for every relevant vessel.

Neuroendocrine Tumors and Other Solid Neoplasms

Pancreatic Neuroendocrine Tumors

Pancreatic neuroendocrine tumors, arising from the pancreas's islet cell population, typically present a strikingly different imaging pattern from adenocarcinoma: a well-defined, often round mass demonstrating intense arterial phase hyperenhancement reflecting the tumor's characteristically hypervascular architecture, in direct contrast to adenocarcinoma's hypovascular pattern, and this arterial hyperenhancement, together with restricted diffusion and, in a meaningful subset, cystic or necrotic change in larger tumors, forms the core recognition pattern for this entity. Functional neuroendocrine tumors, producing a clinically apparent hormonal syndrome such as hyperinsulinemic hypoglycemia from an insulinoma or the Zollinger-Ellison syndrome from a gastrinoma, are generally detected while still small given the clinical symptoms prompting earlier imaging, whereas nonfunctional neuroendocrine tumors, comprising the majority of cases in current practice, are more often detected incidentally or at a larger size once local mass effect or metastatic disease produces symptoms, a distinction relevant to counseling patients and referring clinicians about the circumstances of diagnosis and the tumor's likely biologic behavior.

Grading, Metastatic Potential, and Other Solid Neoplasms

Malignant potential in pancreatic neuroendocrine tumors correlates with tumor grade, determined histologically by mitotic count and the Ki-67 proliferation index rather than by imaging features alone, though larger tumor size, ill-defined margins, and the presence of metastatic disease at diagnosis, most often to the liver where these metastases characteristically share the same hypervascular arterial-phase enhancement pattern as the primary tumor, are imaging findings that correlate with higher-grade, more aggressive disease. Solid pseudopapillary neoplasm, a distinctive tumor occurring predominantly in young women, presents as a well-circumscribed mass with a heterogeneous mixture of solid and cystic or hemorrhagic components, often demonstrating a discrete capsule and, given its frequent internal hemorrhage, an unusually heterogeneous T1 and T2 signal pattern compared to most other pancreatic neoplasms discussed in this chapter, and while it carries low-grade malignant potential, complete surgical resection is generally curative, making its correct recognition, largely on the basis of the characteristic demographic and heterogeneous hemorrhagic imaging pattern, clinically reassuring relative to the adenocarcinoma differential it might otherwise raise given its solid tumor appearance.

Multiple Endocrine Neoplasia Type 1 and Special Population Considerations

Multiple endocrine neoplasia type 1, an autosomal dominant syndrome arising from mutation of the MEN1 tumor suppressor gene, produces a distinctive predisposition to multiple, often multifocal pancreatic neuroendocrine tumors together with parathyroid adenomas and pituitary adenomas, and its recognition, whether from a known family history or from the identification of multiple discrete pancreatic neuroendocrine tumors on a single examination, a pattern distinctly unusual for sporadic disease which is typically solitary, carries direct implications for both the affected patient's own surveillance strategy and genetic counseling and screening recommendations for first-degree relatives. Surveillance imaging in a known multiple endocrine neoplasia type 1 patient typically begins at a young age and continues at regular intervals throughout life given the syndrome's near-complete penetrance for pancreatic neuroendocrine tumor development by mid-adulthood, and MRI's lack of ionizing radiation makes it a particularly suitable modality for this lifelong surveillance requirement compared to CT-based alternatives. In the pediatric population, pancreatic neuroendocrine tumors and pancreatic neoplasms generally are rare, and a pancreatic mass identified in a child should prompt consideration of the specific differential diagnosis relevant to this age group, including pancreatoblastoma and solid pseudopapillary neoplasm, the latter sharing its predilection for a young, predominantly female population with the neuroendocrine tumor differential discussed throughout this section, rather than assuming the adult-population differential discussed elsewhere in this chapter applies unchanged.

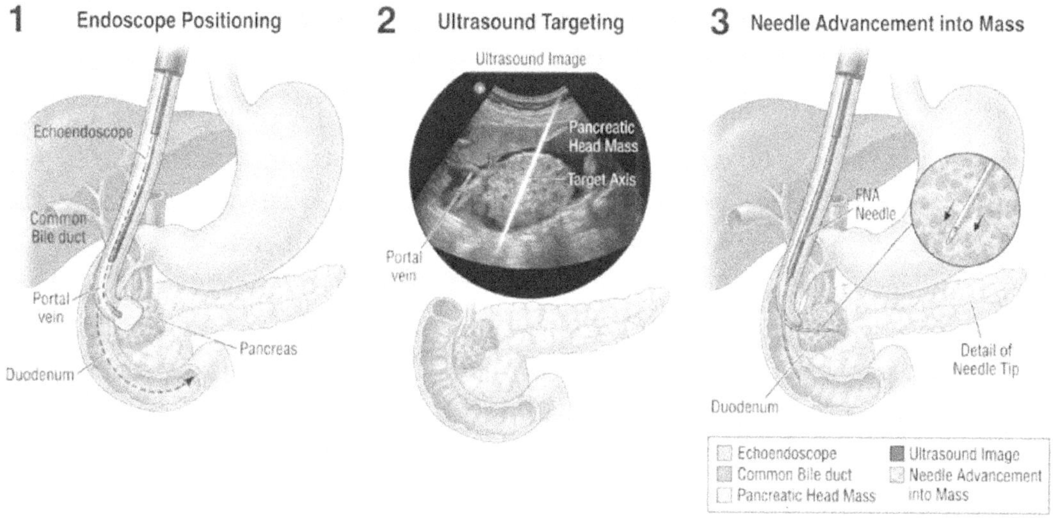

Figure 8.3: Endoscopic Ultrasound-Guided Fine-Needle Aspiration of a Pancreatic Head Mass.

Clinical Case Presentations

Case 1. A 66-year-old woman undergoes MRI for an incidentally discovered 2.8-centimeter branch duct cyst in the pancreatic tail, communicating with a normal-caliber main pancreatic duct. No mural nodule, significant duct dilation, or other worrisome feature is identified, and the radiologist categorizes the lesion as low-risk intraductal papillary mucinous neoplasm, recommending surveillance MRI at the guideline-defined interval rather than immediate further evaluation. The report explicitly documents the specific measurements and absence of each individual worrisome feature and high-risk stigma, providing a clear baseline against which future surveillance examinations can be directly compared for interval change.

Case 2. A 71-year-old man with painless jaundice undergoes MRI demonstrating diffuse pancreatic enlargement with a smooth, sausage-shaped contour and a thin, hypoenhancing peripancreatic capsule-like rim, without a discrete focal mass. Recognizing this as the classic diffuse pattern of autoimmune pancreatitis rather than adenocarcinoma, the radiologist recommends serum IgG4 testing and correlation with any biliary findings before proceeding to biopsy, and the patient's serum IgG4 returns markedly elevated; a subsequent corticosteroid trial produces dramatic clinical and radiographic improvement on follow-up imaging, confirming the diagnosis and sparing the patient an unnecessary pancreaticoduodenectomy that a mistaken adenocarcinoma diagnosis could have prompted.

Case 3. A 59-year-old man with new-onset painless jaundice and a fifteen-pound unintentional weight loss undergoes MRI demonstrating a 2.4-centimeter ill-defined, hypovascular mass in the pancreatic head with abrupt pancreatic duct cutoff and upstream dilation, along with mild common bile duct dilation consistent with a double duct pattern. The mass demonstrates approximately ninety degrees of contact with the superior mesenteric vein, without arterial contact, and the radiologist categorizes this as resectable pancreatic ductal adenocarcinoma, explicitly documenting the specific degree of venous contact and confirming no evidence of hepatic or peritoneal metastatic disease elsewhere in the examination, directly supporting the surgical team's decision to proceed with pancreaticoduodenectomy rather than neoadjuvant therapy.

Case 4. A 34-year-old man with a known family history of multiple endocrine neoplasia type 1 undergoes surveillance MRI demonstrating two discrete, well-defined, arterial-phase hyperenhancing masses within the pancreatic body and tail, the larger measuring 1.6 centimeters, without evidence of hepatic metastatic disease. Recognizing the multifocal pattern as atypical for sporadic pancreatic neuroendocrine tumor and consistent with his known hereditary syndrome, the radiologist recommends correlation with parathyroid and pituitary surveillance imaging already scheduled as part of his multiple endocrine neoplasia type 1 management program, and documents both lesions' precise size and location to guide the endocrine surgery team's discussion of enucleation versus a more extensive resection. The multidisciplinary team elects close interval MRI surveillance for the smaller lesion given its size below the general threshold for intervention in a syndromic patient, while proceeding with enucleation of the larger lesion, illustrating how the size-based management thresholds applied to sporadic pancreatic neuroendocrine tumors are adapted, rather than applied unchanged, in the multifocal syndromic context.

THE SIGNAL-TO-CATEGORY DECISION SYSTEM — Pancreatic Lesion Triage Arc

The Signal Pattern: This chapter's patterns span the full pancreatic risk spectrum, from a cystic lesion whose mural nodule must be confirmed as truly enhancing, to a solid mass whose duct relationship must be confirmed as penetrating versus obliterative.

Category Signature: Cystic lesions are categorized as low-risk, worrisome, or high-risk based on precisely defined size, duct dilation, and confirmed mural nodule criteria; solid masses are categorized as favoring adenocarcinoma or favoring mass-forming pancreatitis based on margin character, duct relationship, and interval behavior.

The Decision: Category assignment in this chapter drives among the highest-stakes decisions in this book, ranging from surveillance to major oncologic surgery, and every category should be assigned only after the specific confirmatory feature, true enhancement for a nodule, true obliteration for a duct, has been explicitly verified rather than assumed from overall gestalt impression.

The Trap Logic: Both patterns in this chapter share a common trap: a feature that superficially resembles the category-defining finding, mucin resembling a nodule, chronic inflammation coexisting with and obscuring malignancy, without actually meeting its specific defining criteria on careful, deliberate scrutiny.

Pattern Anchor: In pancreatic imaging more than almost anywhere else in this book, confirm the specific defining feature explicitly before committing to a category; the consequences of both overcalling and undercalling malignancy in the pancreas are unusually severe.

Summary and Key Concepts

Acute pancreatitis is classified by the revised Atlanta system into acute peripancreatic fluid collections and acute necrotic collections, maturing into pseudocysts and walled-off necrosis respectively after four weeks; MRI excels at distinguishing purely fluid from debris-containing collections.

Intraductal papillary mucinous neoplasm is risk-stratified by main versus branch duct involvement, size, duct dilation, and confirmed mural nodule enhancement, using defined worrisome feature and high-risk stigmata criteria.

Serous cystadenoma shows a microcystic, non-duct-communicating architecture with negligible malignant potential; mucinous cystic neoplasm occurs almost exclusively in women and carries meaningful malignant potential warranting resection.

Autoimmune pancreatitis, part of the IgG4-related disease spectrum, presents with diffuse sausage-shaped enlargement and a hypoenhancing capsule-like rim in its classic form, and responds dramatically to corticosteroid therapy, making its recognition essential to avoiding unnecessary resection.

Pancreatic ductal adenocarcinoma is hypovascular, infiltrative, and duct-obliterating; resectability is determined by degree-of-circumferential-contact staging of the superior mesenteric artery, celiac axis, common hepatic artery, and superior mesenteric-portal venous confluence.

The duct-penetrating sign favors mass-forming pancreatitis over adenocarcinoma, but chronic pancreatitis and adenocarcinoma frequently coexist, and persistent suspicion warrants repeat sampling despite a reassuring initial biopsy.

Pancreatic neuroendocrine tumors are typically well-defined and hypervascular, in direct contrast to adenocarcinoma, with malignant potential correlating with grade, size, and the presence of metastatic disease rather than with imaging appearance alone.

CHAPTER 9: SPLENIC DISORDERS

Learning Objectives

1. Assess normal splenic anatomy, size criteria, and the major congenital variants encountered in routine body MRI.
2. Differentiate benign cystic and solid focal splenic lesions using signal characteristics and enhancement pattern.
3. Recognize the imaging patterns of splenic lymphoma, leukemic infiltration, and metastatic disease.
4. Apply a structured approach to splenic trauma grading and identify vascular injuries requiring intervention.
5. Recognize splenic infarction, splenic artery aneurysm, and pseudoaneurysm and relate their imaging features to management urgency.

Clinical Overview

The spleen occupies a comparatively modest share of body MRI teaching relative to the liver, pancreas, and kidneys, yet its disease spectrum spans some of the most diagnostically satisfying pattern recognition in abdominal imaging, from the reliably benign hemangioma to the reliably urgent splenic laceration with active vascular injury, and correctly triaging across this spectrum requires the same disciplined, feature-by-feature approach applied throughout this book rather than a cursory glance dismissing the spleen as an incidental organ. This chapter proceeds from normal anatomy and congenital variants, through the benign and malignant focal lesion spectrum, to trauma and vascular emergencies, closing the hepatobiliary-adjacent organ system coverage before the book turns to the adrenal glands and retroperitoneum in the chapters that follow.

Two instances of the Signal-to-Category Decision System are applied in this chapter, the first to the cystic-versus-solid triage that anchors focal splenic lesion characterization, and the second to distinguishing diffuse malignant splenic infiltration from reactive splenomegaly, a distinction that recurs constantly in oncology and hematology practice and carries direct staging and treatment-response implications.

Splenic Anatomy, Congenital Variants, and Diffuse Splenic Disease

Normal Splenic Anatomy and Imaging Technique

The spleen demonstrates a characteristic heterogeneous, arciform pattern of enhancement on the arterial phase of contrast-enhanced MRI, reflecting differential perfusion rates between the red pulp and white pulp compartments, that resolves to homogeneous enhancement on delayed phase imaging, a normal physiologic pattern that must not be mistaken for a diffuse infiltrative or ischemic process when encountered on arterial-phase-only or single-phase imaging; recognizing this transient heterogeneity as a normal variant, rather than pursuing it as a pathologic finding, is one of the most basic yet most frequently mismanaged interpretive pitfalls in splenic imaging for trainees new to the organ. On precontrast sequences, the spleen demonstrates signal intensity similar to or slightly greater than normal liver parenchyma on T1-weighted imaging and greater signal intensity than liver on T2-weighted imaging, a baseline relationship worth deliberately confirming on every examination since deviation from this expected relationship, whether from diffuse infiltrative disease elevating T2 signal or iron deposition lowering it, is itself a diagnostically useful observation addressed further below.

Splenic Size Assessment and Splenomegaly

Splenomegaly is most reliably assessed using splenic length in the craniocaudal dimension on coronal imaging, with an upper limit of normal generally cited around thirteen centimeters in an average-sized adult, though this threshold requires adjustment for patient body habitus and height, and volumetric assessment, while more precise and increasingly feasible with modern segmentation tools, remains less commonly performed in routine clinical practice than the simpler linear measurement. Splenomegaly itself is a nonspecific finding with an extensive differential diagnosis spanning portal hypertension, discussed extensively in the liver chapters of this book, hematologic malignancy and myeloproliferative disease, infection, and infiltrative and storage disease, such that the radiologist's role is generally not to determine the cause of splenomegaly from morphology alone but rather to characterize any associated focal lesion, diffuse signal abnormality, or ancillary finding, such as varices or ascites suggesting portal hypertension, that meaningfully narrows this differential for the referring clinician.

Congenital Variants: Accessory Spleen, Splenosis, and Polysplenia and Asplenia Syndromes

Accessory spleen, a common congenital variant present in a meaningful minority of the population, appears as a small, round nodule, most often located near the splenic hilum, that demonstrates identical signal intensity and enhancement pattern to the main spleen on every sequence, a matching-signal feature that is the single most reliable discriminator from a pathologic lymph node or other soft tissue mass in this location and should be specifically sought and confirmed before an incidental perisplenic nodule is characterized as indeterminate. Splenosis, the autotransplantation of splenic tissue following prior splenic trauma or splenectomy, produces similar small, splenic-signal-matching nodules but in atypical locations throughout the peritoneal cavity, and a clinical history of prior splenic injury or splenectomy is essential context for correctly attributing these nodules to splenosis rather than pursuing an unnecessary workup for peritoneal metastatic disease. Polysplenia and asplenia syndromes, part of the heterotaxy spectrum of congenital malformations, present with multiple small splenic remnants or complete splenic absence respectively, each frequently associated with other visceral malposition anomalies including cardiac malformations, intestinal malrotation, and abnormalities of the inferior vena cava and azygos venous system, such that identification of abnormal splenic number or position should prompt a deliberate search for these associated anomalies elsewhere in the examination.

Diffuse Splenic Signal Change and Systemic Disease Correlation

Diffuse splenic iron deposition, most commonly encountered in the context of chronic transfusion therapy or hereditary hemochromatosis discussed in the liver disease chapter of this book, produces markedly decreased splenic signal intensity on T2-weighted and particularly gradient-echo sequences, generally paralleling, though not always in exact proportion to, hepatic iron overload in the same patient, and quantitative splenic R2 or R2-star mapping, while less standardized and less frequently reported than hepatic iron quantification, can provide supplementary information in select clinical contexts. Gaucher disease and other lysosomal storage disorders characteristically produce marked splenomegaly with diffuse, sometimes heterogeneous signal change and, in a meaningful subset of patients, discrete low T2 signal nodules representing Gaucher cells, or so-called Gaucher nodules, a finding that, in the appropriate clinical context of a known or suspected storage disease, should be recognized as a disease-specific manifestation rather than pursued as an indeterminate focal lesion requiring biopsy.

Splenic Signal Change in Sickle Cell Disease and Autosplenectomy

Sickle cell disease produces a distinctive and predictable trajectory of splenic change over a patient's lifetime that the radiologist should recognize as expected disease natural history rather than an incidental or concerning new finding. In early childhood, the spleen is typically enlarged from recurrent vaso-occlusive sequestration episodes, but repeated splenic infarction from recurrent sickling within the splenic microvasculature progressively destroys functional splenic tissue, such that by adulthood the spleen is characteristically small, densely calcified, and often barely identifiable on imaging, a state termed autosplenectomy that leaves the patient functionally asplenic with the associated infection risk discussed below despite the anatomic spleen remaining technically present as a small calcified remnant. Diffuse low T2 signal from hemosiderin deposition secondary to the repeated microinfarctions, together with the marked size reduction and calcification, forms a recognizable pattern distinct from the iron overload pattern discussed earlier in this section, since the mechanism here is local microvascular infarction rather than systemic iron deposition from transfusion, and recognizing this specific sickle cell pattern avoids an unwarranted additional workup for a separate cause of splenic atrophy in a patient with known sickle cell disease.

Differential Diagnosis of Massive Splenomegaly

Massive splenomegaly, generally defined as splenic length exceeding twenty centimeters or a spleen extending well into the pelvis, carries a more focused differential than the broader splenomegaly differential discussed above, dominated by myeloproliferative neoplasms, particularly chronic myeloid leukemia and primary myelofibrosis, chronic lymphocytic leukemia and other indolent lymphoproliferative disorders, and, in endemic regions, chronic malaria and visceral leishmaniasis, such that the degree of splenomegaly itself provides useful, if imperfect, differential-narrowing information beyond the qualitative presence or absence of enlargement alone. Massive splenomegaly carries its own distinct clinical considerations independent of the underlying cause, including a substantially elevated risk of spontaneous or minor-trauma-related splenic rupture given the markedly increased splenic mass and altered capsular tension, and mechanical symptoms from mass effect on adjacent structures, including early satiety from gastric compression and, less commonly, ureteral or venous compression, considerations the radiologist's report can usefully flag for the referring clinician beyond simply documenting the measured splenic dimensions.

Benign Focal Splenic Lesions

Epidemiology and Clinical Context of Benign Splenic Lesions

Focal splenic lesions are identified incidentally on a meaningful minority of abdominal cross-sectional imaging examinations performed for unrelated indications, and the overwhelming majority of these incidental lesions, particularly small lesions under two centimeters in an otherwise asymptomatic patient without a known malignancy history, prove benign on either their classic imaging appearance or subsequent stability on follow-up imaging. This favorable prior probability meaningfully informs the appropriate diagnostic pathway: a small, well-defined lesion demonstrating a classic benign pattern, such as the progressive centripetal enhancement of hemangioma or the simple fluid signal of a cyst, warrants no further workup regardless of the patient's underlying risk profile, while an indeterminate lesion lacking a classic benign pattern warrants a more cautious approach scaled to the patient's individual malignancy risk, with a known active malignancy elsewhere substantially raising the pretest probability that an indeterminate splenic lesion, statistically likely to be benign in an otherwise low-risk patient, instead represents a metastasis or lymphomatous involvement in this specific higher-risk context.

Imaging Technique Considerations for Splenic Lesion Characterization

Diffusion-weighted imaging contributes meaningfully to splenic lesion characterization, with malignant lesions, including lymphoma, metastases, and angiosarcoma, generally demonstrating more pronounced diffusion restriction than benign lesions, though this distinction is imperfect given that cellular benign lesions and areas of infarction or infection can also restrict diffusion, such that diffusion findings should be integrated with, rather than substituted for, the enhancement pattern analysis that remains the primary characterization tool for splenic lesions in this chapter. Because the spleen's normal arterial-phase enhancement heterogeneity, discussed earlier in this chapter, can obscure a genuine focal lesion or, conversely, mimic one where none exists, delayed-phase imaging, obtained after the normal heterogeneity resolves to homogeneous parenchymal enhancement, is essential for confident lesion detection and characterization and should never be omitted from a protocol intended to evaluate the spleen for focal disease, a protocol design principle consistent with the broader phase-timing emphasis introduced in the second chapter of this book.

Splenic Cysts and Pseudocysts

True splenic cysts, lined by epithelium and most often congenital or, less commonly, parasitic in origin from echinococcal infection in endemic regions, demonstrate simple fluid signal, homogeneous marked T2 hyperintensity, low T1 signal, and no internal enhancement, an unambiguous benign pattern requiring no further workup in the absence of internal complexity such as septation, wall thickening, or internal debris that would instead raise concern for infection, hemorrhage, or, rarely, a cystic neoplasm. Pseudocysts, lacking a true epithelial lining and most commonly arising following prior splenic trauma or infarction, are radiologically indistinguishable from true cysts on the basis of signal characteristics alone and share the same benign management implications, such that the distinction, while pathologically meaningful, rarely changes clinical management and need not be forced from imaging alone in the absence of a specific reason to do so.

Hemangioma and Other Vascular Lesions

Splenic hemangioma, the most common benign solid splenic neoplasm, most often demonstrates T2 hyperintensity and a pattern of progressive, centripetal enhancement analogous to hepatic hemangioma discussed earlier in this book, though splenic hemangiomas fill in more variably and less predictably than their hepatic counterparts, such that a splenic lesion demonstrating this classic peripheral nodular, progressively filling-in enhancement pattern can be diagnosed with reasonable confidence while more indeterminate or rapidly, uniformly enhancing lesions warrant a broader differential rather than reflexive hemangioma labeling. Littoral cell angioma, a vascular neoplasm arising specifically from the littoral cells lining the splenic sinuses and essentially unique to the spleen among the vascular tumor differential discussed in this book, typically presents as multiple small, variably enhancing nodules rather than a single dominant mass, and carries an association with systemic disease, including several malignancies and autoimmune conditions, that should prompt clinical correlation and, given its low but nonzero malignant potential, tissue sampling in equivocal cases rather than confident noninvasive characterization.

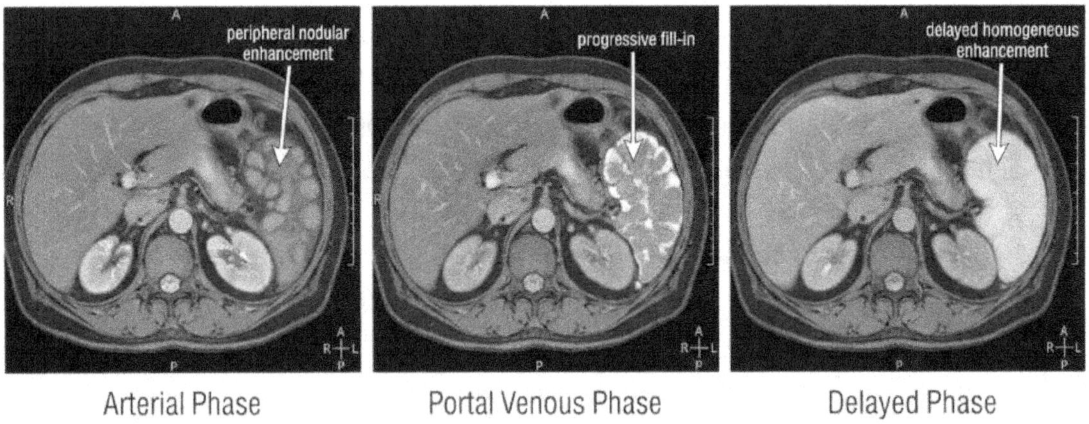

Figure 9.1: Splenic Hemangioma with Progressive Centripetal Enhancement

Hamartoma and Other Benign Solid Lesions

Splenic hamartoma, a rare benign lesion composed of disorganized red pulp elements, typically presents as a solid, variably enhancing mass that can closely mimic both hemangioma and, more concerningly, a malignant solid lesion on imaging alone given its nonspecific enhancement pattern, such that a solid splenic mass lacking the classic hemangioma enhancement pattern generally warrants further characterization with biopsy or resection rather than confident imaging-based benign labeling, particularly in a patient without a clinical context favoring a specific benign diagnosis. Sclerosing angiomatoid nodular transformation, an uncommon benign vascular lesion demonstrating a distinctive multinodular architecture with characteristic radiating fibrous septa best appreciated on delayed postcontrast imaging, can be suggested when this specific morphologic pattern is present but, like hamartoma, is frequently confirmed only after biopsy or resection given the overlap of its imaging features with both benign and malignant alternatives in less than classic presentations.

THE SIGNAL-TO-CATEGORY DECISION SYSTEM — Cystic versus Solid Splenic Lesion Triage

---

The Signal Pattern: A focal splenic lesion is identified, and the reader must first determine whether it is cystic or solid before applying any lesion-specific differential.

Category Signature: A lesion with simple, homogeneous marked T2 hyperintensity, low T1 signal, and no internal enhancement on any postcontrast phase is categorized as a simple cyst or pseudocyst; a lesion demonstrating any measurable postcontrast enhancement, however subtle, is categorized as solid and requires further characterization by its specific enhancement pattern.

The Decision: Cystic lesions meeting the simple criteria require no further workup in the absence of a clinical indication such as suspected echinococcal infection; solid lesions proceed to further categorization by enhancement pattern, most productively by assessing for the classic progressive centripetal filling-in pattern of hemangioma, with lesions lacking this classic pattern warranting biopsy or resection given the broader and more consequential differential this category carries.

Trap Logic: A hemorrhagic or proteinaceous cyst can demonstrate elevated T1 signal and heterogeneous internal signal that superficially suggests a solid lesion; the discriminating step is confirming the complete absence of true postcontrast enhancement, since internal signal complexity without enhancement remains consistent with a complicated but still benign cystic lesion, while any genuine enhancement, however subtle, reclassifies the lesion as solid regardless of its precontrast signal characteristics.

Pattern Anchor: The cystic-versus-solid branch point is decided by postcontrast enhancement alone, not by precontrast signal complexity; confirm true enhancement before abandoning the cystic category for a hemorrhagic or proteinaceous cyst.

KEY POINT: A small, incidentally discovered splenic lesion with a classic benign enhancement pattern requires no further workup regardless of patient risk profile; an indeterminate lesion should be evaluated against the patient's individual malignancy risk rather than a uniform threshold applied to every patient.

Malignant and Infiltrative Splenic Disease

Imaging Response Assessment in Splenic Lymphoma Following Therapy

Response assessment in splenic lymphoma following systemic therapy relies substantially on interval change in splenic size and the resolution or persistence of any discrete focal lesion identified at baseline, generally interpreted in conjunction with the Lugano classification framework applied to nodal and other extranodal disease sites throughout the staging examination rather than through splenic-specific criteria in isolation. A meaningful reduction in splenic size following therapy is generally reassuring, though residual, modest splenomegaly can persist even after successful treatment and should not automatically be interpreted as residual disease in the absence of a discrete residual mass or other concerning feature, an important calibration point given the clinical and psychological significance patients and referring clinicians often place on a still-enlarged spleen on a post-treatment examination. Conversely, new or enlarging splenic lesions, or new splenomegaly following a period of treatment response, should be regarded with the same concern for disease progression or relapse as a new or enlarging nodal mass elsewhere in the body, and the radiologist's report should explicitly compare current splenic size and any focal lesion characteristics against the relevant baseline and interval examinations rather than reporting splenic findings in isolation without this comparative context.

EVIDENCE: The Lugano classification, the current standard framework for lymphoma response assessment on cross-sectional imaging, incorporates splenic size and the presence or resolution of discrete splenic lesions as part of its integrated organ-by-organ response criteria rather than applying isolated, organ-specific thresholds.

Primary Splenic Lymphoma Versus Secondary Splenic Involvement

Primary splenic lymphoma, in which the spleen and splenic hilar lymph nodes are the sole or clearly dominant site of disease at presentation, is considerably less common than secondary splenic involvement by a systemic lymphoma already diagnosed or concurrently identified at other nodal or extranodal sites, and this distinction, while ultimately established through the full extent of disease demonstrated on staging imaging together with any prior diagnostic history rather than through splenic imaging features alone, carries prognostic and treatment-planning relevance that the radiologist's report should support by clearly and specifically documenting every site of disease identified on the examination rather than a summary statement of splenic involvement alone. Hodgkin lymphoma splenic involvement, when present, most often demonstrates a nodular pattern of discrete, well-defined masses, whereas non-Hodgkin lymphoma more frequently produces the diffuse or miliary patterns discussed above, a general tendency that, while not absolute, can help calibrate the reader's expectation for lesion conspicuity and detection difficulty based on the specific lymphoma subtype under evaluation when this information is available from the clinical history.

Post-Splenectomy and Functional Asplenia: Imaging and Clinical Implications

The postsplenectomy abdomen, whether from surgical splenectomy performed for trauma, hypersplenism, or as part of an oncologic procedure, or from functional asplenia as seen in the sickle cell autosplenectomy discussed earlier in this chapter, presents specific interpretive considerations of its own. Splenosis, discussed earlier in this chapter as a source of splenic-signal-matching peritoneal nodules following prior splenic injury or splenectomy, should be specifically distinguished from peritoneal metastatic disease in any postsplenectomy patient undergoing oncologic surveillance imaging, since misattribution in either direction carries meaningful consequences, either an unnecessary biopsy of benign splenosis or a missed peritoneal metastasis incorrectly dismissed as splenosis, making careful attention to matching signal intensity and enhancement across every phase, together with correlation with the specific surgical and oncologic history, essential in this population. Clinically, both surgical and functional asplenia carry a lifelong increased risk of fulminant infection from encapsulated organisms, a risk that, while not directly assessed by imaging, is relevant context the radiologist should be aware of when a postsplenectomy or functionally asplenic patient presents with fever or sepsis of unclear source, since this population's threshold for aggressive infectious workup and empiric treatment is appropriately lower than in an immunocompetent patient with an intact, functioning spleen.

Lymphoma and Leukemic Infiltration

The spleen is the organ most commonly and most diversely involved by lymphoma among the abdominal viscera, presenting in one of several distinct imaging patterns: diffuse splenic enlargement without a discrete focal lesion, the most common pattern and one that can be radiologically indistinguishable from benign splenomegaly without additional context, a miliary pattern of numerous tiny, subtle nodules that can be genuinely difficult to detect against normal background splenic signal heterogeneity, and, least commonly but most readily recognized, a solitary dominant mass or a small number of larger, discrete nodules. Given the frequent subtlety of miliary and diffuse infiltrative lymphomatous involvement, splenic size itself, together with any other sites of nodal or extranodal disease identified elsewhere in a staging examination, often carries as much diagnostic weight as the splenic parenchymal appearance alone, and a normal-sized spleen with normal parenchymal signal in a patient with lymphoma elsewhere provides reasonably reassuring, though not absolute, evidence against splenic involvement.

Splenic Metastases and Angiosarcoma

Splenic metastatic disease is comparatively uncommon relative to the frequency of metastatic involvement of the liver and other abdominal organs, a discrepancy attributed to the spleen's unique intraparenchymal blood flow architecture that is thought to be relatively resistant to tumor cell seeding and implantation, but when present most commonly originates from melanoma, breast carcinoma, lung carcinoma, and ovarian carcinoma, typically presenting as one or more solid, variably enhancing lesions similar in general appearance to hepatic metastases from the same primary. Primary splenic angiosarcoma, a rare but highly aggressive malignant vascular neoplasm, presents as a large, heterogeneous, hemorrhagic mass with irregular, avidly enhancing solid components and a marked propensity for both splenic rupture, which can be the presenting event, and early hematogenous metastatic spread most often to the liver and lungs, such that a large, heterogeneous, hemorrhagic splenic mass, particularly one demonstrating disproportionately aggressive behavior on interval imaging, should prompt urgent consideration of this specific and prognostically poor diagnosis rather than reflexive attribution to a more common benign hemorrhagic process.

Sarcoidosis and Other Infiltrative Disease

Splenic sarcoidosis, part of the same multisystem granulomatous disease process discussed in the context of hepatic involvement earlier in this book, produces a similar pattern of splenomegaly with multiple small, hypoenhancing, T2-hypointense nodules representing non-caseating granulomas, and, as with hepatic sarcoid, the correct diagnosis is most confidently established through the combination of characteristic imaging pattern, other sites of disease such as mediastinal and hilar lymphadenopathy, and clinical and serologic correlation rather than from splenic imaging in isolation. Extramedullary hematopoiesis, a compensatory response to marrow failure or increased hematopoietic demand most often seen in myelofibrosis and severe chronic hemolytic anemias, produces splenomegaly with variable signal characteristics reflecting the specific hematopoietic tissue composition present, and recognizing extramedullary hematopoiesis as the underlying process, generally through correlation with the patient's known hematologic disease and, when present, similar paraspinal or hepatic involvement, avoids an unnecessary and potentially misleading pursuit of a primary splenic neoplasm.

THE SIGNAL-TO-CATEGORY DECISION SYSTEM — Diffuse Splenic Infiltration versus Reactive Splenomegaly

The Signal Pattern: An enlarged spleen is identified in a patient with known or suspected malignancy, and the reader must determine whether the enlargement reflects malignant infiltration or a reactive, non-neoplastic process.

Category Signature: Splenomegaly with a discrete dominant mass, a miliary nodular pattern, or signal heterogeneity distinctly different from the patient's baseline is categorized as favoring malignant infiltration; splenomegaly with homogeneous, otherwise normal parenchymal signal and an identifiable alternative explanation, such as portal hypertension or a systemic infectious or inflammatory process, is categorized as favoring reactive splenomegaly.

The Decision: Findings favoring infiltration prompt correlation with other staging findings and consideration of biopsy or interval imaging following treatment to assess response; findings favoring reactive splenomegaly are managed according to the underlying identified cause, with splenic size itself used as one of several markers of response or progression on subsequent surveillance imaging.

Trap Logic: Splenic size alone correlates imperfectly with the presence or absence of malignant infiltration, since a normal-sized spleen can still harbor microscopic or miliary lymphomatous involvement below the resolution of size-based assessment, and a markedly enlarged spleen can reflect purely reactive change from portal hypertension or infection without any malignant infiltration whatsoever; the discriminating step is integrating splenic size with parenchymal signal homogeneity and the full pattern of disease elsewhere in the examination rather than relying on size in isolation.

Pattern Anchor: Splenic size alone is an unreliable discriminator of malignant infiltration; integrate parenchymal signal homogeneity and disease pattern elsewhere in the study before assigning the reactive-versus-infiltrative category.

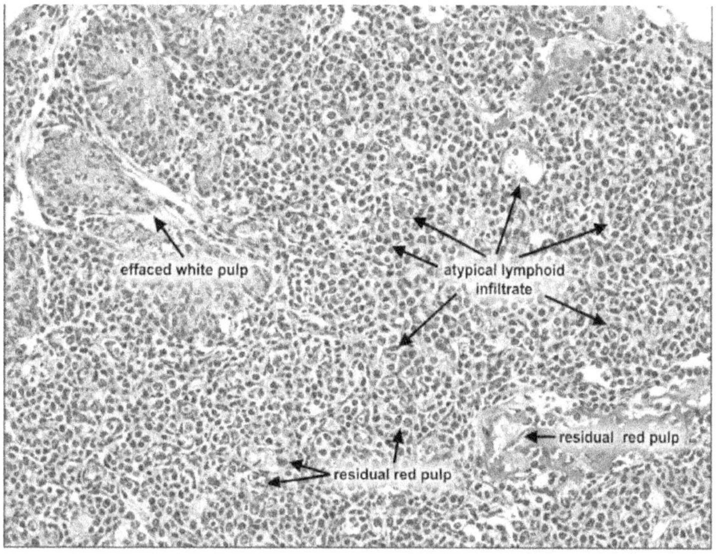

Figure 9.2: Splenic Lymphomatous Infiltration Histopathology

Splenic Trauma, Infarction, and Vascular Disorders

Splenic Vascular Anatomy Relevant to Trauma and Intervention

The spleen receives its blood supply from the splenic artery, a branch of the celiac axis coursing along the superior border of the pancreas before dividing into segmental branches at the splenic hilum, an anatomic relationship that explains the mechanistic link between severe pancreatitis, discussed in the preceding chapter, and splenic vascular complications including splenic artery pseudoaneurysm and splenic vein thrombosis. Venous drainage occurs through the splenic vein, which courses posterior to the pancreatic body before joining the superior mesenteric vein to form the portal vein, an anatomic relationship equally relevant to understanding both pancreatitis-related splenic vein thrombosis and the pattern of sinistral portal hypertension it produces, discussed in the preceding chapter. Familiarity with this segmental arterial anatomy is particularly relevant to interventional and surgical planning, since splenic-artery embolization, increasingly favored over splenectomy for hemodynamically stable trauma patients with vascular injury, can be performed selectively at the level of an individual segmental branch to control bleeding while preserving splenic function supplied by the remaining, non-embolized segments.

Splenic Trauma Grading and the AAST Injury Scale

Splenic trauma is graded using the American Association for the Surgery of Trauma organ injury scale, which stratifies injury severity from grade one, a subcapsular hematoma or laceration involving less than one centimeter of parenchymal depth, through grade five, representing a shattered spleen or complete hilar devascularization, with intermediate grades defined by progressively deeper lacerations, larger hematomas, and increasing vascular involvement, and while this grading system was developed primarily from surgical and CT-based experience, the same grading criteria apply directly to MRI when it is used for splenic trauma assessment, most often in the subacute setting or when CT is contraindicated. Active contrast extravasation, appearing as a focus of contrast pooling that increases in size or intensity between sequential postcontrast phases, is a critical finding independent of the underlying AAST grade, since its presence indicates active, ongoing hemorrhage requiring urgent intervention, typically angiographic embolization, regardless of the anatomic injury grade, and its absence, conversely, supports a trial of nonoperative management even for a comparatively high-grade injury in a hemodynamically stable patient.

Figure 9.3: Splenic Arterial Segmental Anatomy

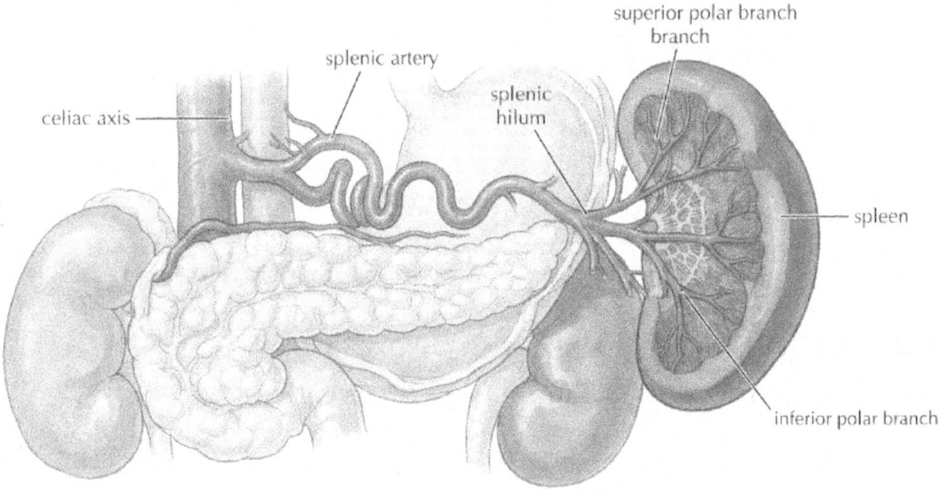

AAST Grade	Injury Description	Typical Management
I	Subcapsular hematoma or laceration less than 1 cm parenchymal depth	Nonoperative management, observation
II	Subcapsular hematoma 10-50% surface area; laceration 1-3 cm depth	Nonoperative management if hemodynamically stable
III	Laceration greater than 3 cm depth or involving trabecular vessels	Nonoperative management or embolization based on extravasation
IV	Laceration involving segmental or hilar vessels with major devascularization	Embolization or surgery depending on stability and extravasation
V	Shattered spleen or complete hilar devascularization	Surgery in most cases; embolization in select stable patients

Nonoperative Management Criteria and Follow-Up Imaging After Splenic Trauma

Nonoperative management has become the preferred approach for the majority of splenic trauma patients, reflecting an appreciation of the spleen's important immunologic function and a desire to avoid the lifelong infection risk associated with splenectomy, and is generally appropriate for a hemodynamically stable patient without active contrast extravasation, peritonitis, or another indication for immediate laparotomy, regardless of anatomic injury grade in isolation, since grade alone, as emphasized earlier in this section, is a less reliable predictor of nonoperative management failure than the presence or absence of active extravasation. Follow-up imaging after a splenic injury is generally reserved for patients with clinical deterioration, a high-grade injury under closer surveillance protocols, or before resumption of contact sports or strenuous activity in an appropriate timeframe following injury, rather than performed routinely on every patient regardless of clinical trajectory, and delayed splenic rupture, while uncommon, remains a recognized complication that should be specifically considered in a patient presenting with new or worsening left upper quadrant pain even at a substantial interval following the initial injury and an unremarkable early follow-up examination.

Splenic Infarction and Vascular Thrombosis

Splenic infarction, arising from embolic occlusion, most often cardioembolic or from a hypercoagulable state, or from direct splenic artery thrombosis or dissection, presents as a wedge-shaped or, in the case of global infarction, more diffuse region of non-enhancing parenchyma, typically peripherally based given the end-organ nature of splenic segmental arterial supply, with the characteristic wedge morphology and its involvement of the splenic capsule generally distinguishing infarction from a mass lesion on morphology alone even before considering the absence of enhancement. Splenic infarction is managed conservatively in the overwhelming majority of cases, with analgesia for the frequently significant associated pain and treatment directed at the underlying embolic or hypercoagulable etiology, reserving splenectomy for the uncommon complications of infected or abscessed infarction or, rarely, delayed splenic rupture, such that the radiologist's role extends beyond simple infarction identification to actively screening for these specific complications, including gas within the infarcted segment suggesting superimposed infection, on any follow-up imaging.

Splenic Artery Aneurysm and Pseudoaneurysm

Splenic artery aneurysm, the most common visceral artery aneurysm encountered in clinical practice, is generally an incidental finding in an asymptomatic patient and, unlike the pseudoaneurysm discussed in the trauma and pancreatitis contexts elsewhere in this book, represents a true aneurysm involving all three layers of the arterial wall rather than a contained rupture; management is generally guided by size, with intervention, typically endovascular embolization or coil placement, considered for aneurysms exceeding a defined size threshold or in specific higher-risk populations, most notably women of childbearing age given an associated risk of rupture during pregnancy that is disproportionate to the aneurysm's size alone. Splenic artery pseudoaneurysm, by contrast, most often arising from trauma or, as discussed in the preceding chapter, pancreatitis-related vascular injury, carries a substantially higher rupture risk than a true aneurysm of comparable size and generally warrants more urgent intervention once identified, such that the radiologist's distinction between a true aneurysm and a pseudoaneurysm, based on wall morphology and clinical context, meaningfully influences the urgency of the recommended management pathway.

Figure 9.4: Endovascular Coil Embolization of Splenic Artery Pseudoaneurysm

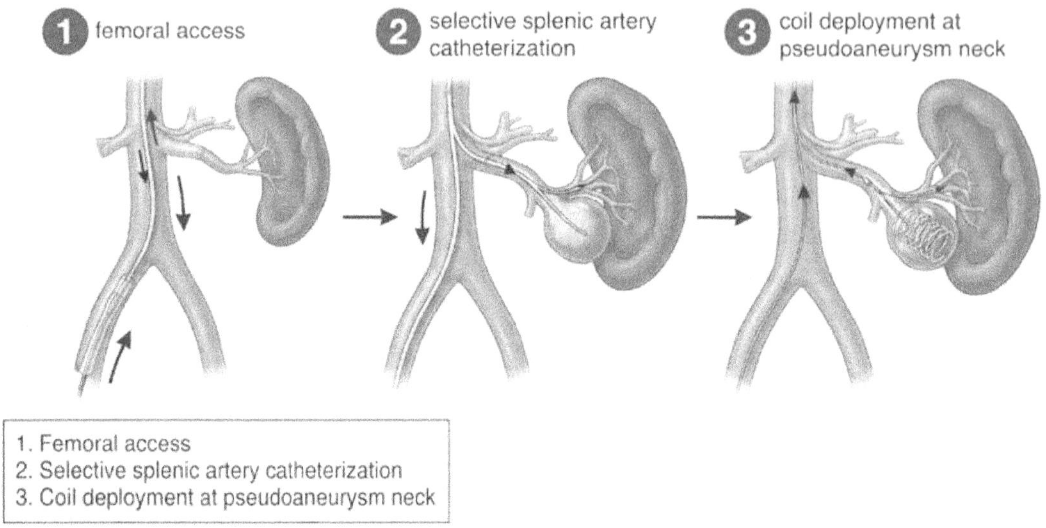

Epidemiology and Risk Factors for Splenic Artery Aneurysm

Splenic artery aneurysm demonstrates a marked female predominance, with several proposed contributing mechanisms including the hemodynamic effects of pregnancy and hormonally mediated changes in arterial wall composition, and additional recognized risk factors include portal hypertension, in which increased splenic arterial flow contributes to aneurysmal degeneration, multiparity, and fibromuscular dysplasia, a systemic arteriopathy discussed in relation to the renal arteries elsewhere in this book that can similarly affect the splenic artery. The pregnancy-associated rupture risk noted earlier in this chapter is disproportionately concentrated in the third trimester, and carries a notably high maternal and fetal mortality when rupture occurs, a risk profile that has led some authorities to recommend a lower intervention size threshold in women of childbearing age, and particularly in those planning pregnancy, than the threshold generally applied to an incidentally discovered splenic artery aneurysm in an asymptomatic man or postmenopausal woman, illustrating how patient-specific factors beyond aneurysm size alone appropriately inform the management threshold in this specific population.

CAUTION: Active contrast extravasation on a splenic trauma examination mandates urgent communication to the trauma team regardless of the anatomic AAST injury grade; a low-grade laceration with active extravasation carries greater immediate management urgency than a high-grade laceration without it.

Clinical Case Presentations

Case 1. A 45-year-old woman undergoes MRI for an incidentally discovered 3.2-centimeter splenic lesion. The lesion demonstrates marked T2 hyperintensity, peripheral nodular enhancement on arterial phase imaging, and progressive centripetal fill-in on delayed phase imaging, a classic pattern for splenic hemangioma. The radiologist categorizes the lesion as a definite benign hemangioma given the classic enhancement pattern and recommends no further workup, sparing the patient an unnecessary biopsy of a deeply located, vascular organ where sampling carries meaningful bleeding risk.

Case 2. A 58-year-old man with known follicular lymphoma undergoes restaging MRI demonstrating a spleen measuring 14.5 centimeters in length, mildly enlarged from a prior baseline of 12 centimeters, with homogeneous parenchymal signal and no discrete focal lesion or miliary nodularity. Given the homogeneous signal, absence of a discrete mass, and the modest, gradual nature of the size change, the radiologist categorizes this as indeterminate for early infiltrative involvement versus reactive change and recommends correlation with the patient's other staging findings and interval follow-up rather than an immediate change in management based on splenic size alone, illustrating the limited standalone specificity of splenic size discussed in this chapter's Rhythm Layer.

Case 3. A 24-year-old man involved in a motor vehicle collision undergoes trauma MRI, obtained after an initial equivocal ultrasound examination, demonstrating a grade three splenic laceration extending through the parenchyma with an associated subcapsular hematoma but no evidence of active contrast extravasation and a hemodynamically stable presentation throughout the examination. Given the absence of active extravasation, the trauma and interventional radiology teams elect nonoperative management with close clinical monitoring rather than angiographic embolization, and the patient is discharged after an uneventful observation period with follow-up imaging confirming stable, resolving injury.

Case 4. A 67-year-old woman with a remote history of severe acute pancreatitis presents with vague left upper quadrant discomfort, and MRI demonstrates a 2.1-centimeter rounded, avidly enhancing structure contiguous with the splenic artery near the pancreatic tail, distinct from the adjacent pancreatic parenchyma and not present on imaging performed at the time of her pancreatitis episode two years earlier. Recognizing this as a splenic artery pseudoaneurysm rather than a true aneurysm given both its interval development and the relevant pancreatitis history, the radiologist recommends urgent interventional radiology consultation given the pseudoaneurysm's elevated rupture risk, and the patient undergoes successful endovascular coil embolization the same day.

Case 5. A 9-year-old boy with known sickle cell disease undergoes surveillance MRI as part of his hematology follow-up, demonstrating a markedly small, densely low-signal spleen measuring 3.1 centimeters with diffuse low T2 signal, unchanged from imaging performed one year earlier. Recognizing this as the expected autosplenectomy pattern of longstanding sickle cell disease rather than a new or concerning finding, the radiologist documents the stable appearance and specifically notes the patient's resulting functional asplenia and associated infection risk for the referring hematology team, reinforcing the ongoing importance of the pneumococcal and other encapsulated-organism vaccination and prophylaxis measures already in place for this patient.

THE SIGNAL-TO-CATEGORY DECISION SYSTEM — Splenic Lesion Triage Arc

The Signal Pattern: This chapter's patterns span the full splenic risk spectrum, from a focal lesion whose cystic-versus-solid status must be confirmed before further characterization, to diffuse splenomegaly whose infiltrative-versus-reactive status must be confirmed by integrating size with parenchymal signal and systemic disease pattern.

Category Signature: Focal lesions are categorized as cystic or solid based on confirmed postcontrast enhancement; diffuse splenic enlargement is categorized as favoring malignant infiltration or reactive change based on parenchymal signal homogeneity and the broader pattern of disease elsewhere in the examination.

The Decision: Category assignment in this chapter ranges from reassuring no-further-workup outcomes for a classic hemangioma or simple cyst to urgent interventional referral for active extravasation or pseudoaneurysm, and every category should be assigned only after the specific confirmatory feature, true enhancement, active extravasation, or systemic disease correlation, has been explicitly verified.

The Trap Logic: Both patterns in this chapter share a common trap: relying on a single feature, splenic size alone or precontrast signal alone, without integrating the full pattern of enhancement and systemic context that this chapter's framework requires.

Pattern Anchor: Splenic size and precontrast signal alone are insufficient for confident categorization anywhere in this chapter; confirm enhancement pattern and systemic context before committing to a final category.

Summary and Key Concepts

The spleen demonstrates normal transient arterial-phase heterogeneous enhancement that resolves on delayed imaging and must not be mistaken for diffuse pathology; splenomegaly is generally assessed by craniocaudal length with an upper limit near thirteen centimeters.

Accessory spleen and splenosis demonstrate splenic-matching signal on every sequence, the key discriminator from pathologic nodal or peritoneal disease; polysplenia and asplenia are part of the heterotaxy spectrum with associated visceral anomalies.

Simple splenic cysts and pseudocysts show homogeneous T2 hyperintensity with no enhancement and require no further workup; hemangioma shows classic progressive centripetal fill-in, while hamartoma and other solid lesions frequently require biopsy given nonspecific enhancement.

Splenic lymphoma presents as diffuse enlargement, a miliary nodular pattern, or a dominant mass; splenic size alone correlates imperfectly with malignant infiltration and must be integrated with parenchymal signal and disease pattern elsewhere in the examination.

Splenic angiosarcoma presents as a large, heterogeneous, hemorrhagic, aggressive mass with rupture and metastatic potential and should be distinguished from more common benign hemorrhagic processes.

Splenic trauma is graded by the AAST organ injury scale, but active contrast extravasation, independent of anatomic grade, is the critical finding mandating urgent intervention.

Splenic artery pseudoaneurysm, most often related to trauma or pancreatitis, carries a substantially higher rupture risk than a true splenic artery aneurysm of comparable size and generally warrants more urgent intervention.

CHAPTER 10: ADRENAL IMAGING AND INCIDENTALOMA CHARACTERIZATION

Learning Objectives

1. Apply chemical-shift imaging to distinguish lipid-rich adenoma from other adrenal lesions and recognize the limitations of this technique for lipid-poor adenoma.
2. Recognize the imaging features of adrenocortical carcinoma and adrenal metastasis and distinguish them from benign adenoma using size, growth rate, and washout characteristics.
3. Recognize pheochromocytoma on MRI and understand the safety implications of an unrecognized pheochromocytoma before biopsy or intravenous contrast administration.
4. Apply a structured incidentaloma management algorithm integrating size, imaging phenotype, and interval growth.
5. Recognize adrenal hyperplasia and its major functional subtypes and their distinguishing clinical and imaging correlates.

Clinical Overview

The adrenal incidentaloma, an adrenal mass discovered on imaging performed for an unrelated indication, has become one of the most frequently encountered interpretive challenges in body imaging as cross-sectional imaging utilization has expanded, and correctly triaging this common finding, the overwhelming majority of which prove to be benign, nonfunctioning adenoma, without either dismissing a genuinely concerning lesion or subjecting a benign finding to unnecessary further workup, is the organizing task of this chapter. This chapter proceeds from the chemical-shift technique that anchors adrenal lesion characterization, through adrenocortical carcinoma and metastatic disease, to pheochromocytoma and its unique safety implications, and closes with adrenal hyperplasia and a structured, evidence-based incidentaloma management algorithm.

Two instances of the Signal-to-Category Decision System are applied in this chapter, the first to the chemical-shift signal-drop triage that anchors adenoma characterization, and the second to the safety-critical distinction between an indeterminate adrenal mass and a pheochromocytoma that has not yet been biochemically excluded, a distinction with direct implications for whether intravenous contrast and biopsy can be safely performed.

Adrenal Anatomy and the Chemical-Shift Approach to Adrenal Lesion Characterization

Normal Adrenal Anatomy and Function

The adrenal glands, paired retroperitoneal structures situated superomedial to each kidney with the right gland typically more triangular in configuration and positioned slightly more cephalad than the elongated, crescentic left gland, comprise a cortex, responsible for glucocorticoid, mineralocorticoid, and androgen production across its three histologically distinct zones, and a medulla, responsible for catecholamine production and the site of origin for pheochromocytoma discussed later in this chapter. This anatomic and functional division underlies the organizing logic of this chapter's lesion differential, since cortical lesions, spanning benign adenoma through adrenocortical carcinoma, and medullary lesions, principally pheochromocytoma, present distinct imaging phenotypes and carry entirely different safety and management implications, such that establishing whether a lesion's imaging phenotype favors a cortical or medullary origin is frequently the first meaningful branch point in adrenal mass characterization.

Chemical-Shift Imaging Technique and Physiologic Basis

Chemical-shift imaging exploits the differential resonant frequency of protons in water- and fat-bound molecules to detect microscopic intracellular lipid, a feature characteristic of the steroid-hormone-producing cells that comprise the majority of benign adrenal adenomas, by acquiring paired in-phase and opposed-phase gradient-echo sequences and comparing signal intensity between them: a lesion containing microscopic fat demonstrates measurable signal drop on the opposed-phase sequence relative to the in-phase sequence, since water and fat protons within the same voxel are out of phase and their signals partially cancel, while a lesion lacking microscopic fat shows no such signal drop. This physiologic basis, detecting intracellular lipid content within the adenoma's steroid-producing cells rather than the gross, macroscopic fat detected by conventional fat-suppression techniques, is a distinct mechanism from the myelolipoma fat-signal characterization discussed later in this chapter and should not be conflated with it despite both ultimately relating to adrenal lesion fat content in different forms.

Quantifying and Reporting Chemical-Shift Signal Drop

Signal drop can be assessed qualitatively, by visual comparison of lesion signal intensity between the in-phase and opposed-phase sequences relative to a reference tissue such as spleen, or quantitatively, using a calculated adrenal signal intensity index or a relative percentage signal-drop formula comparing lesion signal on both sequences, with quantitative assessment generally preferred for borderline cases where qualitative visual assessment is genuinely ambiguous between reader impressions. A signal drop exceeding a validated threshold, generally cited in the range of a sixteen and one-half percent relative signal loss though specific thresholds vary somewhat across validated formulas and should be confirmed against the specific formula in use at the interpreting institution, is diagnostic of a lipid-rich adenoma with high specificity, and the report should state the specific quantitative signal-drop value used to reach this conclusion in borderline cases rather than a purely qualitative visual impression, both for the referring clinician's confidence in the interpretation and for direct comparison on any future examination.

Adrenal Vascular Anatomy and Its Relevance to Sampling and Hemorrhage

Adrenal venous drainage follows an asymmetric pattern with direct clinical relevance to both adrenal venous sampling and the pattern of adrenal hemorrhage: the right adrenal vein drains directly and often quite short-course into the inferior vena cava, an anatomic arrangement that makes right-sided selective adrenal vein catheterization technically more demanding than the left side during the adrenal venous sampling procedure discussed later in this chapter, while the left adrenal vein drains into the left renal vein, providing a longer, more reliably catheterizable venous approach. This same right-sided venous anatomy is invoked to explain the relative predominance of right-sided adrenal hemorrhage in certain clinical contexts, including some series of trauma-related and neonatal adrenal hemorrhage, since the short, direct right adrenal vein is thought to transmit acutely elevated central venous pressure more directly to the right adrenal gland than the longer, more buffered left-sided venous pathway, though this proposed mechanism remains an area of some ongoing physiologic discussion rather than a fully settled explanation.

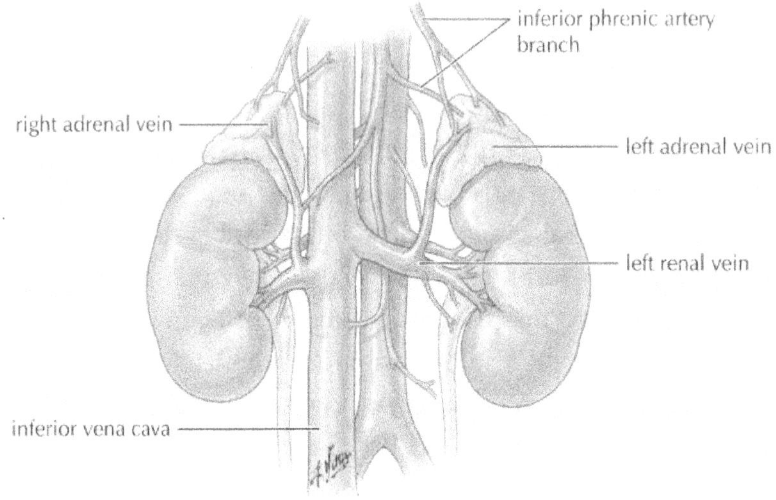

Figure 10.1: Adrenal Arterial and Venous Anatomy

Adrenal Adenoma and the Lipid-Poor Adenoma Problem

Epidemiology and Prevalence of Adrenal Incidentaloma

Adrenal incidentaloma is identified on a meaningful proportion of abdominal cross-sectional imaging examinations performed for unrelated indications, with prevalence rising substantially with advancing age such that autopsy series suggest a considerably higher lifetime prevalence than the imaging-detected rate alone would suggest, reflecting both the imaging-detection threshold and the fact that many small, clinically silent adenomas are never imaged during a patient's lifetime. This high background prevalence, dominated overwhelmingly by benign, nonfunctioning adenoma, is the essential epidemiologic context underlying the size-and-behavior-based management algorithm presented later in this chapter, since a management approach calibrated to this favorable prior probability, reserving aggressive further workup for lesions with specific concerning features rather than applying it uniformly to every incidentally discovered adrenal nodule, avoids both the unnecessary patient anxiety and downstream cost of overtesting a population where true malignancy is a distinct minority of cases.

Lipid-Rich Adenoma: The Chemical-Shift-Positive Pattern

The lipid-rich adenoma, demonstrating unambiguous signal drop on chemical-shift imaging as described above, represents the majority of adrenal adenomas and can be diagnosed with high confidence on this single technique alone without further workup in most clinical contexts, reflecting one of the genuine diagnostic triumphs of body MRI given the technique's simplicity, speed, and complete avoidance of intravenous contrast or ionizing radiation. This confident, noninvasive characterization is precisely why chemical-shift imaging occupies such a central role in the adrenal protocol discussed in the second chapter of this book, and its omission from a dedicated adrenal MRI protocol, or its omission from a general abdominal protocol in a patient with a known adrenal lesion requiring characterization, represents a meaningful and avoidable protocol design failure given how much diagnostic work this single technique reliably performs.

Lipid-Poor Adenoma: A Persistent Diagnostic Challenge

A meaningful minority of adrenal adenomas, generally cited around thirty percent in most series, contain insufficient microscopic intracellular lipid to produce a detectable signal drop on chemical-shift imaging, a category termed lipid-poor adenoma that represents one of the more persistently vexing diagnostic problems in adrenal imaging, since these lesions cannot be confidently distinguished from metastasis or other malignant lesions on chemical-shift imaging alone despite being benign. Additional characterization tools for the lipid-poor adenoma include washout characteristics on delayed postcontrast CT, which remains, somewhat paradoxically, a more validated technique for this specific indication than any single MRI sequence, restricted diffusion, which is generally less pronounced in lipid-poor adenoma than in metastasis though with meaningful overlap limiting its standalone reliability, and, most powerfully, lesion stability on interval imaging over a sufficient follow-up period, which remains one of the most clinically decisive tools available for a genuinely indeterminate lipid-poor lesion when the pretest probability of malignancy is not high enough to warrant immediate biopsy.

Myelolipoma and Other Benign Adrenal Lesions

Adrenal myelolipoma, a benign lesion composed of mature adipose tissue admixed with hematopoietic elements, demonstrates unambiguous macroscopic fat on conventional fat-suppressed sequences, a bulk fat signature entirely distinct from the microscopic intracellular lipid detected by chemical-shift imaging in adenoma, and this macroscopic fat signal, when clearly present, is essentially diagnostic of myelolipoma and requires no further workup regardless of lesion size, a specific and important exception to the general size-based incidentaloma management thresholds discussed later in this chapter. Adrenal cyst and adrenal hemorrhage, the latter most often related to trauma, anticoagulation, or, in the neonate, a difficult delivery, each present with their own characteristic signal patterns, simple fluid signal without enhancement for a cyst and evolving blood-product signal characteristics paralleling the hemorrhage-aging pattern discussed elsewhere in this book for hemorrhage, and both are generally managed conservatively once correctly recognized, reserving further workup for atypical features such as a thickened or irregular cyst wall or a hemorrhagic lesion that fails to evolve or resolve as expected on follow-up imaging.

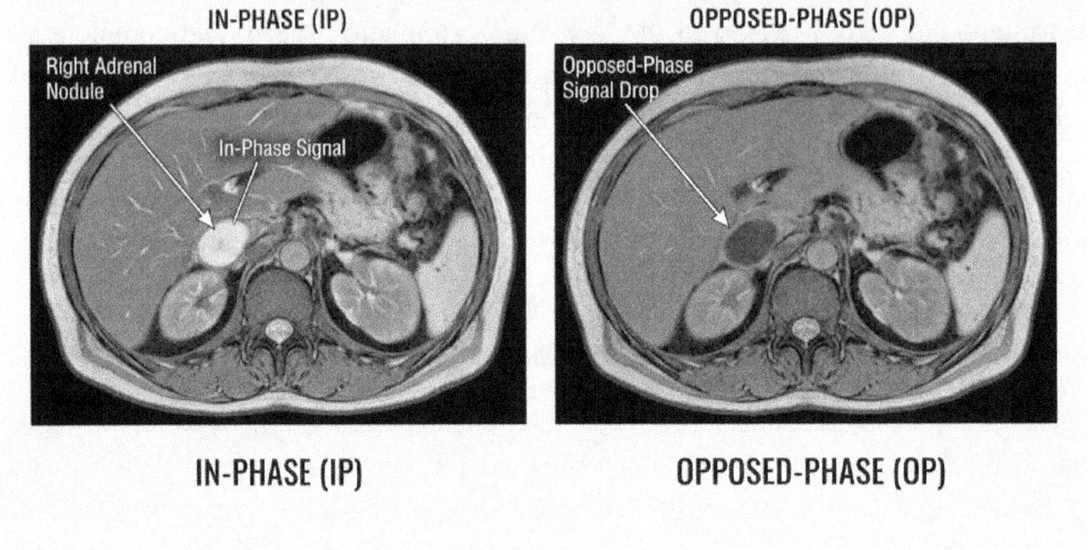

FIGURE 10.2: CHEMICAL-SHIFT ADRENAL ADENOMA CHARACTERIZATION

THE SIGNAL-TO-CATEGORY DECISION SYSTEM — Chemical-Shift Signal Drop Adenoma Triage

The Signal Pattern: An adrenal lesion is identified on cross-sectional imaging, and in-phase and opposed-phase chemical-shift sequences are acquired to assess for microscopic intracellular lipid.

Category Signature: A lesion demonstrating unambiguous signal drop exceeding the validated quantitative threshold is categorized as a lipid-rich adenoma; a lesion demonstrating macroscopic fat on conventional fat-suppressed imaging is categorized separately as myelolipoma; a lesion demonstrating no meaningful signal drop is categorized as lipid-poor and indeterminate, requiring further characterization.

The Decision: Lipid-rich adenoma and myelolipoma require no further workup in most clinical contexts; a lipid-poor, indeterminate lesion proceeds to further evaluation with washout assessment, diffusion-weighted imaging, or, most decisively, interval stability follow-up, with the specific pathway selected according to the patient's malignancy risk profile and the lesion's other imaging characteristics.

Trap Logic: A hemorrhagic or heterogeneous adenoma can demonstrate an atypical or falsely negative chemical-shift pattern despite being a genuinely benign, lipid-rich adenoma on histology, and conversely, a small metastasis can rarely demonstrate an equivocal signal change that could be misread as a positive adenoma pattern; the discriminating step in an atypical or unexpected chemical-shift result is correlating with the lesion's morphology, clinical context, and, when genuinely discordant with the clinical picture, proceeding to additional characterization rather than accepting an unexpected chemical-shift result in isolation.

Pattern Anchor: Chemical-shift signal drop reliably identifies lipid-rich adenoma but cannot exclude malignancy in a lipid-poor lesion; a negative chemical-shift result is not equivalent to a benign result and must proceed to further characterization.

Diagnostic Workup Sequencing: When to Add CT Washout or PET Correlation

When a lesion remains indeterminate after chemical-shift MRI, the choice of the next diagnostic step should be guided by the specific clinical context rather than applying a single reflexive pathway to every lipid-poor lesion: dedicated adrenal protocol CT with delayed washout assessment remains a well-validated complementary technique, particularly useful when the patient will require CT for another indication in the same evaluation, avoiding a duplicated separate MRI-based washout assessment that adds limited incremental value over the already-available chemical-shift result. Positron emission tomography with fluorodeoxyglucose, by contrast, is most productively reserved for the patient with a known or strongly suspected malignancy elsewhere, where the adrenal lesion's metabolic activity relative to background can be interpreted in the context of the broader staging examination, rather than used as a first-line indeterminate-lesion tool in a patient without a malignancy context, given the meaningful false-positive rate posed by metabolically active but benign adrenal lesions, including some adenomas and inflammatory processes, in a lower pretest probability population.

KEY POINT: Given the high background prevalence of benign adenoma among incidentally discovered adrenal nodules, further workup should be reserved for lesions with specific concerning features, size, growth, or a functional syndrome, rather than applied reflexively to every incidental finding.

Adrenal Malignancy: Adrenocortical Carcinoma and Metastasis

Epidemiology and Risk Factors for Adrenocortical Carcinoma

Adrenocortical carcinoma is a rare malignancy with an annual incidence measured in a small number of cases per million population, demonstrating a bimodal age distribution with peaks in early childhood and again in the fourth through sixth decades of adult life, and while the majority of cases are sporadic without an identifiable predisposing syndrome, a meaningful minority arise in the context of hereditary cancer syndromes including Li-Fraumeni syndrome, related to germline TP53 mutation, and Beckwith-Wiedemann syndrome in the pediatric population, such that a family history of early-onset malignancy or a personal history of other syndrome-associated tumors should prompt consideration of an underlying hereditary predisposition when an adrenocortical carcinoma is diagnosed, particularly in a younger patient. The rarity of this malignancy relative to the very high background prevalence of benign adenoma discussed above underscores why the specific concerning imaging features emphasized throughout this section, large size, heterogeneous necrotic morphology, and absent chemical-shift signal drop, rather than adrenal mass detection alone, are what should trigger the diagnostic concern and further workup pathway for this specific, comparatively rare diagnosis.

Complications, Prognosis, and the Weiss Criteria

Prognosis in adrenocortical carcinoma correlates strongly with stage at diagnosis and completeness of surgical resection, with disease confined to the adrenal gland at diagnosis carrying a substantially more favorable outlook than disease with local invasion, nodal involvement, or distant metastasis, most often to the liver and lungs, underscoring the importance of the careful staging assessment, including specific evaluation for venous tumor thrombus and regional lymphadenopathy, emphasized throughout this section. Histologic confirmation of malignancy in a resected adrenocortical lesion relies on the Weiss criteria, a multi-parameter histologic scoring system assessing features including nuclear grade, mitotic rate, atypical mitoses, and capsular or vascular invasion that, while an entirely pathologic rather than radiologic determination, underscores why imaging characterization in this chapter functions as a probability assessment guiding the surgical and biopsy decision rather than a definitive tissue diagnosis, with the Weiss criteria applied only after resection or biopsy has provided tissue for this histologic evaluation.

Adrenocortical carcinoma, a rare but aggressive malignancy, typically presents as a large mass, generally exceeding four to six centimeters at diagnosis, with heterogeneous signal reflecting internal hemorrhage and necrosis, irregular or indistinct margins, and absent or minimal chemical-shift signal drop given its lipid-poor cellular composition, a size-based and morphologic pattern that stands in general contrast to the smaller, well-defined, homogeneous appearance typical of benign adenoma even before considering chemical-shift results specifically. Local invasion of adjacent structures, including the inferior vena cava, where direct tumoral extension into the venous lumen produces a distinctive enhancing intraluminal filling defect analogous to the tumor thrombus pattern discussed in the hepatocellular carcinoma context earlier in this book, and regional lymphadenopathy are important staging features to specifically assess and document, since their presence meaningfully alters both prognosis and surgical planning for what is, when resectable, a disease generally requiring complete surgical excision as the primary curative modality.

Functional Adrenocortical Carcinoma and Hormonal Syndromes

A meaningful proportion of adrenocortical carcinomas are functional, most commonly producing cortisol excess and a resulting Cushing syndrome, though androgen-secreting and, less commonly, mixed-hormone-secreting tumors also occur, and the specific hormonal syndrome, when present, provides useful clinical correlation supporting the adrenocortical carcinoma diagnosis over an adrenal metastasis, which is not typically hormonally functional. Virilization or other rapid-onset, pronounced hormonal symptoms in a patient with a large adrenal mass should specifically raise concern for adrenocortical carcinoma over a functioning adenoma, since benign functioning adenomas, while capable of producing hormonal syndromes of their own, particularly Cushing syndrome from a cortisol-producing adenoma, do so more gradually and rarely to the same clinical severity or in combination with androgen excess as seen with a functional carcinoma.

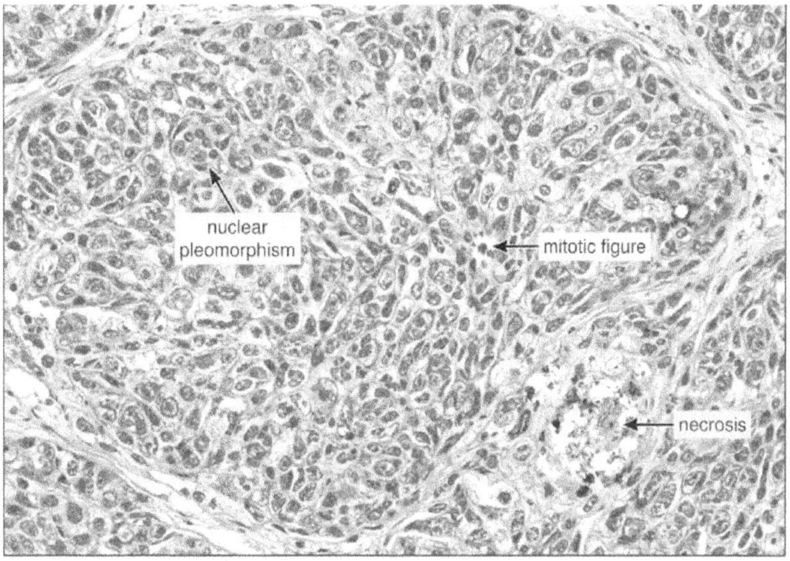

Figure 10.3 — Histopathological Image: Adrenocortical Carcinoma

Adrenal Metastasis

The adrenal gland is a common site of metastatic disease, most often from lung carcinoma, but also breast carcinoma, renal cell carcinoma, melanoma, and lymphoma among others, and a new adrenal lesion in a patient with a known primary malignancy elsewhere carries a substantially elevated pretest probability of representing metastatic disease compared to the general population incidentaloma risk profile, a context-dependent probability shift that should meaningfully lower the threshold for further characterization or biopsy of an indeterminate lesion in this specific population. Adrenal metastases typically demonstrate lipid-poor, chemical-shift-negative signal characteristics similar to adrenocortical carcinoma and can be genuinely difficult to distinguish from a lipid-poor adenoma or, in a large lesion, from adrenocortical carcinoma on morphology alone, such that the full clinical context, including the specific primary malignancy's known metastatic pattern and any other sites of metastatic disease identified on the same staging examination, is frequently as diagnostically useful as the adrenal lesion's imaging features considered in isolation.

Bilateral Adrenal Masses and Adrenal Insufficiency

Bilateral adrenal masses carry a distinct differential from the unilateral incidentaloma discussed throughout most of this chapter, favoring metastatic disease, lymphoma, infection such as tuberculosis or histoplasmosis in endemic regions or immunocompromised patients, or bilateral hemorrhage, most often related to severe physiologic stress, anticoagulation, or, classically, meningococcemia in the Waterhouse-Friderichsen syndrome, over the bilateral simultaneous occurrence of two sporadic benign adenomas, which, while possible, is statistically less likely than a unifying bilateral process when both glands are involved by a mass of similar size and morphology. Bilateral adrenal involvement, particularly from hemorrhage, infection, or infiltrative metastatic replacement of both glands, carries the additional risk of adrenal insufficiency if enough functional cortical tissue is destroyed, a life-threatening complication that may not be clinically apparent until a physiologic stressor such as illness or surgery unmasks the inadequate cortisol reserve, such that the radiologist identifying substantial bilateral adrenal replacement or destruction should explicitly flag the possibility of adrenal insufficiency for the referring clinician's consideration rather than reporting the anatomic finding without this clinically important functional correlation.

PATIENT EDUCATION: Patients undergoing evaluation for a pheochromocytoma should understand that biochemical testing is a required safety step before any biopsy, that surgery is generally curative when the tumor is confined to the adrenal gland, and that a period of blood-pressure medication before surgery is a standard and important part of safe surgical preparation.

Feature	Benign Adenoma	Adrenocortical Carcinoma	Metastasis
Typical size	Usually under 3 cm	Usually over 4-6 cm at diagnosis	Variable, often correlates with primary
Chemical-shift signal drop	Present if lipid-rich; absent if lipid-poor	Absent	Absent
Margins	Well-defined, homogeneous	Irregular, heterogeneous, necrotic	Variable, often irregular
Growth on interval imaging	Stable	Progressive, often rapid	Progressive, correlates with primary
Clinical context	Often asymptomatic, incidental	May be hormonally functional	Known malignancy elsewhere

Pheochromocytoma and Functional Adrenal Tumors

Epidemiology and Genetics of Pheochromocytoma and Paraganglioma

Pheochromocytoma and paraganglioma together represent a rare cause of secondary hypertension, but their identification carries outsized clinical importance given both the potentially curable nature of the resulting hypertension following resection and the acute perioperative and procedural risks discussed below if the diagnosis is missed before an invasive intervention. Contemporary genetic testing has revealed that a substantial minority, now estimated in some series to approach or exceed a third of apparently sporadic cases, actually harbor an identifiable germline mutation in one of more than a dozen recognized susceptibility genes, including the succinate dehydrogenase subunit genes most strongly associated with extra-adrenal paraganglioma and an elevated malignant potential, RET associated with multiple endocrine neoplasia type 2, and the VHL gene associated with von Hippel-Lindau disease, a syndrome also associated with the renal and central nervous system findings discussed elsewhere in this book, such that current guidelines generally recommend genetic counseling and testing be offered to essentially all patients diagnosed with pheochromocytoma or paraganglioma rather than reserved only for those with an overt syndromic or family history.

Pheochromocytoma: Imaging Features and Clinical Presentation

Pheochromocytoma, arising from the chromaffin cells of the adrenal medulla, classically presents with marked, homogeneous T2 hyperintensity, sometimes described using the traditional but imprecise light bulb descriptor reflecting the lesion's strikingly bright T2 signal relative to surrounding tissue, together with avid, often heterogeneous postcontrast enhancement and an absence of chemical-shift signal drop given its non-adrenocortical, medullary cellular origin, though this classic T2-hyperintense pattern is present in only a subset of cases and its absence does not exclude the diagnosis in a patient with an otherwise compatible clinical and biochemical picture. Clinically, pheochromocytoma classically produces the paroxysmal triad of headache, diaphoresis, and palpitations related to episodic catecholamine release, together with hypertension that may be sustained or, characteristically, paroxysmal and refractory to standard antihypertensive management, though a meaningful proportion of pheochromocytomas, particularly smaller incidentally discovered lesions, are biochemically silent or minimally symptomatic at diagnosis, underscoring why biochemical screening, rather than symptoms alone, is the appropriate gate before any adrenal mass proceeds to biopsy or, in some protocols, intravenous contrast administration.

Safety Implications: Contrast, Biopsy, and the Ten Percent Tumor

An unrecognized pheochromocytoma undergoing biopsy or, per some historical and institution-specific protocols, certain contrast administration carries a risk of precipitating a hypertensive crisis from acute catecholamine release, a risk that has driven the widespread adoption of biochemical screening, typically plasma-free or urinary fractionated metanephrines, before percutaneous biopsy of any adrenal mass with imaging features that cannot confidently exclude pheochromocytoma, and this safety consideration, more than any single imaging feature, should drive the radiologist's threshold for recommending biochemical clearance before proceeding to tissue sampling of an indeterminate adrenal lesion. Pheochromocytoma is traditionally associated with the so-called ten percent rule, referencing the approximate proportion of cases that are bilateral, extra-adrenal, that is, arising from paraganglion tissue elsewhere along the sympathetic chain and termed paraganglioma in this location, malignant, or hereditary, though contemporary series suggest each of these proportions, particularly the hereditary proportion, is meaningfully higher than the traditional teaching once suggested, reflecting more widespread genetic testing revealing hereditary syndromes including multiple endocrine neoplasia type 2, von Hippel-Lindau disease, and succinate dehydrogenase-related hereditary paraganglioma syndromes in a substantial minority of apparently sporadic cases.

THE SIGNAL-TO-CATEGORY DECISION SYSTEM — Indeterminate Adrenal Mass versus Pheochromocytoma Safety Check

The Signal Pattern: An adrenal mass is identified that is being considered for biopsy or further contrast-enhanced characterization, and the reader must assess whether pheochromocytoma has been adequately excluded before either proceeds.

Category Signature: A lesion with marked T2 hyperintensity, avid heterogeneous enhancement, and absent chemical-shift signal drop, particularly in a patient with compatible symptoms or hypertension, is categorized as suspicious for pheochromocytoma; a lesion lacking these features in a patient without compatible clinical findings is categorized as low suspicion, though this categorization does not substitute for biochemical testing when genuine uncertainty remains.

The Decision: A lesion categorized as suspicious for pheochromocytoma should not proceed to biopsy without prior biochemical screening and, if biochemically confirmed, appropriate alpha-blockade before any subsequent intervention; a lesion categorized as low suspicion may generally proceed with standard further workup, though the report should explicitly state that pheochromocytoma has not been definitively excluded by imaging alone when appropriate.

Trap Logic: A pheochromocytoma without the classic marked T2 hyperintensity, an atypical but well-documented presentation, can be mistaken for a lipid-poor adenoma or other indeterminate lesion on imaging alone, and proceeding directly to biopsy of this atypical pheochromocytoma without biochemical clearance risks a hypertensive crisis; the discriminating safety practice is maintaining a low threshold for biochemical screening in any indeterminate adrenal mass being considered for biopsy, rather than relying on the classic imaging phenotype to be reliably present.

Pattern Anchor: Biochemical screening, not imaging phenotype alone, is the definitive safety gate before biopsy of an indeterminate adrenal mass; an atypical pheochromocytoma can mimic a lipid-poor adenoma on imaging.

CAUTION: Before recommending or performing percutaneous biopsy of any indeterminate adrenal mass, confirm that biochemical screening for pheochromocytoma has been performed or explicitly recommend it in the report if it has not, given the risk of a hypertensive crisis from an unrecognized pheochromocytoma undergoing sampling.

Perioperative Management: Alpha-Blockade and Surgical Considerations

Once pheochromocytoma is biochemically confirmed, preoperative alpha-adrenergic blockade, typically initiated with phenoxybenzamine or a selective alpha-1 antagonist over a period of one to two weeks before surgery, is essential to prevent intraoperative hypertensive crisis during tumor manipulation, when mechanical handling of the catecholamine-rich tumor can precipitate a massive, acute catecholamine surge, and beta-blockade, when needed for associated tachycardia, is added only after adequate alpha-blockade has been established, since beta-blockade in the absence of alpha-blockade can paradoxically worsen hypertension through unopposed alpha-adrenergic vasoconstriction. The radiologist's report contributes meaningfully to this perioperative planning process by providing precise tumor size, laterality, and any evidence of local invasion or vascular involvement, since this anatomic detail directly informs the surgical approach, most often laparoscopic adrenalectomy for a smaller, well-defined tumor without evidence of local invasion, reserving an open surgical approach for a larger or more locally invasive tumor where the laparoscopic approach carries a higher risk of tumor capsule rupture and intraoperative catecholamine release.

Adrenal Hyperplasia and Incidentaloma Management Algorithm

Primary Aldosteronism: Clinical Presentation and Screening

Primary aldosteronism, characterized by autonomous, renin-independent aldosterone overproduction, is an increasingly recognized cause of secondary hypertension, with contemporary screening-based series suggesting a substantially higher prevalence among patients with resistant or difficult-to-control hypertension than was traditionally appreciated when the diagnosis relied primarily on the classic but insensitive presentation of hypertension with spontaneous hypokalemia, a combination now recognized to be present in only a minority of confirmed cases. Screening is generally performed using the plasma aldosterone-to-renin ratio, with a confirmatory suppression test, such as an oral sodium loading or saline infusion test, required before proceeding to the adrenal imaging and, where indicated, adrenal venous sampling discussed in this section, since imaging performed before appropriate biochemical confirmation risks both false localization from an incidentally coexisting nonfunctioning nodule and an inappropriate surgical referral based on an anatomic finding that may have no relationship to the patient's aldosterone excess.

Adrenal Hyperplasia and Its Functional Subtypes

Adrenal hyperplasia, an enlargement of one or both adrenal glands without a discrete dominant mass, most often reflects bilateral macronodular or micronodular hyperplasia and can be a source of autonomous cortisol secretion producing a Cushing syndrome phenotype distinct from the more common pituitary-driven or exogenous steroid causes, congenital adrenal hyperplasia, most often from twenty-one-hydroxylase deficiency and typically diagnosed in infancy or childhood through newborn screening and characteristic electrolyte and hormonal abnormalities well before adrenal imaging is obtained, or, less commonly, primary aldosteronism from bilateral adrenal hyperplasia rather than a discrete aldosterone-producing adenoma. Distinguishing bilateral hyperplasia from bilateral nodular disease, and distinguishing a unilateral aldosterone-producing adenoma from bilateral hyperplasia specifically in the primary aldosteronism workup, carries direct surgical planning implications, since a unilateral adenoma is amenable to curative adrenalectomy while bilateral hyperplasia is managed medically, a distinction for which adrenal venous sampling, rather than imaging alone, remains the reference standard given imaging's documented limitations in reliably making this specific lateralization determination.

Structured Incidentaloma Management Algorithm

A structured approach to the adrenal incidentaloma integrates size, chemical-shift phenotype, and interval behavior into a coherent management pathway: a lesion under one centimeter is generally considered too small for reliable characterization and is followed according to general incidentaloma principles without aggressive further workup, a lesion demonstrating a definite lipid-rich adenoma or myelolipoma pattern on chemical-shift or fat-sensitive imaging requires no further workup regardless of size in the absence of a functional syndrome or malignancy risk context, and a lipid-poor, indeterminate lesion is managed according to size and growth, with lesions under four centimeters generally favoring interval follow-up imaging to confirm stability and lesions at or above four centimeters, or any lesion demonstrating interval growth on follow-up, warranting more urgent further evaluation given the size-correlated increase in the probability of adrenocortical carcinoma. This size-and-behavior-based framework should always be adjusted for the individual patient's malignancy risk context, since a known active malignancy elsewhere substantially raises the pretest probability that an indeterminate lesion at any size represents metastatic rather than benign disease, appropriately shifting the threshold toward earlier biopsy or dedicated positron emission tomography correlation rather than routine imaging follow-up alone.

Figure 10.4: Adrenal Venous Sampling for Lateralization of Primary Aldosteronism

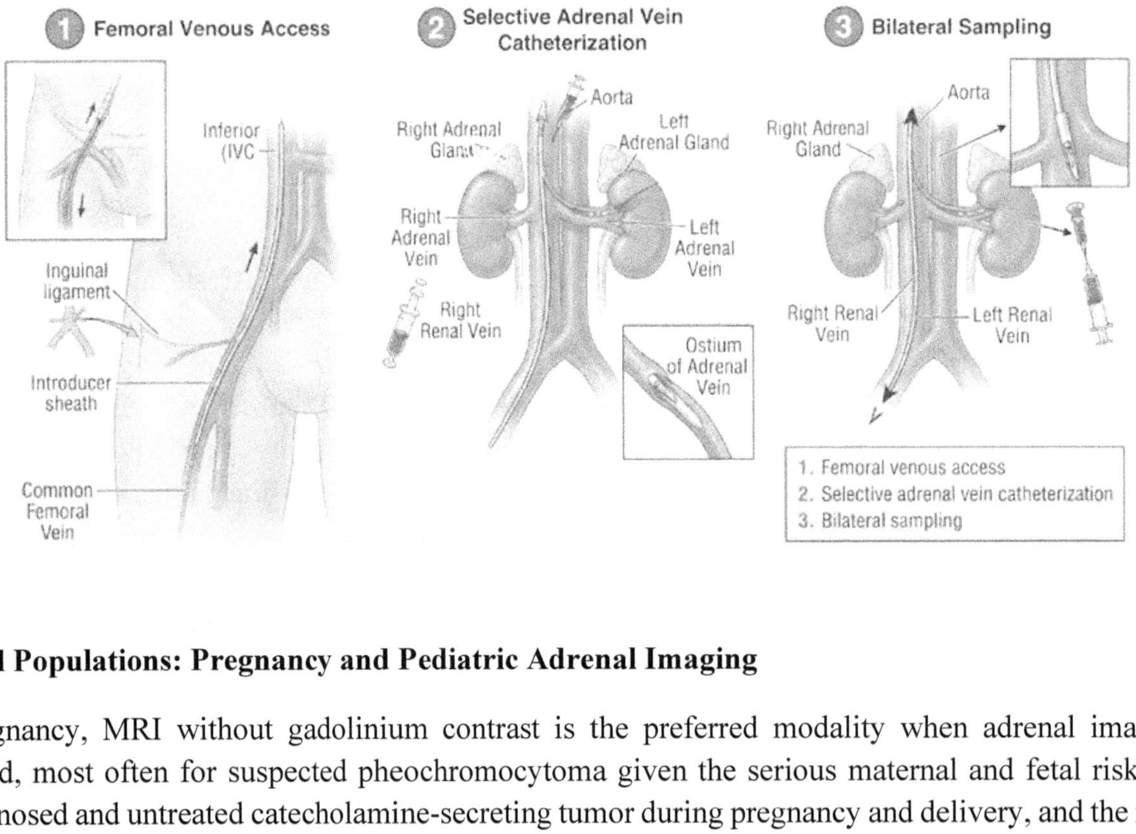

Special Populations: Pregnancy and Pediatric Adrenal Imaging

In pregnancy, MRI without gadolinium contrast is the preferred modality when adrenal imaging is required, most often for suspected pheochromocytoma given the serious maternal and fetal risks of an undiagnosed and untreated catecholamine-secreting tumor during pregnancy and delivery, and the marked T2 hyperintensity characteristic of pheochromocytoma remains reliably assessable on non-contrast sequences, preserving substantial diagnostic value even without gadolinium administration. In the pediatric population, the adrenal mass differential differs meaningfully from the adult incidentaloma-dominated differential discussed throughout this chapter, with neuroblastoma, a malignant tumor of primitive neural crest origin most often presenting in early childhood, and, less commonly, congenital adrenal hemorrhage in the neonate, comprising a substantially larger proportion of the pediatric adrenal mass differential than adenoma, such that a pediatric adrenal mass should generally be approached with a distinct, age-appropriate differential rather than the adult-oriented incidentaloma framework emphasized throughout this chapter applied unchanged to a child.

Clinical Case Presentations

Case 1. A 62-year-old woman undergoes MRI for an incidentally discovered 1.8-centimeter left adrenal nodule. Chemical-shift imaging demonstrates unambiguous signal drop on the opposed-phase sequence relative to the in-phase sequence, with a calculated relative signal-drop percentage well above the validated diagnostic threshold. The radiologist categorizes the lesion as a definite lipid-rich adenoma and recommends no further workup, providing the referring physician with a confident, actionable interpretation from a single noncontrast examination.

Case 2. A 55-year-old man with known non-small cell lung carcinoma undergoes staging MRI demonstrating a new 2.6-centimeter right adrenal nodule without significant chemical-shift signal drop. Given the known active malignancy, the radiologist categorizes the lesion as indeterminate with an elevated pretest probability of metastatic disease in this specific clinical context and recommends dedicated positron emission tomography correlation and, if metabolically active, biopsy given the direct staging implications of confirmed adrenal metastatic involvement for this patient's treatment planning.

Case 3. A 41-year-old woman with episodic headaches, diaphoresis, and poorly controlled hypertension undergoes MRI demonstrating a 3.4-centimeter right adrenal mass with marked T2 hyperintensity and avid heterogeneous enhancement, without chemical-shift signal drop. Recognizing this pattern together with the compatible clinical presentation as highly suspicious for pheochromocytoma, the radiologist explicitly recommends plasma-free metanephrine testing before any biopsy is considered, and the patient's metanephrines return markedly elevated, confirming the diagnosis and allowing appropriate preoperative alpha-blockade before surgical resection.

Case 4. A 68-year-old man undergoes MRI demonstrating a 6.8-centimeter heterogeneous left adrenal mass with irregular margins, internal necrosis, and no chemical-shift signal drop, with associated tumor thrombus extending into the left renal vein. Given the large size, heterogeneous morphology, and vascular invasion, the radiologist categorizes this as highly suspicious for adrenocortical carcinoma rather than a benign or metastatic process and recommends surgical oncology referral, explicitly documenting the venous extension given its direct relevance to surgical planning.

Case 5. A 46-year-old woman with resistant hypertension and hypokalemia undergoes MRI demonstrating bilateral mild adrenal nodularity without a single dominant mass. Recognizing that imaging alone cannot reliably lateralize the source of aldosterone excess between a unilateral microadenoma and bilateral hyperplasia in this bilateral nodular pattern, the radiologist recommends adrenal venous sampling for definitive lateralization before any consideration of unilateral adrenalectomy, correctly deferring to the reference-standard biochemical lateralization technique rather than offering a surgical recommendation based on imaging morphology alone.

Case 6. A 29-year-old woman with a strong family history of paraganglioma undergoes surveillance MRI as part of a known succinate dehydrogenase subunit B mutation screening program, demonstrating a new 1.4-centimeter left adrenal nodule with mild T2 hyperintensity and no definite chemical-shift signal drop. Given her known hereditary predisposition and the specific association of this genetic subtype with an elevated malignant potential, the radiologist categorizes the finding as suspicious for an early pheochromocytoma despite its small size and recommends biochemical testing and short-interval follow-up imaging rather than the longer routine incidentaloma surveillance interval that would apply to a similarly sized nodule in a patient without this specific hereditary context, illustrating how genetic risk stratification appropriately modifies the standard management algorithm presented in this chapter.

THE SIGNAL-TO-CATEGORY DECISION SYSTEM — Adrenal Mass Triage Arc

The Signal Pattern: This chapter's patterns span the full adrenal risk spectrum, from a lesion whose lipid content must be confirmed by chemical-shift signal drop, to a mass whose medullary origin and biochemical status must be confirmed before any invasive procedure is undertaken.

Category Signature: Lesions are categorized as lipid-rich adenoma, myelolipoma, lipid-poor indeterminate, or suspicious for malignancy based on chemical-shift signal, size, and morphology; a separate safety-oriented categorization determines whether pheochromocytoma has been adequately excluded before proceeding to biopsy.

The Decision: Category assignment in this chapter ranges from no-further-workup outcomes for a classic adenoma to urgent surgical referral for adrenocortical carcinoma, and, uniquely in this chapter, a safety-gating decision that determines whether an invasive procedure can proceed at all.

The Trap Logic: Both patterns in this chapter share a common trap: an atypical presentation, a hemorrhagic adenoma with falsely negative chemical shift, or a pheochromocytoma without classic T2 hyperintensity, that could lead to a mischaracterization with either diagnostic or, in the pheochromocytoma case, genuine safety consequences.

Pattern Anchor: In adrenal imaging, a negative chemical-shift result never independently excludes either malignancy or pheochromocytoma; biochemical and clinical correlation remain essential safety and diagnostic gates throughout this chapter.

Summary and Key Concepts

Chemical-shift imaging detects microscopic intracellular lipid characteristic of adenoma; a signal drop exceeding the validated threshold is diagnostic of lipid-rich adenoma, but roughly thirty percent of adenomas are lipid-poor and chemical-shift-negative.

Myelolipoma demonstrates unambiguous macroscopic fat on fat-suppressed imaging, a distinct mechanism from chemical-shift signal drop, and requires no further workup regardless of size when clearly present.

Adrenocortical carcinoma is typically large, heterogeneous, and lipid-poor with irregular margins and may be hormonally functional; adrenal metastasis shares a similar lipid-poor pattern and carries elevated pretest probability in a patient with known malignancy.

Pheochromocytoma classically shows marked T2 hyperintensity and avid enhancement without chemical-shift signal drop, but atypical presentations occur, and biochemical screening, not imaging phenotype, is the definitive safety gate before biopsy.

The traditional ten percent rule for pheochromocytoma bilaterality, extra-adrenal location, malignancy, and hereditary association understates true rates in contemporary genetically-tested series.

Adrenal hyperplasia includes bilateral macronodular and micronodular forms, congenital adrenal hyperplasia, and hyperplasia-related primary aldosteronism; adrenal venous sampling, not imaging, remains the reference standard for lateralization in primary aldosteronism.

A structured incidentaloma algorithm integrates size, chemical-shift phenotype, and interval growth, adjusted for the individual patient's malignancy risk context, to guide the surveillance-versus-further-workup decision.

CHAPTER 11: RETROPERITONEAL AND PERITONEAL DISEASE

Learning Objectives

1. Describe retroperitoneal compartmental anatomy and its role in localizing and characterizing retroperitoneal disease.
2. Recognize the imaging features of retroperitoneal fibrosis and distinguish idiopathic from malignancy-related and IgG4-related forms.
3. Characterize primary retroperitoneal neoplasms, including liposarcoma and leiomyosarcoma, and apply a fat-content-based triage to fat-containing retroperitoneal masses.
4. Recognize the imaging patterns of peritoneal carcinomatosis and mesothelioma and distinguish malignant from benign peritoneal disease.
5. Characterize ascites, peritoneal fluid collections, and abdominal wall hernias relevant to body MRI interpretation.

Clinical Overview

The retroperitoneum and peritoneal cavity, spaces defined by their relationship to the peritoneal lining rather than by a single organ system, present a unifying interpretive challenge distinct from the organ-based chapters preceding this one: disease here is characterized as much by its location and spread pattern relative to these anatomic compartments as by the specific tissue of origin, and a systematic, compartment-based approach is essential to avoiding both missed disease and mischaracterization of its extent. This chapter proceeds from retroperitoneal compartmental anatomy, through retroperitoneal fibrosis and inflammatory disease, primary retroperitoneal neoplasms, and peritoneal carcinomatosis and mesothelioma, closing with ascites, fluid collections, and abdominal wall hernias, completing the coverage of Part III before the book turns to the genitourinary system.

Two instances of the Signal-to-Category Decision System are applied in this chapter, the first to the fat-content-based triage that anchors retroperitoneal mass characterization, distinguishing benign lipoma from well-differentiated and dedifferentiated liposarcoma, and the second to the peritoneal nodularity pattern that distinguishes benign peritoneal thickening from carcinomatosis.

Retroperitoneal Anatomy and Compartments

Retroperitoneal Compartmental Divisions

The retroperitoneum is divided by the anterior and posterior renal fascia, collectively termed Gerota fascia, into three principal compartments: the anterior pararenal space, containing the pancreas, duodenum, and ascending and descending colon, the perirenal space, containing the kidneys, adrenal glands, and perirenal fat, and the posterior pararenal space, containing predominantly fat without a major solid organ, an anatomic framework that directly informs the differential diagnosis of a retroperitoneal mass by its compartmental location, since a mass centered in the posterior pararenal space, for example, is inherently less likely to represent a primary pancreatic or renal process than one centered in the anterior pararenal or perirenal space respectively. These compartments communicate to a variable degree, particularly anteriorly and inferiorly, such that a sufficiently large or aggressive process can span multiple compartments, but establishing the compartment of predominant involvement and, when possible, the specific organ of origin remains the essential first step in retroperitoneal mass characterization, generally more diagnostically productive than proceeding directly to a differential diagnosis based on imaging appearance alone.

The Great Vessels and Their Relevance to Retroperitoneal Disease

The aorta and inferior vena cava traverse the retroperitoneum in close proximity to one another, and several important retroperitoneal disease processes, most notably retroperitoneal fibrosis discussed in the following section, characteristically center on and encase these great vessels, such that assessment of periaortic and paracaval soft tissue, together with any resulting vascular narrowing, ureteral obstruction, or venous compression, is an essential component of retroperitoneal imaging interpretation regardless of the specific disease process ultimately identified. Familiarity with the normal course of the ureters as they descend through the retroperitoneum anterior to the psoas muscles, crossing the iliac vessels near the pelvic brim before entering the pelvis, is similarly essential, since ureteral encasement and obstruction is among the most common and clinically consequential complications of retroperitoneal disease addressed throughout this chapter, from fibrosis to malignant nodal or soft tissue disease.

Retroperitoneal Lymph Node Stations and Their Clinical Relevance

Retroperitoneal lymph nodes are conventionally described by their relationship to the great vessels, paraaortic, paracaval, and interaortocaval, together with the more inferiorly located common, external, and internal iliac chains, an anatomic nomenclature with direct relevance to oncologic staging throughout this book, since specific malignancies drain preferentially to specific nodal stations, testicular malignancy to the paraaortic and interaortocaval nodes near the renal hilum reflecting the testis's embryologic descent, for example, in a pattern distinct from the more caudal nodal drainage of most pelvic malignancies. Retroperitoneal lymphadenopathy carries an extensive differential spanning metastatic disease, lymphoma, and reactive or infectious causes, and while nodal size remains a commonly applied screening threshold, morphologic features including loss of the normal fatty hilum, rounded rather than oval configuration, and, particularly for lymphoma, nodal conglomeration into a bulky, matted mass, contribute meaningfully to distinguishing pathologic from reactive lymphadenopathy beyond size criteria alone.

Psoas Muscle and Paraspinal Considerations in Retroperitoneal Disease

The psoas muscles, coursing through the retroperitoneum from their origin along the lumbar vertebral bodies to their insertion on the lesser trochanter of the femur, are a common site for both primary and secondary disease processes relevant to this chapter, including direct extension of vertebral osteomyelitis or discitis into a psoas abscess, a complication most reliably characterized by the combination of adjacent vertebral marrow and disc signal abnormality with a rim-enhancing psoas fluid collection, and hematoma, most often related to anticoagulation or trauma, which can be substantial in volume given the psoas compartment's capacity and can present with femoral neuropathy from compression of the femoral nerve as it courses within or adjacent to the muscle belly. Retroperitoneal sarcoma and lymphadenopathy not infrequently involve or abut the psoas muscle, and documenting this specific relationship, together with any resulting muscle displacement, invasion, or denervation change, contributes meaningfully to surgical planning given the psoas muscle's functional importance in hip flexion and gait.

Retroperitoneal Hemorrhage and Its Causes

Spontaneous retroperitoneal hemorrhage, most commonly related to anticoagulation therapy, a bleeding diathesis, or a ruptured underlying vascular or renal lesion, including a bleeding angiomyolipoma discussed in the renal chapters later in this book, presents with evolving blood-product signal characteristics on MRI paralleling the hemorrhage-aging pattern discussed elsewhere in this book, and its identification should prompt a deliberate search for an underlying structural cause, including a renal or adrenal mass, rather than attributing the hemorrhage to anticoagulation alone even in a patient with a clear anticoagulation history, since anticoagulation more often unmasks bleeding from an underlying structural lesion than causes hemorrhage from an entirely normal retroperitoneum. Traumatic retroperitoneal hemorrhage, most often related to renal, adrenal, or great vessel injury, is addressed in the broader trauma imaging context, but active contrast extravasation within a retroperitoneal hematoma, regardless of the underlying cause, carries the same urgent management implication discussed for splenic and hepatic hemorrhage elsewhere in this book, mandating prompt communication to the clinical team given the potential need for angiographic or surgical intervention.

Retroperitoneal Fibrosis and Inflammatory Disease

Epidemiology and Clinical Presentation of Retroperitoneal Fibrosis

Retroperitoneal fibrosis is an uncommon disease demonstrating a male predominance and typically presenting in the fifth through seventh decades of life, with clinical presentation often insidious and nonspecific, including vague back or flank pain, and frequently delayed until progressive ureteral obstruction produces declining renal function or, in a substantial minority of cases, until the disease is discovered incidentally on imaging performed for an unrelated indication before symptoms of obstruction have developed. Recognized associations beyond the IgG4-related and malignancy-related etiologies discussed below include certain medications, most classically ergot-derived compounds and, less commonly, some dopamine agonists, prior radiation therapy, and, rarely, an association with inflammatory aortic aneurysm, termed perianeurysmal retroperitoneal fibrosis, in which the fibrotic soft tissue specifically surrounds an aneurysmal rather than normal-caliber aortic segment, a distinct subtype recognized by this specific vascular relationship.

Idiopathic Retroperitoneal Fibrosis

Idiopathic retroperitoneal fibrosis, historically termed Ormond disease, presents as periaortic and paracaval soft tissue thickening, typically centered around the infrarenal aorta and extending to encase the ureters, producing the characteristic medial ureteral deviation that is one of the most specific ancillary findings supporting this diagnosis over an alternative process, together with a variable degree of hydronephrosis reflecting the ureteral obstruction that is frequently the presenting clinical finding prompting the initial imaging evaluation. Signal characteristics evolve with disease activity and chronicity: active, cellular, inflammatory fibrosis demonstrates intermediate to high T2 signal and measurable postcontrast enhancement, while mature, burned-out fibrosis demonstrates low T2 signal with minimal enhancement reflecting its predominantly acellular, densely collagenous composition, a distinction with direct treatment implications since active, enhancing disease is generally more responsive to immunosuppressive or corticosteroid therapy than mature, densely fibrotic, non-enhancing disease, for which surgical ureterolysis is more often required to relieve obstruction.

IgG4-Related and Malignancy-Related Retroperitoneal Fibrosis

A meaningful proportion of retroperitoneal fibrosis cases previously classified as idiopathic are now recognized as part of the IgG4-related disease spectrum discussed throughout this book in the contexts of the pancreas, biliary tree, and other organs, and identifying this specific etiology, most reliably through serum IgG4 elevation together with any other sites of IgG4-related organ involvement identified on the same examination, carries treatment relevance given this subtype's characteristic corticosteroid responsiveness paralleling the pattern described for autoimmune pancreatitis in the preceding chapter. Malignancy-related retroperitoneal fibrosis, whether from a desmoplastic response to an underlying retroperitoneal or pelvic malignancy or from a paraneoplastic fibrotic process, should be specifically considered before a fibrotic-appearing periaortic soft tissue process is labeled idiopathic, particularly when the soft tissue extends anteriorly displacing rather than encasing the aorta, a pattern termed the reverse or anterior displacement sign that favors a malignant rather than idiopathic process and should prompt biopsy rather than presumptive treatment for benign fibrosis.

Treatment Response Assessment in Retroperitoneal Fibrosis

Following initiation of corticosteroid or other immunosuppressive therapy for retroperitoneal fibrosis, interval imaging is used to assess treatment response, with a reduction in soft tissue bulk, decreasing T2 signal, and, importantly, improvement or resolution of ureteral obstruction and hydronephrosis representing favorable response, while the periaortic soft tissue thickness itself can, somewhat counterintuitively, persist or even appear stable in overall bulk despite genuine and clinically meaningful biochemical and symptomatic improvement, reflecting the transition from active, edematous, inflammatory tissue to quiescent, stable fibrotic tissue that occupies similar physical space, such that ureteral and renal function assessment should be weighted at least as heavily as soft tissue bulk alone when characterizing treatment response on interval imaging. Persistent or progressive ureteral obstruction despite adequate medical therapy generally prompts consideration of ureteral stenting or surgical ureterolysis, in which the ureters are surgically freed from the encasing fibrotic tissue and repositioned, often with an intraperitonealization technique to reduce the risk of recurrent retroperitoneal encasement, an intervention whose planning benefits from the radiologist's precise documentation of the length and location of ureteral involvement on the pretreatment and interval imaging.

KEY POINT: Anterior displacement of the aorta by periaortic soft tissue, rather than the more typical encasement pattern of idiopathic retroperitoneal fibrosis, should raise concern for an underlying malignant process and generally warrants biopsy before presumptive treatment for benign fibrosis.

Feature	Idiopathic/IgG4-Related Fibrosis	Malignancy-Related Fibrosis
Aortic relationship	Encasement, vessel not displaced	Anterior displacement (reverse sign)
Margin	Smooth, symmetric	Irregular, asymmetric
Associated findings	Other IgG4-related organ involvement, elevated serum IgG4	Known or occult primary malignancy elsewhere
Response to corticosteroids	Often favorable	Generally absent or minimal

Primary Retroperitoneal Neoplasms

Epidemiology and Risk Factors for Retroperitoneal Sarcoma

Primary retroperitoneal sarcomas are rare, comprising a small minority of all soft tissue sarcomas despite the retroperitoneum's substantial volume, and typically present in mid to late adulthood, often reaching a considerable size before diagnosis given the retroperitoneum's capacity to accommodate a slowly growing mass without producing symptoms until substantial local mass effect, organ compression, or, less commonly, a palpable abdominal mass develops, a delayed-presentation pattern that distinguishes retroperitoneal sarcoma from extremity soft tissue sarcoma, where a palpable mass is typically noticed and evaluated at a considerably smaller size. Recognized predisposing conditions include prior radiation therapy, particularly relevant in patients with a distant history of radiation for another malignancy, and neurofibromatosis type 1 specifically for malignant peripheral nerve sheath tumor as discussed above, though the substantial majority of retroperitoneal sarcomas arise sporadically without an identifiable predisposing condition or exposure.

Liposarcoma: The Dominant Primary Retroperitoneal Malignancy

Liposarcoma is the most common primary retroperitoneal malignancy, presenting across a spectrum from well-differentiated liposarcoma, demonstrating predominantly macroscopic fat signal with only subtle internal septation or nodularity distinguishing it from a benign lipoma, to dedifferentiated liposarcoma, in which a discrete non-fatty, more aggressive-appearing soft tissue component develops within or adjacent to a fat-containing mass, to the fat-poor pleomorphic and myxoid subtypes that lack the fat-predominant signature entirely and present a greater diagnostic challenge given their nonspecific soft tissue mass appearance. Well-differentiated liposarcoma, despite its comparatively indolent behavior relative to the dedifferentiated and pleomorphic subtypes, still carries a substantial risk of local recurrence following resection and, in the retroperitoneum specifically, is managed with wide surgical excision when feasible given the space available in this location, unlike the extremity liposarcomas where limb-sparing considerations more heavily constrain the surgical approach, a location-based management distinction relevant to interpreting retroperitoneal liposarcoma literature and outcomes.

Leiomyosarcoma and Other Non-Fatty Retroperitoneal Sarcomas

Leiomyosarcoma, the second most common primary retroperitoneal sarcoma, most often arises from the wall of the inferior vena cava or from retroperitoneal smooth muscle elsewhere, presenting as a large, heterogeneous, non-fatty mass with variable degrees of necrosis and hemorrhage, and when centered on or clearly arising from the inferior vena cava wall, with resulting luminal narrowing or occlusion, this specific vascular relationship should be explicitly documented given its direct implications for the surgical approach, which may require vascular reconstruction. Other primary retroperitoneal sarcomas, including malignant peripheral nerve sheath tumor, often arising in association with neurofibromatosis type 1 and demonstrating the target sign of central low and peripheral high T2 signal shared with its benign neurofibroma counterpart though generally with a larger size and more heterogeneous, rapidly growing appearance favoring malignant transformation, and solitary fibrous tumor, demonstrating characteristic low T2 signal reflecting its dense collagenous stroma together with prominent flow voids from its hypervascularity, together comprise the remaining minority of the primary retroperitoneal sarcoma differential.

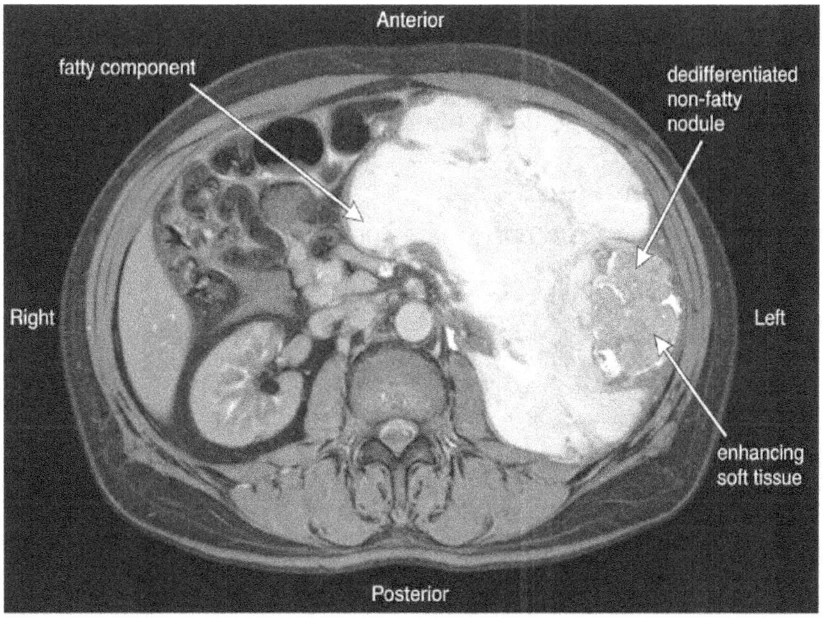

Figure 11.1 Axial Postcontrted post contrzatienxe, dedifferentiated retroperitoneal liposarcoma.

THE SIGNAL-TO-CATEGORY DECISION SYSTEM — Fat-Containing Retroperitoneal Mass Triage

The Signal Pattern: A retroperitoneal mass containing macroscopic fat signal is identified, and the reader must determine whether internal architecture favors a benign lipoma or a well-differentiated to dedifferentiated liposarcoma.

Category Signature: A mass composed of homogeneous, uncomplicated macroscopic fat without septation, nodularity, or a non-fatty soft tissue component is categorized as favoring lipoma; a mass with thick or nodular internal septation, or any discrete non-fatty soft tissue component, however small, is categorized as favoring well-differentiated to dedifferentiated liposarcoma.

The Decision: A mass categorized as favoring lipoma in the retroperitoneum still generally warrants at least a period of surveillance imaging or biopsy given the comparatively higher pretest probability of liposarcoma over simple lipoma in this specific location relative to more common lipoma locations elsewhere in the body; a mass categorized as favoring liposarcoma proceeds to biopsy and surgical oncology referral.

Trap Logic: A retroperitoneal lipoma is a genuinely uncommon diagnosis relative to well-differentiated liposarcoma, such that even a fat-predominant retroperitoneal mass without an obvious non-fatty component should not be reflexively labeled benign lipoma without careful, deliberate scrutiny for subtle septal thickening or nodularity, features that can be genuinely difficult to appreciate against the surrounding normal retroperitoneal fat if the search is not conducted deliberately.

Pattern Anchor: In the retroperitoneum specifically, a fat-containing mass should be treated as liposarcoma until proven otherwise; true retroperitoneal lipoma is comparatively rare and this location shifts the pretest probability meaningfully compared to fat-containing masses elsewhere in the body.

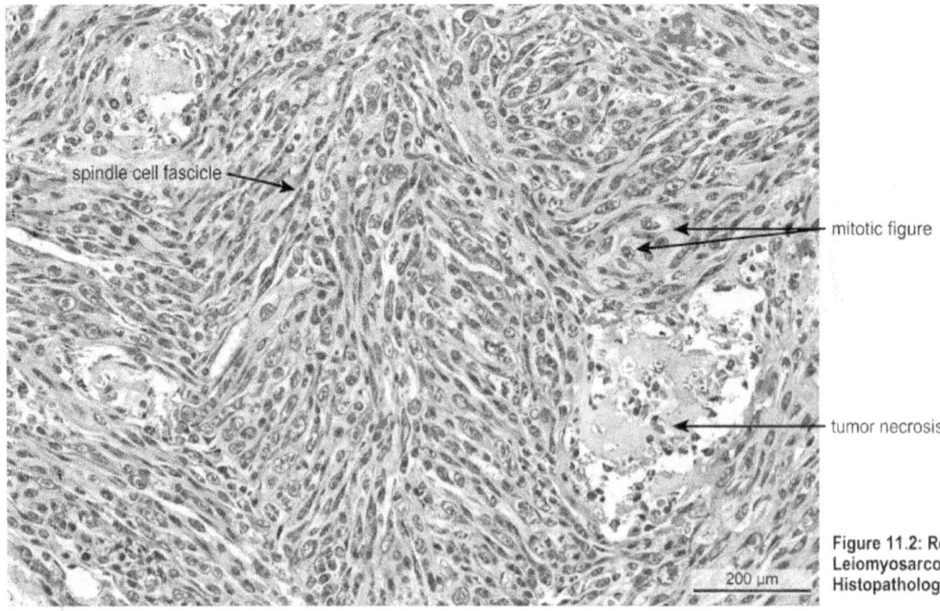

Figure 11.2: Retroperitoneal Leiomyosarcoma Histopathology

Surgical Margins, Recurrence, and Prognosis in Retroperitoneal Sarcoma

Complete surgical resection with negative margins offers the only realistic curative pathway for primary retroperitoneal sarcoma, but achieving negative margins is frequently constrained by the retroperitoneum's proximity to critical structures including the great vessels, kidneys, and bowel, such that resection often requires en bloc removal of adjacent, potentially uninvolved organs, most commonly the ipsilateral kidney and colon, to achieve an adequate margin around the tumor, a radical surgical philosophy the radiologist's report should support by precisely delineating the tumor's relationship to each adjacent organ and structure rather than a general statement of adjacency. Local recurrence, rather than distant metastasis, is the dominant pattern of treatment failure for well-differentiated and dedifferentiated liposarcoma specifically, occurring in a substantial proportion of cases even after ostensibly complete resection and often years after the original surgery, underscoring the importance of long-term surveillance imaging extending well beyond the shorter-interval follow-up protocols applied to many other malignancies discussed elsewhere in this book, while leiomyosarcoma and the other non-fatty retroperitoneal sarcomas carry a comparatively higher distant metastatic potential, most often to the lungs, warranting periodic chest imaging as part of comprehensive surveillance.

Peritoneal Disease: Carcinomatosis and Mesothelioma

Peritoneal Carcinomatosis: Imaging Patterns and Distribution

Peritoneal carcinomatosis, most commonly arising from ovarian, gastric, colorectal, appendiceal, and pancreatic primary malignancies, presents with a range of imaging findings including nodular or plaque-like peritoneal thickening and enhancement, omental caking, a confluent, often scalloped soft tissue infiltration of the omentum discussed further in the gynecologic and gastrointestinal chapters later in this book, and discrete peritoneal implants, often clustered along characteristic sites of ascitic fluid pooling and peristaltic flow including the pelvic cul-de-sac, right paracolic gutter, and the small bowel mesentery. Diffusion-weighted imaging has assumed an increasingly central role in peritoneal carcinomatosis detection given its high sensitivity for even small-volume peritoneal implants that can be genuinely difficult to detect on conventional anatomic sequences against the background of normal peritoneal fat and adjacent bowel loops, and a dedicated whole-abdomen diffusion-weighted sequence, rather than a bowel-focused, one that limits the field of view, is essential for adequate peritoneal carcinomatosis staging, a protocol design point consistent with the field-of-view emphasis introduced in the second chapter of this book.

Malignant Peritoneal Mesothelioma

Malignant peritoneal mesothelioma, a rare primary peritoneal malignancy with a well-established association with asbestos exposure, though a meaningful minority of cases occur without an identifiable exposure history, presents with a pattern that substantially overlaps with peritoneal carcinomatosis, including diffuse peritoneal thickening, omental involvement, and ascites, such that the correct diagnosis is frequently established only through peritoneal biopsy and immunohistochemistry rather than imaging characterization alone, though a relevant occupational asbestos exposure history in a patient without a known primary malignancy elsewhere should specifically raise this diagnostic consideration and prompt biopsy of the peritoneal disease itself rather than an extensive search for an occult extraperitoneal primary tumor that carcinomatosis would otherwise imply.

THE SIGNAL-TO-CATEGORY DECISION SYSTEM — Peritoneal Nodularity: Benign versus Carcinomatosis Pattern

---

The Signal Pattern: Peritoneal thickening or nodularity is identified, and the reader must determine whether the pattern favors benign reactive change or malignant carcinomatosis.

Category Signature: Smooth, thin, uniform peritoneal enhancement without discrete nodularity, particularly in a patient with a plausible benign cause such as recent surgery, peritoneal dialysis, or infection, is categorized as favoring benign or reactive change; nodular, thickened, or plaque-like peritoneal enhancement, particularly with omental caking or discrete soft tissue implants, is categorized as favoring malignant carcinomatosis.

The Decision: Findings favoring benign or reactive change are managed according to the identified underlying cause with interval imaging as clinically indicated; findings favoring carcinomatosis prompt a search for the primary malignancy if not already known, peritoneal biopsy when the primary is not evident, and, in a patient with a known primary, direct integration into oncologic staging and treatment planning.

Trap Logic: Benign peritoneal processes, including tuberculous peritonitis and, less commonly, other granulomatous or infectious peritonitis, can produce nodular peritoneal thickening that closely mimics carcinomatosis, and this mimicry is a well-recognized diagnostic pitfall particularly in endemic regions or immunocompromised patients; the discriminating step is integrating the peritoneal pattern with clinical context, including relevant exposure or immunocompromise history, and maintaining a lower threshold for biopsy when the clinical context does not clearly favor a malignant process despite a nodular imaging pattern.

Pattern Anchor: Nodular peritoneal thickening is not synonymous with carcinomatosis; tuberculous and other granulomatous peritonitis can produce a closely mimicking pattern, and clinical context should guide the threshold for biopsy in an ambiguous case.

Peritoneal Cancer Index and Surgical Planning for Cytoreduction

The peritoneal cancer index, a standardized scoring system quantifying disease burden across thirteen defined abdominopelvic regions based on the size of the largest implant within each region, is increasingly used to guide patient selection for cytoreductive surgery with hyperthermic intraperitoneal chemotherapy, a combined surgical and regional chemotherapy approach offering meaningful survival benefit in selected patients with peritoneal carcinomatosis from appendiceal, colorectal, and, in some protocols, ovarian primary malignancies, and preoperative MRI, particularly with dedicated thin-section and diffusion-weighted sequences, contributes directly to this scoring by characterizing disease distribution and, critically, identifying small bowel and mesenteric involvement, since extensive small bowel serosal or mesenteric root involvement is among the strongest predictors of incomplete cytoreduction and may exclude a patient from this otherwise potentially beneficial surgical approach. The radiologist's report in this specific surgical planning context benefits from a region-by-region description of disease distribution corresponding to the peritoneal cancer index framework, rather than a general summary statement of peritoneal carcinomatosis, given the direct influence of this granular distribution information on the surgical team's operative candidacy determination.

Special Populations: Pseudomyxoma Peritonei and Appendiceal Mucinous Neoplasms

Pseudomyxoma peritonei, a distinctive form of peritoneal spread arising most often from a ruptured appendiceal mucinous neoplasm, produces copious mucinous ascites with a characteristic scalloped, lobulated appearance as the gelatinous mucin conforms to and displaces adjacent organs including the liver and spleen, a morphologic pattern that, together with the profound T2 hyperintensity of the mucinous material itself, is sufficiently distinctive to suggest this specific diagnosis over conventional carcinomatosis even before the appendiceal or, less commonly, ovarian mucinous primary is definitively identified. This entity's distinctive biology, characterized by widespread intraperitoneal mucin deposition with a comparatively low tendency for the true invasive, destructive tissue infiltration and hematogenous or lymphatic metastasis characteristic of conventional peritoneal carcinomatosis, underlies its comparatively favorable prognosis relative to carcinomatosis from most other primary sites when treated with the same cytoreductive surgery and hyperthermic intraperitoneal chemotherapy approach discussed above, making its correct recognition and distinction from conventional carcinomatosis clinically meaningful beyond simple diagnostic precision.

Response Assessment in Peritoneal Carcinomatosis Following Systemic Therapy

Response assessment in peritoneal carcinomatosis following systemic chemotherapy presents specific challenges relative to the more straightforward size-based response criteria applied to discrete, measurable masses elsewhere in oncologic imaging, since peritoneal disease is frequently diffuse, plaque-like, or composed of numerous small implants that resist the simple linear measurement RECIST-type criteria rely upon, such that qualitative assessment of ascites volume, peritoneal enhancement intensity, and diffusion restriction, integrated with any measurable target lesions that are present, together provide a more complete picture of treatment response than any single quantitative metric applied to peritoneal disease in isolation. A decrease in ascites volume and peritoneal enhancement together with reduced diffusion restriction in previously identified implants generally supports treatment response, while new ascites, new peritoneal nodularity, or increasing diffusion restriction in a previously stable pattern supports disease progression, and the radiologist's report benefits from explicitly addressing each of these components against the relevant baseline or best-response comparison examination rather than a single overall impression statement.

EVIDENCE: Cytoreductive surgery with hyperthermic intraperitoneal chemotherapy has demonstrated meaningful survival benefit in selected patients with peritoneal carcinomatosis from appendiceal and colorectal primary malignancies, with outcomes strongly dependent on achieving complete or near-complete cytoreduction, underscoring the importance of the precise preoperative disease-mapping imaging described in this section.

Ascites, Peritoneal Fluid Collections, and Abdominal Wall Hernias

Characterizing Ascites: Transudative, Exudative, and Hemorrhagic Patterns

Simple ascites, most commonly related to portal hypertension from cirrhosis as discussed extensively in the liver disease chapters of this book, demonstrates simple fluid signal without appreciable internal complexity, while complex ascites, demonstrating internal septation, debris, or loculation, raises concern for infection, malignant seeding, or hemorrhage and warrants closer correlation with the peritoneal enhancement pattern discussed above rather than being dismissed as simple, benign fluid on the basis of overall abdominal distension alone. Hemorrhagic ascites, demonstrating elevated T1 signal reflecting blood products, can arise from a ruptured hepatic or other visceral tumor, anticoagulation, or trauma, and its recognition should prompt a deliberate search for a bleeding source, including a hepatic lesion with a hemoperitoneum pattern similar to that discussed in the hepatocellular carcinoma context earlier in this book, rather than attributing the finding to hemorrhage in isolation without pursuing its underlying cause.

Spontaneous Bacterial Peritonitis and Infected Ascites

Spontaneous bacterial peritonitis, a bacterial infection of preexisting ascites without an identifiable surgical source, occurs predominantly in patients with cirrhotic ascites and carries substantial morbidity and mortality if not promptly recognized and treated, and while the definitive diagnosis relies on ascitic fluid sampling and cell count rather than imaging, certain imaging features, including enhancing, thickened peritoneal or bowel wall segments and loculation of previously simple ascites into a more complex pattern, should raise clinical suspicion and prompt communication to the referring clinician for consideration of diagnostic paracentesis, particularly in a cirrhotic patient presenting with fever, abdominal pain, or unexplained clinical deterioration. Secondary peritonitis, by contrast, arises from a defined surgical source, most often bowel perforation, and is distinguished by the identification of that source, free air, a discrete abscess, or bowel wall discontinuity, together with typically more severe, often loculated and complex fluid collections than the diffuse, generally simpler pattern of spontaneous bacterial peritonitis, a distinction with direct management implications since secondary peritonitis generally requires surgical source control in addition to antibiotic therapy, unlike spontaneous bacterial peritonitis, which is managed medically.

Special Populations: Pregnancy-Related Retroperitoneal and Peritoneal Considerations

In pregnancy, MRI without gadolinium contrast is the preferred modality for evaluating retroperitoneal and peritoneal pathology when imaging is required, most often for suspected appendicitis, adnexal torsion, or, less commonly, retroperitoneal hemorrhage, and the gravid uterus produces predictable anatomic displacement of retroperitoneal and peritoneal structures that should be accounted for when localizing pathology and comparing against non-pregnant anatomic references, since organ position relative to fixed bony landmarks shifts progressively with advancing gestational age. Round ligament varicosities, a benign, pregnancy-related venous dilation that can mimic a hernia or mass clinically given its groin location and can cause a palpable, sometimes tender bulge, should be recognized on imaging by its characteristic serpiginous, vascular morphology and continuity with the round ligament and ovarian venous plexus, avoiding an unnecessary surgical referral for a presumed hernia or mass in this specific and benign pregnancy-related entity.

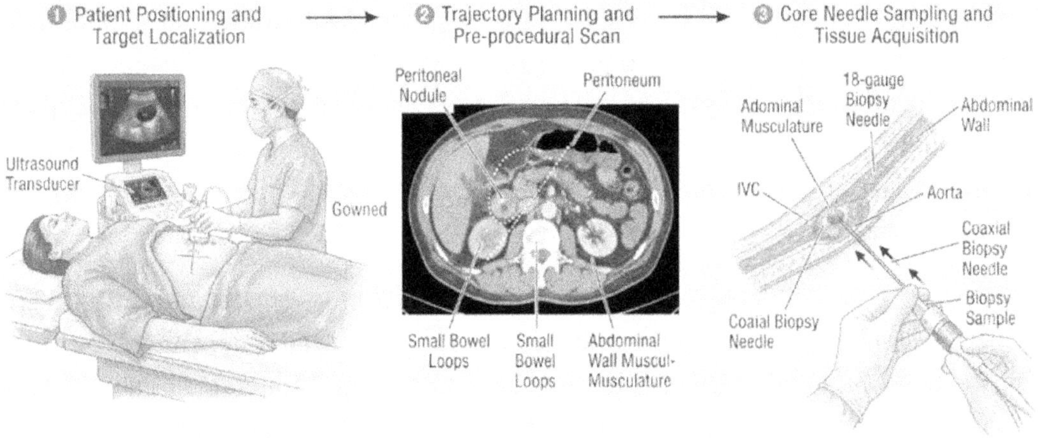

Figure 11.4
Image-Guided Peritoneal Biopsy Technique
1. Patient Positioning and Target Localization
2. Trajectory Planning and Pre-procedural Scan
3. Core Needle Sampling and Tissue Acquisition

Abdominal Wall and Groin Hernias

Abdominal wall and groin hernias, while frequently identified incidentally on body MRI performed for other indications, warrant systematic characterization including hernia type, most commonly inguinal, femoral, umbilical, or incisional in a patient with a prior surgical history, contents, whether omental fat alone or bowel, and, most clinically urgent, any signs of incarceration or strangulation, including bowel wall thickening, mesenteric edema, or reduced enhancement of incarcerated bowel loops, findings that should prompt urgent surgical communication given the risk of bowel ischemia if strangulation is present. Femoral hernias, while less common than inguinal hernias, carry a disproportionately higher risk of incarceration and strangulation given the comparatively rigid, unyielding boundaries of the femoral canal relative to the inguinal canal, such that a femoral hernia, even when asymptomatic at the time of imaging, generally warrants a more proactive surgical referral than an equivalently sized, asymptomatic inguinal hernia given this differential complication risk.

Clinical Case Presentations

Case 1. A 64-year-old man with a remote history of asbestos exposure presents with vague abdominal distension, and MRI demonstrates diffuse nodular peritoneal thickening and omental caking with moderate ascites, without an identifiable primary malignancy elsewhere in the abdomen or pelvis. Given the occupational exposure history and the absence of an identifiable primary, the radiologist recommends image-guided peritoneal biopsy to distinguish malignant peritoneal mesothelioma from an occult primary carcinomatosis, and biopsy confirms mesothelioma, directing the patient to the appropriate specialized surgical oncology and cytoreductive treatment pathway rather than a search for a nonexistent extraperitoneal primary tumor.

Case 2. A 52-year-old woman undergoes MRI for a palpable flank mass, demonstrating a large retroperitoneal fat-containing mass with several regions of thick, nodular internal septation but no discrete non-fatty soft tissue component. Recognizing the septal nodularity as inconsistent with simple lipoma despite the predominantly fatty composition, and applying the elevated pretest probability of liposarcoma in this specific anatomic location, the radiologist categorizes the mass as favoring well-differentiated liposarcoma and recommends biopsy and surgical oncology referral rather than reassurance based on the mass's overall fatty appearance.

Case 3. A 71-year-old man with progressive bilateral lower extremity edema and declining renal function undergoes MRI demonstrating periaortic and paracaval soft tissue thickening centered around the infrarenal aorta with bilateral medial ureteral deviation and moderate bilateral hydronephrosis. Recognizing the classic pattern of retroperitoneal fibrosis, the radiologist recommends serum IgG4 testing given the specific treatment implications of an IgG4-related etiology, and correlates the soft tissue's intermediate T2 signal and measurable enhancement with active, likely treatment-responsive disease rather than mature, burned-out fibrosis, supporting a trial of corticosteroid therapy before considering surgical ureterolysis.

Case 4. A 39-year-old woman with a several-month history of vague abdominal bloating undergoes MRI demonstrating a moderate volume of complex ascites with fine internal septation and diffuse, smooth, mild peritoneal enhancement without discrete nodularity, in the setting of a recent history of peritoneal dialysis catheter placement. Given the benign, uniform enhancement pattern and the clear alternative explanation from recent peritoneal dialysis access, the radiologist categorizes the findings as favoring reactive peritoneal change rather than carcinomatosis and recommends clinical correlation and short-interval follow-up rather than immediate biopsy, illustrating the importance of integrating clinical context into the benign-versus-malignant peritoneal categorization emphasized in this chapter.

Case 5. A 58-year-old man with a known prior incisional hernia repair presents with acute abdominal pain, and MRI demonstrates a recurrent incisional hernia containing a loop of small bowel with associated bowel wall thickening, mesenteric edema, and reduced mural enhancement compared to adjacent nonherniated bowel loops. Recognizing these findings as concerning for incarceration with early ischemia, the radiologist communicates the findings urgently to the surgical team, and the patient proceeds to emergent surgical repair, confirming a strangulated hernia requiring bowel resection, a time-critical outcome that underscores the clinical importance of the specific complication-focused hernia assessment emphasized in this chapter.

Case 6. A 47-year-old woman with a remote history of a ruptured appendix undergoes surveillance MRI demonstrating extensive scalloped, T2-hyperintense mucinous material surrounding the liver and spleen with characteristic mass effect displacing rather than invading adjacent organs, and a moderate volume of similar mucinous material throughout the pelvis. Recognizing this as the characteristic pattern of pseudomyxoma peritonei rather than conventional carcinomatosis, the radiologist provides a region-by-region description of disease distribution consistent with the peritoneal cancer index framework to support the surgical oncology team's evaluation for cytoreductive surgery with hyperthermic intraperitoneal chemotherapy, correctly anticipating the more favorable prognosis this specific entity carries relative to conventional peritoneal carcinomatosis from a non-mucinous primary.

Case 7. A 74-year-old man on warfarin therapy for atrial fibrillation presents with sudden-onset left flank pain and a falling hemoglobin, and MRI demonstrates a large left retroperitoneal hematoma with evolving blood-product signal and a small, fat-containing renal lesion at its presumed epicenter. Recognizing the fat-containing lesion as a likely angiomyolipoma that has bled, rather than attributing the hemorrhage to anticoagulation alone, the radiologist recommends renal-specific correlation and further characterization of the underlying lesion once the acute hemorrhage has been addressed, appropriately directing attention to the structural cause the framework in this chapter specifically emphasizes rather than accepting anticoagulation as a sufficient standalone explanation.

THE SIGNAL-TO-CATEGORY DECISION SYSTEM — Retroperitoneal and Peritoneal Triage Arc

The Signal Pattern: This chapter's patterns span the retroperitoneal and peritoneal risk spectrum, from a fat-containing mass whose septal architecture must be scrutinized before a benign lipoma label is applied, to peritoneal nodularity whose pattern must be integrated with clinical context before a carcinomatosis label is applied.

Category Signature: Fat-containing retroperitoneal masses are categorized as favoring lipoma or liposarcoma based on internal septal architecture and any non-fatty component; peritoneal thickening is categorized as favoring benign or malignant based on nodularity, distribution, and clinical context.

The Decision: Category assignment in this chapter ranges from surveillance for a fat-predominant mass with truly simple architecture to urgent surgical oncology referral for liposarcoma or carcinomatosis, and every category should be assigned only after deliberate scrutiny for the specific discriminating feature this chapter's framework requires.

The Trap Logic: Both patterns in this chapter share a common trap: a reassuringly common-appearing finding, uncomplicated fat or nodular peritoneal thickening, that in this specific location or clinical context carries a materially higher malignant probability than the same finding would carry elsewhere in the body.

Pattern Anchor: Location and clinical context meaningfully shift pretest probability throughout this chapter; apply the retroperitoneum- and peritoneum-specific probability adjustments this chapter's framework establishes rather than a generic, location-independent interpretation.

Summary and Key Concepts

Retroperitoneal compartments, anterior pararenal, perirenal, and posterior pararenal, defined by Gerota fascia, directly inform the differential diagnosis of a retroperitoneal mass by its compartment of predominant involvement.

Idiopathic retroperitoneal fibrosis produces periaortic and paracaval soft tissue with medial ureteral deviation; anterior displacement of the aorta instead favors an underlying malignant process.

In the retroperitoneum, a fat-containing mass should be treated as liposarcoma until proven otherwise given the comparative rarity of true retroperitoneal lipoma; septal nodularity or a non-fatty component favors liposarcoma over lipoma.

Leiomyosarcoma often arises from the inferior vena cava wall, and its specific vascular relationship should be documented given direct surgical planning implications.

Peritoneal carcinomatosis presents with nodular peritoneal thickening, omental caking, and discrete implants along characteristic ascitic fluid flow pathways; diffusion-weighted imaging improves detection of small-volume implants.

Tuberculous and other granulomatous peritonitis can closely mimic carcinomatosis; clinical context and exposure history should lower the threshold for biopsy in an ambiguous nodular peritoneal pattern.

Femoral hernias carry a disproportionately higher incarceration and strangulation risk than inguinal hernias given the rigid femoral canal boundaries, warranting more proactive surgical referral even when asymptomatic.

CHAPTER 12: RENAL MASS CHARACTERIZATION AND THE BOSNIAK CLASSIFICATION

Learning Objectives

1. Distinguish cystic from solid renal masses and apply the Bosniak classification to stratify cystic renal masses by malignant potential.
2. Recognize the major renal cell carcinoma subtypes and their distinguishing imaging features.
3. Distinguish angiomyolipoma from fat-poor renal cell carcinoma using fat detection technique and its limitations.
4. Apply a structured approach to renal mass staging, including venous invasion and nodal assessment relevant to surgical planning.
5. Recognize oncocytoma and other benign solid renal masses and understand the limitations of imaging-based differentiation from renal cell carcinoma.

Clinical Overview

The renal mass, whether cystic or solid, is among the most consequential incidental findings in body imaging, since it sits at the intersection of a very common, largely benign finding, the simple renal cyst, and one of the more common solid organ malignancies encountered in general practice, renal cell carcinoma, such that a disciplined, criteria-based approach to renal mass characterization is essential to correctly triaging across this spectrum. This chapter opens Part IV of this book with renal mass detection and cystic-versus-solid triage, proceeds through the Bosniak classification system for cystic renal masses, solid renal cell carcinoma subtypes, angiomyolipoma and other benign solid masses, and closes with renal mass staging and surgical planning considerations.

Two instances of the Signal-to-Category Decision System are applied in this chapter, the first to Bosniak category assignment, the single most consequential categorization task in renal cystic mass imaging, and the second to the fat-containing renal mass trap that distinguishes angiomyolipoma from the minority of renal cell carcinomas that can mimic it.

Renal Mass Detection and Characterization: Solid Versus Cystic

Multiparametric MRI and Renal Mass Biopsy Technique Considerations

Multiparametric renal mass MRI, incorporating diffusion-weighted imaging and, in some protocols, arterial spin labeling perfusion in addition to the standard multiphase postcontrast sequences discussed throughout this chapter, has an expanding but still evolving role in noninvasive renal cell carcinoma subtype prediction and grade estimation, with lower apparent diffusion coefficient values generally correlating with higher tumor grade across several validated series, though this correlation remains probabilistic rather than diagnostic and does not yet substitute for histologic grading in routine clinical practice. When percutaneous biopsy is pursued for a solid or complex cystic renal mass, image guidance, most often with ultrasound or CT given their real-time or near-real-time feedback and wide availability, targets the solid, enhancing component of the lesion specifically, avoiding necrotic or cystic regions that yield nondiagnostic tissue at a disproportionately high rate, and coaxial technique with multiple core samples improves diagnostic yield and subtype concordance with the eventual surgical specimen relative to a single-pass sampling approach.

Imaging Technique for Renal Mass Characterization

Renal mass characterization on MRI relies fundamentally on the comparison of precontrast and multiphase postcontrast imaging to establish true enhancement, the single most important determinant separating a solid or complex cystic mass requiring further workup from a simple cyst requiring none, and, as emphasized in the protocol design chapter of this book, subtraction imaging, in which the precontrast sequence is digitally subtracted from each postcontrast phase, is particularly valuable for confirming true enhancement in a renal lesion with high intrinsic T1 signal, such as a hemorrhagic or proteinaceous cyst, where enhancement can be genuinely difficult to distinguish from high baseline signal on visual inspection of the postcontrast image alone. Corticomedullary, nephrographic, and excretory phase imaging each contribute distinct information: the corticomedullary phase best depicts the renal vasculature and a hypervascular mass, the nephrographic phase, obtained once the entire renal parenchyma enhances homogeneously, is generally the most sensitive phase for detecting a renal mass against the enhancing background parenchyma, and the excretory phase depicts the collecting system, relevant to assessing collecting system invasion by a central mass and to the urothelial pathology discussed further in the following chapter.

The Simple Renal Cyst

The simple renal cyst, among the most common incidental findings in abdominal imaging at any age and increasing in prevalence with advancing age, demonstrates homogeneous, marked T2 hyperintensity, low T1 signal, a thin or imperceptible wall, and no measurable enhancement on any postcontrast phase, a definitively benign pattern, formally corresponding to Bosniak category I discussed in the following section, that requires no further workup or follow-up regardless of size once these strict criteria are confirmed. Establishing true absence of enhancement is the critical, sometimes technically demanding step in confidently assigning this most reassuring category, since a small, partially volume-averaged cyst adjacent to enhancing renal parenchyma can produce a spurious impression of enhancement on a single sequence, making careful correlation across all postcontrast phases, ideally with subtraction imaging as discussed above, essential before a cystic renal lesion is confidently labeled simple.

Epidemiology of Renal Masses and the Incidentaloma Context

Renal masses, both cystic and solid, are identified with increasing frequency as incidental findings on cross-sectional imaging performed for unrelated indications, mirroring the broader incidentaloma trend discussed for the adrenal gland in the preceding chapter, and simple renal cysts in particular demonstrate a prevalence that rises steadily with advancing age, present in a substantial proportion of the population by the seventh and eighth decades of life, such that an isolated simple cyst in an older adult is an expected, essentially universal finding rather than a notable one. Solid renal masses, by contrast, carry a meaningfully higher malignant probability even when small, with a substantial majority of small, incidentally discovered solid enhancing renal masses ultimately proving to be renal cell carcinoma on pathology, a probability distinction from the cystic mass differential that appropriately drives the generally more assertive characterization and workup pathway applied to solid renal lesions throughout this chapter relative to the more permissive approach applied to a simple or minimally complex cyst.

Hemorrhagic and Complicated Renal Cysts

A hemorrhagic or proteinaceous renal cyst, demonstrating elevated T1 signal from blood products or high protein content, can closely mimic a solid enhancing mass on a single postcontrast sequence evaluated without careful attention to precontrast signal, making subtraction imaging, discussed earlier in this chapter, particularly essential for this specific scenario to confirm the genuine absence of enhancement that would support a benign, complicated but ultimately Bosniak category II or IIF cyst rather than a solid or complex mass requiring more assertive workup. Infected renal cyst, presenting with a thickened, sometimes irregularly enhancing wall together with internal debris and, in the appropriate clinical context, fever and flank pain, can similarly mimic a more concerning Bosniak category III lesion on imaging alone, and correlating imaging findings with the clinical presentation, together with short-interval follow-up imaging after treatment to confirm resolution of the wall thickening, helps avoid an unnecessary surgical referral for a lesion that resolves entirely once the underlying infection is treated.

The Bosniak Classification System for Renal Cystic Masses

Bosniak Categories I Through IV: Criteria and Malignant Potential

The Bosniak classification stratifies cystic renal masses into five categories based on wall thickness, septation, calcification, and, most decisively, the presence and character of enhancing soft tissue components: category I, the simple cyst discussed above, carries essentially no malignant potential; category II, a minimally complex cyst with a few thin, hairline-thin septa or fine calcification without measurable enhancement of the septa or wall, similarly carries minimal malignant potential and requires no follow-up; category IIF, an intermediate category introduced specifically to capture cysts with slightly more complexity than category II but not yet meeting category III criteria, including a greater number of thin septa or minimal, smooth wall or septal thickening, carries a small but nonnegligible malignant potential and requires follow-up imaging rather than either dismissal or immediate intervention; category III, demonstrating thickened, irregular, or multiple enhancing septa or walls, carries a substantially elevated malignant potential, historically cited around fifty percent, that generally warrants surgical or ablative intervention or, in select cases, active surveillance rather than routine follow-up alone; and category IV, demonstrating a discrete enhancing soft tissue component or nodule beyond simple septal or wall thickening, carries the highest malignant potential of the cystic categories and is managed as a renal malignancy essentially by default.

The MRI-Specific Bosniak Classification Version 2019

The Bosniak classification was originally developed and validated using contrast-enhanced CT, and the more recently developed MRI-specific version of the classification, published in 2019, adapts the original CT-based criteria to account for MRI's distinct enhancement detection sensitivity and its superior soft tissue contrast for characterizing septal and wall thickness, incorporating MRI-specific quantitative and qualitative enhancement thresholds together with more explicit guidance for characterizing septal number, thickness, and nodularity than the original CT-based scheme provided. This MRI-specific version should be applied when reporting a renal cystic mass characterized on MRI rather than directly translating the original CT-based criteria, since meaningful differences exist between the two versions, particularly around the specific enhancement threshold used to distinguish measurable true enhancement from pseudoenhancement or noise, and using the version matched to the imaging modality in hand improves both the accuracy and the inter-reader reproducibility of the final assigned category.

THE SIGNAL-TO-CATEGORY DECISION SYSTEM — Bosniak Category Assignment

The Signal Pattern: A cystic renal mass is identified, and the reader must systematically assess its wall and septal thickness, number of septa, presence of calcification, and, most critically, the presence and character of any enhancing component.

Category Signature: A mass with a hairline-thin wall and no septa or enhancement is categorized as I; a mass with a few hairline-thin, non-enhancing septa is categorized as II; a mass with more numerous thin septa or minimal smooth thickening is categorized as IIF; a mass with thickened or irregular enhancing septa or walls is categorized as III; a mass with a discrete enhancing soft tissue nodule is categorized as IV.

The Decision: Categories I and II require no follow-up; category IIF requires follow-up imaging at defined intervals to confirm stability; category III generally proceeds to surgical or ablative intervention, or active surveillance in select patients; category IV is managed as renal malignancy.

Trap Logic: The distinction between a thickened, irregular, enhancing septum, category III, and a discrete enhancing nodule, category IV, is a frequent source of inter-reader disagreement, since a sufficiently thick or bulbous septal thickening can be genuinely difficult to distinguish from a true nodule; the discriminating step, per the 2019 MRI-specific criteria, is assessing whether the enhancing component demonstrates a convex, bulging, mass-like morphology protruding beyond the expected plane of a septum, which favors a true category IV nodule, versus a thickened but still fundamentally linear, septum-conforming morphology, which favors category III.

Pattern Anchor: Category assignment hinges on confirmed true enhancement and, at the III-versus-IV boundary, on convex nodular morphology versus linear septal thickening; apply the MRI-specific 2019 criteria rather than translating CT-based criteria directly.

Management and Surveillance Intervals by Bosniak Category

Category IIF surveillance is generally recommended at defined intervals, commonly at six months and then annually thereafter for a period of approximately five years, with progression to a higher category, development of a new enhancing component, or interval growth prompting reclassification and, generally, surgical or ablative referral, while a category IIF lesion demonstrating sustained stability over the full surveillance period can generally be considered to have effectively excluded clinically significant malignant potential and surveillance discontinued.

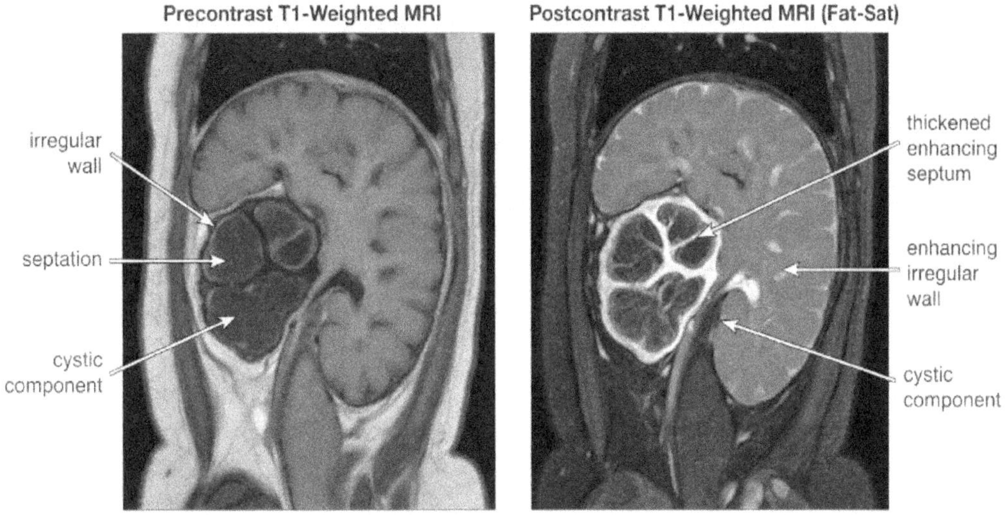

Figure 12.1: Bosniak Category III Cystic Renal Mass with Enhancing Septa

Category III lesions, given their substantially elevated malignant potential, are more often managed with either surgical resection, generally partial nephrectomy given the nephrometry principles discussed later in this chapter, percutaneous ablation for a smaller lesion or a patient who is a poor surgical candidate, or, increasingly in an appropriately selected and counseled patient, active surveillance with closer-interval imaging than the IIF protocol, reflecting an evolving appreciation that not every category III lesion harbors aggressive malignancy and that some patients, particularly older patients with significant comorbidity, may reasonably prefer surveillance over intervention for a lesion carrying meaningful but not universal malignant potential.

Bosniak Category	Malignant Potential	Typical Management
I	Essentially none	No follow-up
II	Minimal	No follow-up
IIF	Low but nonnegligible	Surveillance imaging at defined intervals
III	Substantially elevated (historically ~50%)	Surgery, ablation, or active surveillance

IV	Highest	Managed as renal malignancy

Solid Renal Mass Characterization and Renal Cell Carcinoma Subtypes

Epidemiology and Risk Factors for Renal Cell Carcinoma

Renal cell carcinoma incidence has risen over recent decades, a trend attributed substantially to the increasing detection of small, incidentally discovered tumors on cross-sectional imaging performed for unrelated indications rather than a true rise in disease-specific mortality, which has remained comparatively stable, reflecting the generally more favorable prognosis of the smaller, earlier-stage tumors now more frequently detected. Established modifiable risk factors include cigarette smoking, obesity, and hypertension, each independently associated with an elevated risk across large epidemiologic studies, while acquired cystic kidney disease, occurring in patients with long-standing end-stage renal disease and dialysis dependence, carries a substantially elevated renal cell carcinoma risk that warrants a specifically heightened index of suspicion for any new or growing solid component within a background of numerous renal cysts in this specific dialysis-dependent population, a population in whom baseline renal imaging surveillance protocols differ meaningfully from the general population given this elevated risk.

Hereditary Renal Cell Carcinoma Syndromes

A meaningful minority of renal cell carcinoma cases arise in the context of a hereditary syndrome, and recognizing a pattern suggestive of hereditary disease, most classically multiple, often bilateral renal masses at a comparatively young age, carries direct implications for genetic counseling and, in some cases, altered surgical management favoring nephron-sparing approaches given the elevated likelihood of additional tumors developing over the patient's lifetime. Von Hippel-Lindau disease, associated with multiple clear cell renal cell carcinomas together with the pancreatic, adrenal, and central nervous system findings discussed elsewhere in this book, and hereditary leiomyomatosis and renal cell carcinoma syndrome, associated with an aggressive papillary renal cell carcinoma subtype requiring a lower size threshold for intervention than sporadic renal cell carcinoma given its disproportionately aggressive behavior even at small size, are among the more clinically significant hereditary syndromes the radiologist should recognize when a suggestive multiplicity or family history pattern is encountered.

Clear Cell Renal Cell Carcinoma

Clear cell renal cell carcinoma, the most common renal cell carcinoma subtype, typically presents as a heterogeneous, hypervascular mass demonstrating avid arterial-phase enhancement with washout on delayed phases, a hemodynamic pattern reflecting its rich capillary vascularity, together with a propensity for internal necrosis, hemorrhage, and, in a subset of cases, macroscopic fat when calcification is also present within the mass, a specific combination that, unlike fat without calcification favoring angiomyolipoma as discussed below, can actually be seen in clear cell renal cell carcinoma and should not be used in isolation to exclude malignancy. This hypervascular, washout-demonstrating pattern is the imaging correlate of clear cell carcinoma's characteristically aggressive biology relative to the other renal cell carcinoma subtypes discussed below, and its recognition, together with the tumor's size and any evidence of local invasion or venous extension discussed later in this chapter, contributes to risk stratification even before histologic confirmation is available.

Papillary and Chromophobe Renal Cell Carcinoma

Papillary renal cell carcinoma, the second most common subtype, typically demonstrates a more homogeneous, comparatively hypovascular enhancement pattern relative to clear cell carcinoma, often with restricted diffusion and, in a meaningful subset, susceptibility signal loss from hemosiderin deposition, and this comparatively hypovascular pattern, together with a generally more indolent clinical behavior than clear cell carcinoma, together form a recognizable, if imperfect, noninvasive discriminator between these two most common subtypes. Chromophobe renal cell carcinoma, the third most common subtype, presents as a well-circumscribed, homogeneously enhancing mass that can be genuinely difficult to distinguish from oncocytoma, discussed later in this chapter, given substantial imaging overlap between these two entities, though chromophobe carcinoma's segmental enhancement inversion pattern, in which the tumor demonstrates a spoke-wheel enhancement pattern radiating from a central scar that can enhance more intensely on delayed relative to arterial phase imaging, has been proposed as a discriminating feature in select cases, albeit with imperfect reliability that generally still necessitates biopsy or resection for definitive distinction from oncocytoma.

Renal Medullary Carcinoma and Collecting Duct Carcinoma

Renal medullary carcinoma, a rare but highly aggressive subtype occurring almost exclusively in patients with sickle cell trait or, less commonly, sickle cell disease, typically presents as an infiltrative, centrally located mass with ill-defined margins, often with associated caliectasis and regional lymphadenopathy at diagnosis given its characteristically advanced stage at presentation, and its recognition in a patient with known sickle cell trait, together with prompt oncologic referral given its aggressive natural history and generally poor prognosis even with treatment, distinguishes it sharply from the far more common and considerably more indolent renal cell carcinoma subtypes discussed elsewhere in this chapter. Collecting duct carcinoma, another rare and aggressive subtype arising from the medullary collecting ducts, similarly presents as an infiltrative, centrally located mass with a comparatively poor prognosis, and while imaging cannot reliably distinguish these rare aggressive subtypes from one another or from a centrally infiltrative presentation of urothelial carcinoma discussed in the following chapter, the combination of central location, infiltrative margins, and a clinical presentation atypical for the more common renal cell carcinoma subtypes should prompt consideration of this less common but prognostically important differential category.

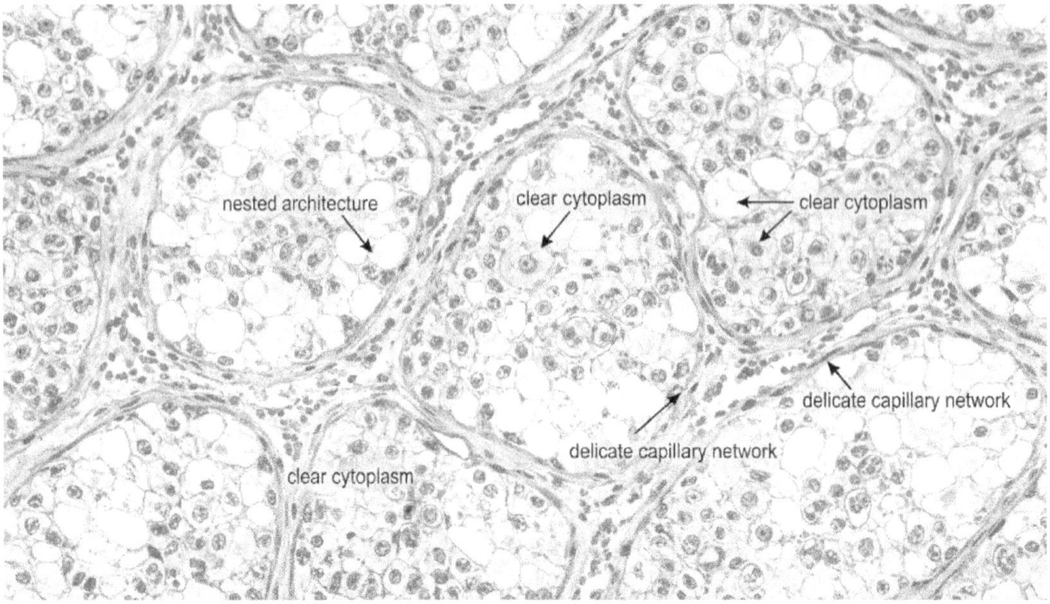

CAUTION: A hemorrhagic or proteinaceous renal cyst can closely mimic a solid enhancing mass on a single postcontrast sequence; always confirm true enhancement with subtraction imaging or careful precontrast comparison before assigning a higher Bosniak category or recommending biopsy.

Angiomyolipoma and Other Benign Solid Renal Masses

Classic Angiomyolipoma: Macroscopic Fat Detection

Classic angiomyolipoma, a benign renal tumor composed of variable proportions of mature fat, smooth muscle, and abnormal thick-walled blood vessels, is diagnosed with high confidence when macroscopic fat is confidently identified within a renal mass on fat-suppressed sequences, a finding that, in the overwhelming majority of cases, essentially excludes renal cell carcinoma and requires no further workup beyond, in larger lesions, monitoring for the size-related hemorrhage risk discussed below, making fat detection one of the most decisively reassuring findings in the entire renal mass differential covered in this chapter. Signal dropout on opposed-phase chemical-shift imaging, the same technique introduced in the adrenal chapter of this book, can supplement conventional fat-suppressed sequence assessment for detecting fat within a renal mass, though conventional frequency-selective fat suppression generally remains the primary technique given its greater sensitivity for the sometimes small or admixed fat volumes encountered in angiomyolipoma relative to the different signal mechanism assessed by chemical-shift imaging.

Fat-Poor Angiomyolipoma and the Renal Cell Carcinoma Mimicry Problem

A meaningful minority of angiomyolipomas contain minimal or no detectable macroscopic fat on conventional imaging, a category termed fat-poor angiomyolipoma that presents one of the most challenging differential problems in solid renal mass imaging, since these lesions can closely mimic renal cell carcinoma, particularly the hypervascular pattern of clear cell carcinoma, without the reassuring fat signature that would otherwise allow confident benign characterization. Certain ancillary features have been proposed to favor fat-poor angiomyolipoma over renal cell carcinoma, including homogeneous, marked T2 hypointensity relative to renal cortex reflecting the lesion's dense smooth muscle composition, and a specific pattern on precontrast T1 and T2 imaging sometimes described as demonstrating a hypointense rim, but none of these ancillary features carries sufficient individual or even combined reliability to substitute for biopsy in a genuinely indeterminate solid renal mass lacking definitive macroscopic fat, such that biopsy, rather than imaging-based presumptive characterization, remains the appropriate pathway for most fat-poor lesions that cannot be confidently characterized by other means.

THE SIGNAL-TO-CATEGORY DECISION SYSTEM — Fat-Containing Renal Mass: Angiomyolipoma versus Fat-Poor RCC Trap

---

The Signal Pattern: A renal mass with signal characteristics suggesting possible fat content is identified, and the reader must confirm whether the fat is truly macroscopic, intracellular microscopic, or absent before assigning a category.

Category Signature: A mass with unambiguous macroscopic fat, confirmed on conventional fat-suppressed sequences, without an associated calcification, is categorized as classic angiomyolipoma; a mass with fat and calcification together, an unusual but recognized combination, is categorized as indeterminate given the rare but real possibility of renal cell carcinoma with fat; a mass without confident macroscopic fat is categorized as fat-poor and indeterminate.

The Decision: Classic angiomyolipoma without calcification requires no further workup beyond size-based hemorrhage risk monitoring discussed below; a fat-and-calcification mass or a fat-poor mass proceeds to biopsy for definitive characterization given the inadequate reliability of imaging-based ancillary features alone.

Trap Logic: Renal cell carcinoma engulfing or growing adjacent to a small volume of perinephric or sinus fat can produce a spurious impression of intratumoral fat if the fat is not confirmed to be genuinely intralesional on every imaging plane and sequence; the discriminating step is confirming that the fat signal is unambiguously contained within, rather than merely adjacent to or engulfed by, the mass on multiplanar review before applying the reassuring classic angiomyolipoma category.

Pattern Anchor: Confirm fat is genuinely intralesional, not merely adjacent or engulfed, before applying the reassuring angiomyolipoma category; fat combined with calcification is an indication for further workup, not reassurance.

Angiomyolipoma Hemorrhage Risk and Management

Angiomyolipoma carries a size-dependent risk of spontaneous hemorrhage related to the abnormal, aneurysm-prone vasculature within the lesion, with a size threshold, generally cited around four centimeters, above which the hemorrhage risk rises meaningfully and prophylactic intervention, typically selective arterial embolization, is often considered even in an asymptomatic patient, a size-based management threshold distinct from and substantially smaller than the size thresholds applied to most other renal mass categories in this chapter given angiomyolipoma's specific vascular hemorrhage mechanism rather than malignant potential. Angiomyolipoma occurs with increased frequency and multiplicity in tuberous sclerosis complex, a genetic syndrome also associated with the cerebral, cardiac, and pulmonary findings addressed in other imaging contexts, such that multiple or bilateral angiomyolipomas, particularly in a younger patient, should prompt consideration of this underlying syndrome and correlation with the relevant clinical and other-organ imaging findings.

Oncocytoma and Other Benign Solid Renal Masses

Renal oncocytoma, a benign epithelial tumor, classically demonstrates a central stellate scar and a well-circumscribed, homogeneously enhancing appearance, but, as discussed above in the chromophobe carcinoma context, this appearance overlaps substantially with chromophobe renal cell carcinoma and, to a lesser degree, with other renal cell carcinoma subtypes, such that oncocytoma cannot be reliably diagnosed by imaging features alone despite the classic central scar description that persists in some older teaching, and biopsy or resection remains necessary for a solid renal mass suspected of representing oncocytoma given the genuinely inadequate specificity of any single or combined imaging feature for this specific diagnosis. This imaging overlap between oncocytoma and renal cell carcinoma, more pronounced than for almost any other benign-versus-malignant distinction addressed in this book, is an important limitation the radiologist's report should transparently acknowledge, generally recommending biopsy for a solid, enhancing renal mass without macroscopic fat rather than offering a confident imaging-based benign oncocytoma diagnosis that current evidence does not support.

Epithelioid Angiomyolipoma and Malignant Potential

Epithelioid angiomyolipoma, a rare, biologically distinct variant containing minimal or no fat and composed predominantly of epithelioid cells, carries genuine malignant potential with a recognized capacity for local invasion and, uncommonly, metastatic spread, distinguishing it sharply from the classic, entirely benign angiomyolipoma discussed above despite sharing the same broader angiomyolipoma family designation, and this entity, lacking the reassuring macroscopic fat signature of classic angiomyolipoma, generally presents as an indeterminate, fat-poor solid renal mass indistinguishable from renal cell carcinoma on imaging, appropriately funneling into the same biopsy-based workup pathway as other fat-poor lesions discussed earlier in this chapter rather than being separable from the renal cell carcinoma differential by any reliable imaging feature. This malignant-potential subtype underscores why the fat-poor angiomyolipoma category should never be presumptively treated as benign on clinical grounds alone, since even a lesion that ultimately proves to be an angiomyolipoma variant on biopsy can, in the epithelioid subtype specifically, warrant oncologic management rather than the observation appropriate for classic angiomyolipoma.

Figure 12.3: Renal Collecting System and Vascular Anatomy

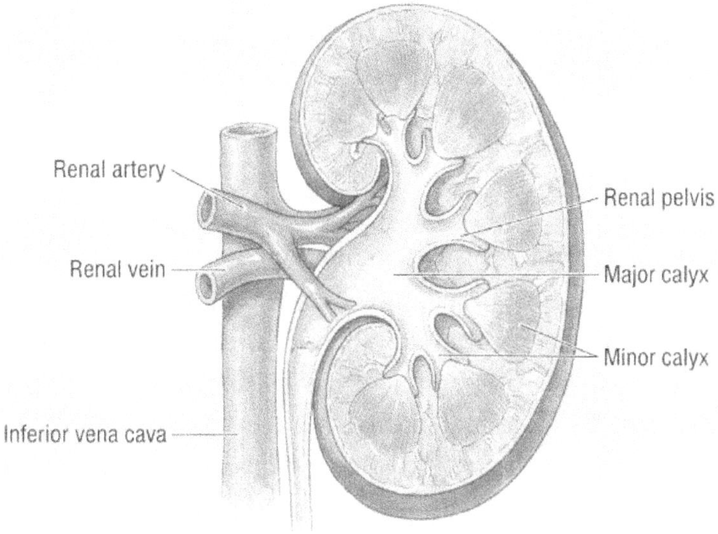

Renal Mass Staging and Surgical Planning

Venous Invasion and Tumor Thrombus

Renal cell carcinoma demonstrates a distinctive propensity for venous invasion, with tumor thrombus extending from the renal vein into the inferior vena cava, and occasionally as far cephalad as the right atrium, in a meaningful minority of cases, and precise documentation of the cephalad extent of tumor thrombus, using a standardized level classification distinguishing thrombus confined to the renal vein, thrombus extending into the infrahepatic, intrahepatic, or suprahepatic inferior vena cava, and thrombus extending into the right atrium, is essential surgical planning information, since each level carries a progressively more complex surgical approach, potentially requiring cardiopulmonary bypass for the most cephalad extent of thrombus. Distinguishing bland, non-tumoral thrombus from true tumor thrombus, when both coexist or when the distinction is otherwise ambiguous, relies on identifying enhancement within the thrombus itself, confirming its vascularized, tumoral nature, versus a non-enhancing, avascular bland clot, a distinction with meaningful implications for the surgical approach and for whether anticoagulation, appropriate for bland thrombus, is an appropriate component of management.

Nephron-Sparing Surgery and Partial Nephrectomy Planning

Partial nephrectomy, preserving functional renal parenchyma relative to radical nephrectomy, has become the preferred surgical approach for many localized renal masses, particularly smaller tumors, and preoperative imaging plays a central planning role through structured scoring systems, most widely the R.E.N.A.L. nephrometry score, which incorporates tumor radius, exophytic-versus-endophytic location, nearness to the collecting system, anterior-versus-posterior location, and location relative to the polar lines, to predict surgical complexity and guide the choice between a partial and radical nephrectomy approach. The radiologist's report contributes most productively to this planning process by explicitly addressing each of these nephrometry components, tumor size, depth of endophytic extension, proximity to the renal sinus and collecting system, and precise anatomic location, rather than a general descriptive statement of tumor location, since this granular, standardized detail is what the surgical planning nephrometry framework specifically requires.

Nodal and Distant Metastatic Staging

Regional lymph node assessment in renal cell carcinoma centers on the renal hilar and retroperitoneal paraaortic and paracaval nodal stations, discussed in their broader retroperitoneal context in the preceding chapter, with nodal involvement, while less common than hematogenous spread as the dominant pattern of metastatic dissemination for this specific malignancy, still carrying meaningfully adverse prognostic implications that should be assessed and documented using the same morphologic criteria, size together with loss of normal fatty hilum and rounded configuration, discussed for retroperitoneal lymphadenopathy generally in the preceding chapter. Distant metastatic disease from renal cell carcinoma demonstrates a distinctive predilection for the lungs, bone, liver, and, less commonly but with a recognized association, the pancreas, where a renal cell carcinoma metastasis can present as a solitary, sometimes markedly hypervascular pancreatic lesion that can be genuinely difficult to distinguish from a primary pancreatic neuroendocrine tumor discussed in an earlier chapter of this book without the relevant clinical history of a prior or concurrent renal cell carcinoma diagnosis, underscoring the importance of a thorough clinical history review whenever an unexpectedly hypervascular pancreatic lesion is encountered.

Active Surveillance for Small Renal Masses

Active surveillance, involving serial imaging without immediate intervention, has emerged as an appropriate management option for a select subset of patients with a small renal mass, generally under two to three centimeters, particularly older patients or those with significant comorbidity for whom the competing mortality risk from other conditions may exceed the comparatively low metastatic potential of a small, indolent renal cell carcinoma over their expected remaining lifespan, reflecting a broader appreciation that not every small renal mass, even when biopsy-confirmed as malignant, requires immediate intervention in every patient. Growth rate on serial surveillance imaging, generally assessed as the change in maximum diameter over a defined interval, is the primary metric guiding continued surveillance versus conversion to active intervention, with a rapid growth rate or a mass approaching a size threshold associated with meaningfully increased metastatic potential prompting reconsideration of surgical or ablative therapy, such that the radiologist's precise, reproducible measurement technique on each surveillance examination, ideally using the same imaging plane and measurement method as the baseline study, is essential to this management pathway's reliability.

Figure 12.4: Robotic-Assisted Partial Nephrectomy Technique.

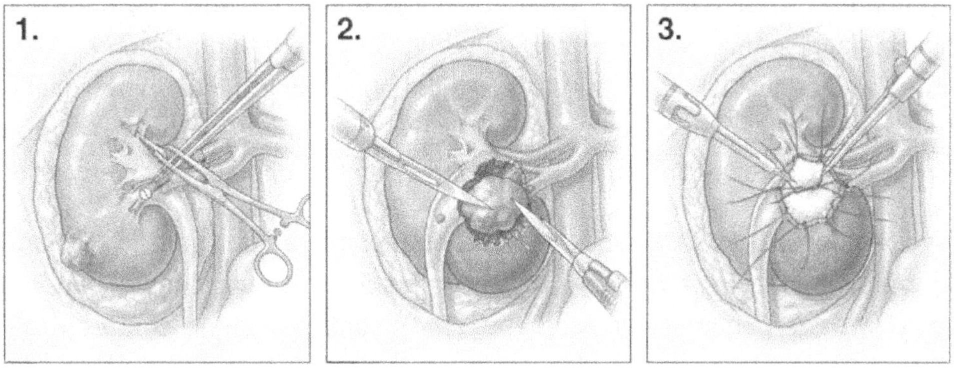

1. Hilar Vascular Control 2. Tumor Excision 3. Renorrhaphy Closure

1 — Hilar Vascular Control
2 — Tumor Excision

Clinical Case Presentations

Case 1. A 56-year-old woman undergoes MRI for an incidentally discovered 2.1-centimeter right renal cystic lesion demonstrating a hairline-thin wall, two thin, non-enhancing septa, and no measurable enhancement of any component. The radiologist categorizes the lesion as Bosniak category II and recommends no follow-up, applying the 2019 MRI-specific criteria to confidently exclude the need for further imaging or intervention.

Case 2. A 63-year-old man undergoes MRI demonstrating a 3.8-centimeter cystic renal mass with several thickened, irregular septa demonstrating clear, unambiguous enhancement on subtraction imaging, without a discrete nodular component. The radiologist categorizes the mass as Bosniak category III, distinguishing the linear, septum-conforming thickening from a true category IV nodule per the trap logic emphasized in this chapter's Rhythm Layer, and recommends urology referral for consideration of surgical resection or active surveillance.

Case 3. A 48-year-old woman undergoes MRI for flank pain, incidentally revealing a 5.2-centimeter left renal mass containing unambiguous macroscopic fat on fat-suppressed sequences without associated calcification, confirmed as genuinely intralesional on multiplanar review. The radiologist categorizes the lesion as classic angiomyolipoma and, given its size above the four-centimeter hemorrhage-risk threshold, recommends interventional radiology consultation for consideration of prophylactic embolization rather than watchful waiting alone.

Case 4. A 67-year-old man undergoes MRI demonstrating a 6.5-centimeter heterogeneous, hypervascular right renal mass with washout on delayed imaging and tumor thrombus extending from the renal vein into the infrahepatic inferior vena cava, with enhancement confirmed within the thrombus itself. The radiologist categorizes the mass as clear cell renal cell carcinoma with level I tumor thrombus per the standardized venous extension classification and explicitly documents the thrombus's enhancing, tumoral nature and its precise cephalad extent to support the urologic and cardiac surgery teams' joint operative planning.

Case 5. A 39-year-old woman undergoes MRI for an incidentally discovered 2.4-centimeter solid, homogeneously enhancing right renal mass without macroscopic fat, demonstrating a subtle central scar. Recognizing that this appearance cannot reliably distinguish oncocytoma from chromophobe renal cell carcinoma despite the classic scar description, the radiologist recommends percutaneous biopsy rather than presumptive benign characterization, appropriately declining to offer a confident noninvasive oncocytoma diagnosis given the documented imaging overlap this chapter's framework emphasizes.

Case 6. A 79-year-old man with significant cardiopulmonary comorbidity is found to have a 1.8-centimeter solid, mildly enhancing renal mass on imaging performed for an unrelated indication, without macroscopic fat. Given the patient's advanced age, significant competing comorbidity, and the mass's small size and comparatively low associated metastatic potential, the multidisciplinary team elects active surveillance with serial MRI at defined intervals rather than immediate biopsy or intervention, and the radiologist documents precise, reproducible baseline measurements using a consistent imaging plane to support reliable growth-rate assessment on subsequent surveillance examinations.

Case 7. A 34-year-old man with known sickle cell trait presents with gross hematuria and flank pain, and MRI demonstrates an infiltrative, ill-defined central right renal mass with associated caliectasis and enlarged retroperitoneal lymph nodes. Recognizing the combination of the patient's sickle cell trait status, the infiltrative central morphology, and advanced nodal involvement as highly suspicious for renal medullary carcinoma rather than a more common and indolent renal cell carcinoma subtype, the radiologist recommends urgent oncologic referral given this entity's aggressive natural history, appropriately flagging the atypical, higher-risk pattern this chapter's framework specifically distinguishes from the far more common renal cell carcinoma differential.

THE SIGNAL-TO-CATEGORY DECISION SYSTEM — Renal Mass Triage Arc

The Signal Pattern: This chapter's patterns span the full renal mass risk spectrum, from a cystic lesion whose septal and wall enhancement must be systematically assessed for Bosniak category assignment, to a solid mass whose fat content must be confirmed as truly intralesional before the reassuring angiomyolipoma category is applied.

Category Signature: Cystic masses are categorized I through IV based on wall and septal thickness, number, and enhancement character; solid masses are categorized as angiomyolipoma, indeterminate fat-poor, or favoring a specific renal cell carcinoma subtype based on fat content, vascularity, and morphology.

The Decision: Category assignment in this chapter ranges from no-further-workup outcomes for a simple cyst or classic angiomyolipoma to complex multidisciplinary surgical planning for a mass with venous tumor thrombus, and every category should be assigned only after the specific confirmatory feature, true enhancement, genuinely intralesional fat, or confirmed thrombus enhancement, has been explicitly verified.

The Trap Logic: Both patterns in this chapter share a common trap: a feature that superficially resembles the category-defining finding, engulfed perinephric fat resembling intratumoral fat, or thickened septa resembling a true nodule, without actually meeting its specific defining criteria on careful, deliberate multiplanar scrutiny.

Pattern Anchor: In renal mass imaging, confirm the specific defining feature, true enhancement, genuinely intralesional fat, or true nodular morphology, explicitly before committing to a final category; superficial resemblance is not sufficient.

Summary and Key Concepts

True enhancement, best confirmed with subtraction imaging, is the central determinant of renal mass characterization; the simple renal cyst shows no enhancement and requires no further workup.

The Bosniak classification stratifies cystic renal masses into categories I through IV based on wall and septal thickness, number, and enhancement character; the 2019 MRI-specific version should be applied to MRI-characterized masses.

Clear cell renal cell carcinoma is typically hypervascular with washout; papillary carcinoma is comparatively hypovascular; chromophobe carcinoma overlaps substantially with oncocytoma on imaging.

Classic angiomyolipoma with unambiguous, genuinely intralesional macroscopic fat and no calcification requires no further workup; fat-poor angiomyolipoma cannot be reliably distinguished from renal cell carcinoma by imaging alone and generally requires biopsy.

Angiomyolipoma hemorrhage risk rises meaningfully above a four-centimeter size threshold, prompting consideration of prophylactic embolization; multiple or bilateral angiomyolipomas suggest tuberous sclerosis complex.

Oncocytoma cannot be reliably distinguished from chromophobe renal cell carcinoma on imaging despite the classic central scar description, and biopsy or resection remains necessary for definitive diagnosis.

Precise documentation of tumor thrombus level and confirmed enhancement within the thrombus, together with structured nephrometry scoring, directly informs surgical planning for renal cell carcinoma.

CHAPTER 13: RENAL PARENCHYMAL AND COLLECTING SYSTEM DISEASE

Learning Objectives

1. Recognize the MRI findings of diffuse medical renal disease and correlate parenchymal signal change with underlying pathophysiology.
2. Distinguish acute pyelonephritis from renal abscess and recognize their major complications.
3. Recognize urothelial carcinoma of the collecting system and distinguish it from stone and clot as causes of a filling defect.
4. Apply a systematic approach to hydronephrosis and obstruction, including congenital anomalies of the collecting system.
5. Recognize autosomal dominant polycystic kidney disease and other renal cystic disease syndromes and their major extrarenal manifestations.

Clinical Overview

Beyond the focal renal mass differential addressed in the preceding chapter, the kidney and its collecting system present a distinct disease spectrum organized around diffuse parenchymal processes, infection, urothelial neoplasia, obstruction, and inherited cystic disease, each with its own interpretive framework and each carrying meaningfully different management urgency, from the reassuring surveillance appropriate for stable medullary sponge kidney to the urgent decompression required for an infected, obstructed collecting system. This chapter proceeds from diffuse medical renal disease, through pyelonephritis and renal infection, urothelial carcinoma and collecting system neoplasms, hydronephrosis and congenital anomalies, and closes with the major inherited renal cystic disease syndromes.

Two instances of the Signal-to-Category Decision System are applied in this chapter, the first to the acute pyelonephritis-versus-abscess triage that determines whether percutaneous drainage is required, and the second to the collecting system filling defect trap that distinguishes urothelial tumor from the far more common stone or clot.

Diffuse Renal Parenchymal Disease and Medical Renal Disease

Normal Renal Parenchymal Signal and Corticomedullary Differentiation

Normal renal parenchyma demonstrates preserved corticomedullary differentiation on T1-weighted imaging, with the cortex, containing the glomeruli and proximal convoluted tubules, demonstrating relatively higher T1 signal than the medulla, containing the loops of Henle and collecting ducts, a differentiation pattern that becomes more pronounced on early postcontrast imaging when the cortex, receiving the bulk of renal blood flow, enhances substantially more intensely than the comparatively hypovascular medulla during the corticomedullary phase discussed in the preceding chapter. Loss of this normal corticomedullary differentiation, appearing as a more homogeneous, less distinctly layered parenchymal signal pattern, is a nonspecific but clinically useful marker of diffuse renal parenchymal disease, whether from chronic medical renal disease, acute tubular injury, or infection, and while this loss of differentiation cannot by itself specify the underlying cause, its presence should prompt correlation with the patient's renal function and clinical history to guide further characterization.

Chronic Kidney Disease and Diffuse Parenchymal Signal Change

Chronic kidney disease of any etiology produces a generally predictable, if nonspecific, imaging pattern of progressive parenchymal thinning, reduced overall renal size, and increasingly indistinct corticomedullary differentiation as the disease advances, with the specific underlying cause, whether diabetic nephropathy, hypertensive nephrosclerosis, glomerulonephritis, or another etiology, generally not distinguishable by imaging alone and instead established through clinical, laboratory, and, when indicated, renal biopsy correlation, such that the radiologist's role in this context is generally to characterize the degree and symmetry of parenchymal involvement, exclude an obstructive or structural cause potentially amenable to a distinct treatment pathway, and provide baseline renal size and morphology for future comparison rather than to render a specific medical renal disease diagnosis from imaging features alone. Asymmetric renal size or parenchymal involvement, by contrast, should prompt a specific search for a unilateral process such as renal artery stenosis, chronic unilateral obstruction, or reflux nephropathy, since bilateral symmetric medical renal disease is the more common pattern and an asymmetric finding meaningfully narrows this differential toward a more specific, and sometimes correctable, unilateral cause.

Renal Artery Stenosis and Renovascular Disease

Renal artery stenosis, most commonly related to atherosclerotic disease at the vessel origin in an older patient or fibromuscular dysplasia, characteristically producing a beaded, string-of-beads appearance from alternating areas of stenosis and poststenotic dilation in a younger patient, most often a woman, is assessed with contrast-enhanced MR angiography as part of a comprehensive renal MRI protocol, and hemodynamically significant stenosis can produce a smaller, poorly enhancing kidney on the affected side together with delayed and diminished nephrographic and excretory phase enhancement relative to the contralateral kidney. Renal artery stenosis carries direct clinical relevance beyond the vascular finding itself, since it represents a correctable cause of secondary hypertension and can contribute to progressive renal function decline if unaddressed, and precise documentation of stenosis severity, location, and any poststenotic dilation supports the interventional or surgical revascularization decision, though the specific patient selection criteria for intervention, generally reserved for more severe stenosis with correlating clinical findings, extend beyond the imaging characterization discussed in this chapter.

Epidemiology of Chronic Kidney Disease and Common Etiologies

Chronic kidney disease affects a substantial proportion of the adult population globally, with diabetic nephropathy and hypertensive nephrosclerosis together accounting for the majority of cases in most developed-world populations, and its rising prevalence, tracking the broader rise in diabetes and obesity discussed in the context of other organ systems throughout this book, has made incidental identification of chronic parenchymal changes on body MRI performed for unrelated indications an increasingly routine occurrence that the radiologist should recognize and characterize even when renal disease is not the primary indication for the examination. Glomerulonephritis, encompassing a diverse group of immune-mediated and other inflammatory processes affecting the glomerulus, produces a similarly nonspecific pattern of parenchymal signal change and, in more advanced or rapidly progressive cases, can present with normal or even enlarged kidney size despite significantly impaired function, a pattern termed the discordant kidney that should prompt consideration of an acute or subacute inflammatory process rather than the more chronic, atrophic pattern typical of longstanding diabetic or hypertensive nephropathy.

Acute Kidney Injury: Imaging Correlates

Acute kidney injury, an abrupt decline in renal function from a variety of causes including prerenal hypoperfusion, intrinsic renal injury such as acute tubular necrosis, and postrenal obstruction, produces variable and often subtle imaging findings that generally cannot reliably distinguish among these mechanisms on morphology alone, such that imaging's primary contribution in acute kidney injury evaluation is typically to exclude a postrenal obstructive cause, readily identified as hydronephrosis, rather than to characterize the specific intrinsic renal injury mechanism, which remains a clinical and laboratory diagnosis. Renal size and cortical thickness on the acute kidney injury evaluation carry some prognostic value, since normal-sized kidneys with preserved cortical thickness suggest a potentially reversible acute process, while small, atrophic kidneys with cortical thinning suggest a superimposed chronic component less likely to fully recover, a distinction relevant to the referring clinician's counseling about the anticipated trajectory of renal function recovery.

Pyelonephritis and Renal Infection

Epidemiology and Risk Factors for Pyelonephritis

Acute pyelonephritis demonstrates a marked female predominance related to the comparatively short female urethra facilitating ascending infection from the bladder, with additional recognized risk factors including diabetes mellitus, which independently predisposes to more severe and complicated infection including an elevated risk of the emphysematous and xanthogranulomatous variants discussed below, urinary tract obstruction or stasis from any cause, vesicoureteral reflux, and pregnancy, during which physiologic ureteral dilation and compression by the gravid uterus both contribute to an elevated pyelonephritis risk relative to the nonpregnant state. Recurrent pyelonephritis, particularly in a child or young adult, should prompt evaluation for an underlying structural or functional predisposing cause, most often vesicoureteral reflux discussed later in this chapter or an anatomic anomaly such as a duplicated collecting system, rather than being attributed to recurrent, unrelated sporadic infection alone, since identifying and addressing a correctable underlying cause can meaningfully reduce the risk of future episodes and the cumulative renal scarring recurrent infection can produce.

Xanthogranulomatous Pyelonephritis

Xanthogranulomatous pyelonephritis, a rare, destructive chronic granulomatous infection most often associated with a long-standing obstructing staghorn calculus and recurrent infection, typically in a patient with diabetes, produces a markedly enlarged, nonfunctioning kidney with multiple dilated, debris-filled calyces demonstrating a characteristic bear-paw appearance, together with a central staghorn calculus and variable extension of the inflammatory process into the perinephric space, a pattern that can closely mimic a complex or infiltrative renal neoplasm on imaging alone given its destructive, mass-like appearance. Correctly recognizing this specific inflammatory entity, most reliably through the combination of a central staghorn calculus, the bear-paw calyceal pattern, and a compatible clinical history of chronic infection, is important both because the treatment, generally nephrectomy given the extensive parenchymal destruction and infection typically present, differs from oncologic surgical planning, and because misdiagnosis as malignancy can lead to inappropriate anxiety or unnecessary additional oncologic workup before the correct inflammatory diagnosis is established, usually only definitively at the time of surgical pathology.

Acute Pyelonephritis: Imaging Features

Acute pyelonephritis on MRI demonstrates one or more wedge-shaped or striated areas of reduced enhancement, most conspicuous on the nephrographic phase, reflecting focal areas of decreased perfusion related to the inflammatory process, together with perinephric fat stranding and, frequently, mild ipsilateral renal enlargement, a pattern that, while classically described using contrast-enhanced CT in most clinical guidelines, translates directly to MRI's multiphase postcontrast technique with comparable diagnostic performance and the added advantage of avoiding ionizing radiation in a population, often young women, for whom repeated imaging over a lifetime of recurrent urinary tract infections is a genuine consideration. Diffusion-weighted imaging contributes meaningfully to pyelonephritis detection and characterization, with the inflamed, infected renal parenchyma typically demonstrating restricted diffusion that can be more conspicuous than the corresponding postcontrast enhancement changes in some cases, making a diffusion-weighted sequence an important complementary component of a renal infection protocol rather than an optional addition.

Renal and Perinephric Abscess

Renal abscess, representing a more advanced, localized complication of pyelonephritis in which the infected parenchyma undergoes frank liquefactive necrosis, presents as a discrete, rim-enhancing fluid collection with central non-enhancing, typically diffusion-restricting contents, a pattern that, once identified, carries direct treatment implications since an abscess of sufficient size, generally cited around three centimeters though clinical judgment and the patient's response to medical therapy alone also factor into this threshold, generally requires percutaneous drainage in addition to antibiotic therapy, unlike uncomplicated pyelonephritis, which is managed with antibiotics alone. Perinephric abscess, in which infection extends beyond the renal capsule into the perinephric space, most often as a complication of an underlying obstructing stone or a delayed or inadequately treated intrarenal abscess, similarly requires drainage in most cases and should prompt a specific search for an underlying obstructing calculus, since source control of any contributing obstruction is essential to definitive treatment and failure to identify and address an obstructing stone risks recurrent or persistent infection despite adequate drainage and antibiotic therapy.

THE SIGNAL-TO-CATEGORY DECISION SYSTEM — Acute Pyelonephritis versus Renal Abscess Triage

---

The Signal Pattern: A patient with clinical signs of urinary tract infection undergoes MRI demonstrating wedge-shaped or striated areas of reduced renal enhancement, and the reader must determine whether the process remains uncomplicated pyelonephritis or has progressed to a drainable abscess.

Category Signature: Wedge-shaped or striated areas of reduced enhancement without a discrete, well-defined fluid collection are categorized as uncomplicated acute pyelonephritis; a discrete, rim-enhancing fluid collection with non-enhancing central contents, particularly exceeding approximately three centimeters, is categorized as abscess requiring drainage.

The Decision: Uncomplicated pyelonephritis is managed with antibiotic therapy alone, generally with clinical and, if needed, imaging follow-up to confirm response; abscess proceeds to percutaneous drainage in addition to antibiotics, with a specific search for and treatment of any underlying obstructing calculus.

Trap Logic: An early, small, or immature abscess can appear as a poorly marginated area of reduced enhancement without the fully developed rim-enhancing, discrete fluid collection morphology of a mature abscess, closely resembling uncomplicated pyelonephritis on a single examination; the discriminating step in a patient failing to improve clinically despite appropriate antibiotic therapy is short-interval follow-up imaging to reassess for interval abscess formation, rather than assuming the initial uncomplicated categorization remains accurate throughout the treatment course.

Pattern Anchor: A discrete, rim-enhancing, non-enhancing-center fluid collection mandates drainage; clinical non-response to antibiotics in presumed uncomplicated pyelonephritis warrants follow-up imaging to reassess for interval abscess formation.

Emphysematous Pyelonephritis

Emphysematous pyelonephritis, a fulminant, gas-forming necrotizing renal infection occurring almost exclusively in patients with poorly controlled diabetes, represents a true urologic and infectious emergency, with mortality historically substantial in the absence of prompt recognition and aggressive treatment, and its recognition on imaging, most classically as intraparenchymal or collecting system gas producing signal void on MRI sequences, a finding this modality is comparatively less sensitive for than CT given gas's more subtle and sometimes ambiguous MRI signal characteristics relative to its unambiguous CT appearance, underscores one of the relatively few clinical scenarios in body imaging where CT may be specifically preferred over MRI for a time-critical diagnosis if either modality is readily available. Management of emphysematous pyelonephritis has evolved toward a more nephron-sparing approach than the historical default of emergent nephrectomy, with percutaneous drainage combined with aggressive antibiotic therapy and glycemic control now achieving renal preservation in a meaningful proportion of appropriately selected, hemodynamically stable patients, reserving emergent nephrectomy for patients with extensive parenchymal destruction or those failing to stabilize despite maximal medical and percutaneous management, a management evolution the radiologist should be aware of when characterizing the extent of parenchymal gas and destruction to support this specific triage decision.

Figure 13.1: Acute Pyelonephritis with Wedge-Shaped Perfusion Defects

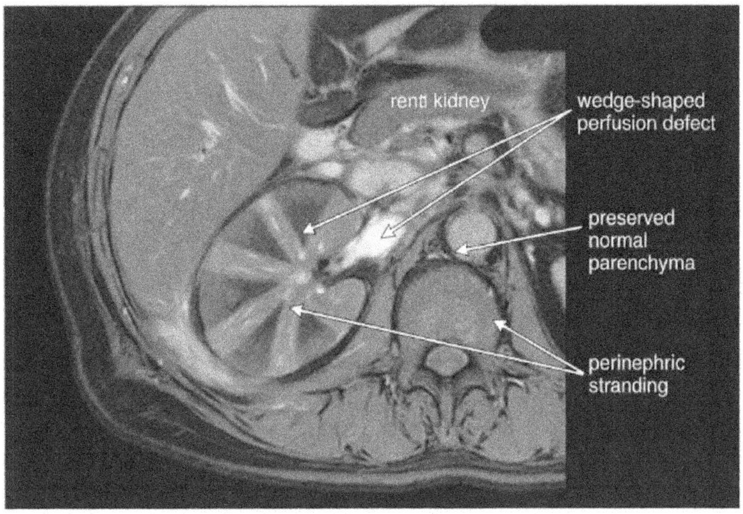

Urothelial Carcinoma and Collecting System Neoplasms

Epidemiology and Risk Factors for Urothelial Carcinoma

Urothelial carcinoma of the upper tract is considerably less common than its bladder counterpart, comprising a small minority of all urothelial malignancies, and shares major risk factors with bladder urothelial carcinoma, most prominently cigarette smoking, the single most consistently identified and modifiable risk factor, together with occupational exposure to aromatic amines and, in specific endemic regions, exposure to aristolochic acid-containing botanical compounds associated with a distinctive nephropathy and markedly elevated upper tract urothelial carcinoma risk. Lynch syndrome, the hereditary colorectal and endometrial cancer syndrome discussed in the pancreatic chapter of this book, carries a specific and disproportionate association with upper tract urothelial carcinoma relative to its considerably lower association with bladder urothelial carcinoma, such that a patient with known or suspected Lynch syndrome presenting with an upper tract urothelial lesion should be recognized as fitting an established hereditary cancer pattern rather than a purely sporadic occurrence, with corresponding implications for genetic counseling and enhanced surveillance of the patient's other Lynch-associated cancer risks.

Bladder Field-Change Considerations and Surveillance Protocol Design

Because the entire urothelium shares a common field-change carcinogenic exposure, a comprehensive upper tract urothelial carcinoma workup and subsequent surveillance protocol must incorporate deliberate, technically adequate visualization of the bladder in addition to the upper tracts, and the excretory phase sequence discussed throughout this chapter, timed to allow adequate bladder distension with excreted contrast, is essential to this complete assessment, since an inadequately distended bladder can obscure a flat or subtle papillary bladder lesion that a well-distended, technically optimized excretory phase acquisition would otherwise reveal. Following treatment of an upper tract urothelial carcinoma, whether by nephroureterectomy or a kidney-sparing endoscopic approach, lifelong bladder surveillance, generally with cystoscopy as the primary surveillance tool given its superior sensitivity for the flat and subtle lesions that cross-sectional imaging can miss, remains essential given the persistent field-change risk, with cross-sectional imaging surveillance of the contralateral upper tract and, when a kidney-sparing approach was used, the treated tract itself, playing a complementary rather than primary surveillance role in this specific clinical context.

Urothelial Carcinoma: Imaging Features and Detection

Urothelial carcinoma of the upper collecting system, arising from the urothelial lining of the renal pelvis or calyces, presents as a soft tissue filling defect within the contrast-opacified collecting system on excretory phase imaging, typically demonstrating measurable enhancement on earlier postcontrast phases that distinguishes it from a non-enhancing stone or blood clot, a distinguishing feature that anchors this chapter's second Rhythm Layer instance and represents one of the most clinically important discriminations in collecting system imaging given the substantially different management pathways each diagnosis triggers. Urothelial carcinoma demonstrates a field-change phenomenon in which the entire urothelium, from the renal pelvis through the ureter to the bladder, carries an elevated risk of synchronous or metachronous tumor development, such that identification of an upper tract urothelial carcinoma should prompt deliberate, complete evaluation of the remaining urothelium, particularly the bladder, using the excretory phase and, when available, dedicated bladder imaging technique discussed in the following chapter, rather than a focused evaluation of the identified lesion alone.

Staging and Grading Considerations

Upper tract urothelial carcinoma staging assesses the depth of invasion into and through the collecting system wall and into the adjacent renal parenchyma or perinephric fat, together with regional lymphadenopathy and distant metastatic disease, using a framework analogous to the depth-of-invasion staging applied to bladder urothelial carcinoma discussed in the following chapter, and this staging assessment directly informs the choice between nephroureterectomy, the standard treatment for higher-stage or higher-grade disease, and a kidney-sparing endoscopic approach appropriate for select low-grade, low-stage, or unifocal disease, particularly in a patient with a solitary kidney or significant baseline renal impairment where preserving renal function carries outsized importance. High-grade upper tract urothelial carcinoma carries a meaningfully worse prognosis than low-grade disease and a greater propensity for invasive, infiltrative growth into the renal parenchyma that can, in advanced cases, produce an appearance overlapping with the centrally infiltrative renal cell carcinoma subtypes discussed in the preceding chapter, underscoring why a central, collecting-system-centered infiltrative renal mass should specifically raise urothelial carcinoma in the differential alongside the renal cell carcinoma subtypes more directly addressed in that chapter.

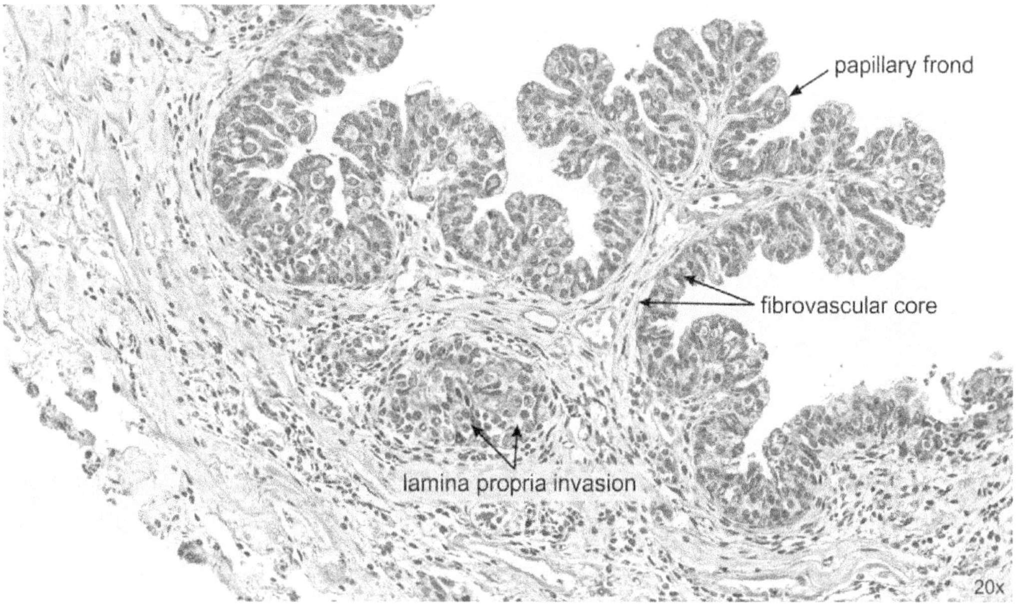

THE SIGNAL-TO-CATEGORY DECISION SYSTEM — Filling Defect in the Collecting System: Urothelial Tumor versus Stone or Clot Trap

The Signal Pattern: A filling defect is identified within the contrast-opacified collecting system on excretory phase imaging, and the reader must determine whether it represents urothelial tumor, stone, or clot before recommending further workup.

Category Signature: A filling defect demonstrating measurable soft tissue enhancement on early postcontrast phases is categorized as favoring urothelial tumor; a filling defect demonstrating no enhancement, particularly with signal characteristics consistent with calcification or blood products on precontrast sequences, is categorized as favoring stone or clot.

The Decision: A filling defect favoring tumor proceeds to urologic referral for ureteroscopic evaluation and biopsy, together with complete urothelial evaluation for field-change disease as discussed above; a filling defect favoring stone or clot is managed according to the relevant benign pathway, with follow-up imaging to confirm resolution or passage when appropriate.

Trap Logic: A small or partially obscured filling defect can be genuinely difficult to assess for enhancement given the confounding effect of adjacent excreted contrast within the collecting system itself, and a blood clot, while classically non-enhancing, can occasionally demonstrate confusing signal characteristics that complicate straightforward categorization; the discriminating step in a genuinely ambiguous filling defect is dedicated delayed or repeat imaging with attention to interval change, since a clot typically diminishes or resolves on follow-up imaging while a tumor persists or grows, providing a time-based discriminator when the single-examination enhancement assessment remains equivocal.

Pattern Anchor: True enhancement, not simply the presence of a filling defect, distinguishes tumor from stone or clot; when enhancement assessment is genuinely equivocal, interval imaging showing persistence versus resolution provides a reliable secondary discriminator.

Hydronephrosis, Obstruction, and Congenital Anomalies

Vesicoureteral Reflux and Reflux Nephropathy

Vesicoureteral reflux, the retrograde flow of urine from the bladder into the ureter and, in more severe grades, into the collecting system itself, is most reliably diagnosed with fluoroscopic or nuclear voiding cystourethrography rather than the cross-sectional imaging emphasized throughout this chapter, but its chronic sequela, reflux nephropathy, produces a distinctive and directly MRI-visible pattern of focal parenchymal scarring, typically most pronounced at the renal poles where the compound papillae are more susceptible to intrarenal reflux, together with corresponding calyceal blunting overlying the scarred segment, a combination that, once recognized, should specifically suggest reflux nephropathy as the underlying chronic process rather than a nonspecific pattern of chronic parenchymal disease. Reflux nephropathy carries long-term implications extending well beyond childhood, including an elevated risk of hypertension and, in more severe or bilateral cases, progressive chronic kidney disease into adulthood, such that its recognition on an adult examination performed for an unrelated indication, even without an antecedent clinical history of childhood urinary tract infection or known reflux, provides clinically useful context for the patient's longitudinal renal function monitoring.

Special Populations: Pediatric and Pregnancy-Related Hydronephrosis

Physiologic hydronephrosis of pregnancy, related to progesterone-mediated ureteral smooth muscle relaxation together with mechanical compression by the gravid uterus, is a normal, expected finding, generally more pronounced on the right side given the uterus's typical rightward dextrorotation and the cushioning effect of the sigmoid colon on the left, and should not be mistaken for pathologic obstruction in the absence of additional concerning features such as significant flank pain, fever, or a visible obstructing calculus, with the degree of physiologic dilation generally most pronounced in the third trimester and resolving following delivery. In the pediatric population, antenatally detected hydronephrosis, increasingly identified on routine prenatal ultrasound, requires postnatal confirmation and, when persistent or high-grade, further evaluation for an underlying cause including ureteropelvic junction obstruction, vesicoureteral reflux, or a posterior urethral valve in a male infant, with MRI, avoiding ionizing radiation entirely, an increasingly favored modality for this specific pediatric evaluation, particularly when functional assessment of differential renal function is also required.

Grading and Characterizing Hydronephrosis

Hydronephrosis is graded by the degree of collecting system dilation, ranging from mild caliectasis alone through severe dilation with associated parenchymal thinning, and while grading systems vary somewhat in their specific terminology, the essential interpretive task is distinguishing a dilated but unobstructed collecting system, as can be seen with vesicoureteral reflux or a prior, now resolved, obstructive episode, from a genuinely obstructed system requiring intervention, a distinction for which MR urography, incorporating heavily T2-weighted sequences that depict the fluid-filled collecting system without requiring intravenous contrast, together with functional assessment when available, contributes meaningfully beyond simple anatomic dilation grading alone. Identifying the specific level and cause of obstruction, whether an intraluminal filling defect as discussed above, an extrinsic mass compressing the ureter, or a stricture, most often at the ureteropelvic or ureterovesical junction, is essential to appropriate management planning, since the treatment approach differs substantially between these etiologies, from simple stone removal to stricture repair to oncologic management of an extrinsic compressing mass.

Ureteropelvic Junction Obstruction

Ureteropelvic junction obstruction, whether congenital, most often identified in childhood or occasionally as an incidental adult finding, or acquired from prior instrumentation, stone disease, or inflammation, produces dilation of the renal pelvis and calyces with an abrupt transition to a normal-caliber, non-dilated ureter at the ureteropelvic junction, a specific anatomic pattern that, once recognized, distinguishes this entity from the more diffuse ureteral dilation seen with a more distal obstruction or with reflux.

Figure 13.3: Collecting System and Ureteral Anatomy

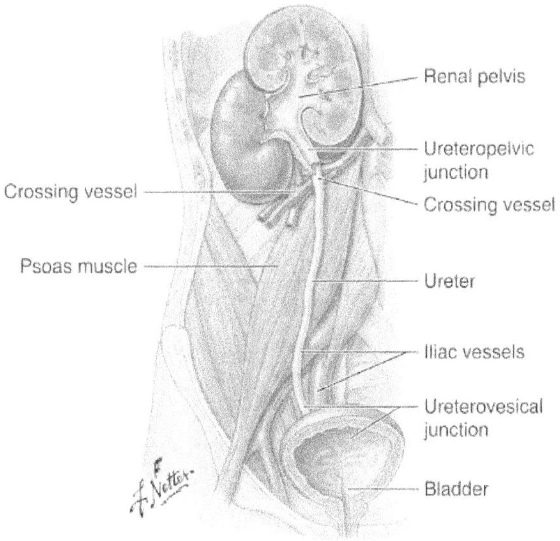

A crossing vessel, most often an accessory or aberrant lower pole renal artery crossing anterior to the ureteropelvic junction, is a recognized contributing or causative factor in a subset of ureteropelvic junction obstruction cases, and its identification on MR angiography carries direct surgical planning relevance, since a pyeloplasty procedure addressing this specific anatomic relationship, transposing the ureter relative to the crossing vessel, differs meaningfully from a standard pyeloplasty performed without this consideration.

Duplicated Collecting Systems and Other Congenital Anomalies

Duplicated collecting system, among the most common congenital urinary tract anomalies, ranges from an incomplete duplication with a single ureter draining both moieties to a complete duplication with two separate ureters draining independently to the bladder, and, per the Weigert-Meyer rule, when complete duplication is present, the upper pole moiety ureter inserts ectopically, often into the bladder inferomedial to the normal orthotopic insertion of the lower pole ureter, or, less commonly, entirely outside the bladder, and is characteristically associated with an obstructing ureterocele, while the lower pole moiety ureter inserts orthotopically but carries an elevated risk of vesicoureteral reflux given its comparatively shortened, more perpendicular submucosal tunnel. Recognizing a duplicated collecting system and correctly assigning findings, hydronephrosis, a ureterocele, or reflux, to the specific upper or lower pole moiety per the Weigert-Meyer rule is essential for coherent, clinically actionable reporting, since the anticipated complication differs by moiety and a report describing findings without this specific moiety attribution provides materially less useful information to the referring urologist than one that does.

Renal Cystic Disease Syndromes

Genetics and Screening in Autosomal Dominant Polycystic Kidney Disease

Autosomal dominant polycystic kidney disease arises predominantly from mutation in one of two genes, PKD1, accounting for the majority of cases and associated with a generally more severe clinical course and earlier progression to end-stage renal disease, and PKD2, associated with a comparatively milder, later-onset disease course, a genotype-phenotype relationship that, together with total kidney volume measurement discussed below, contributes to individualized risk stratification and prognostic counseling for affected patients and their families. Given the autosomal dominant inheritance pattern, at-risk first-degree relatives of an affected patient face a fifty percent inheritance probability, and imaging-based screening in an at-risk relative, most often with ultrasound as the primary, lower-cost screening tool with MRI reserved for equivocal cases or for the detailed volumetric assessment discussed below once the diagnosis is established, follows age-specific diagnostic criteria reflecting the fact that cyst number and size are age-dependent, such that the same cyst burden that would be diagnostic in an older adult may be insufficient to confirm the diagnosis in a young adult still early in the expected disease course.

Syndrome	Inheritance	Key Extrarenal Feature
Autosomal dominant PKD	Autosomal dominant (PKD1, PKD2)	Hepatic cysts, intracranial aneurysm risk
Autosomal recessive PKD	Autosomal recessive	Congenital hepatic fibrosis, biliary ductal plate malformation
Medullary sponge kidney	Generally sporadic	Nephrocalcinosis, stone formation
Tuberous sclerosis complex	Autosomal dominant (TSC1, TSC2)	Multiple bilateral angiomyolipomas, cerebral/cardiac findings

KEY POINT: Total kidney volume in autosomal dominant polycystic kidney disease is a validated prognostic biomarker for renal function decline and should be measured using a consistent, reproducible volumetric technique to support both clinical risk stratification and therapeutic monitoring.

Autosomal Dominant Polycystic Kidney Disease

Autosomal dominant polycystic kidney disease, the most common inherited renal cystic disease, produces progressive bilateral renal enlargement with innumerable cysts of varying size replacing the normal parenchyma, ultimately leading to end-stage renal disease in a substantial proportion of affected individuals, generally in mid to late adulthood, and total kidney volume, measured using semi-automated or manual volumetric technique on MRI, has emerged as a validated prognostic biomarker predicting the rate of subsequent renal function decline, supporting its use in both clinical risk stratification and as an endpoint in therapeutic trials for the disease-modifying medications now available for this condition. Extrarenal manifestations of autosomal dominant polycystic kidney disease, including hepatic cysts, present in a substantial majority of affected patients and generally not affecting hepatic function even when numerous, intracranial aneurysm, carrying a meaningfully elevated prevalence relative to the general population and warranting screening in patients with a family history of aneurysm rupture, and, less commonly, pancreatic and splenic cysts, should be specifically assessed and documented on renal imaging performed for this indication, given their relevance to the patient's comprehensive management beyond the renal findings alone.

Figure 13.4: Percutaneous Nephrostomy Placement for Obstructed Infected Collecting System

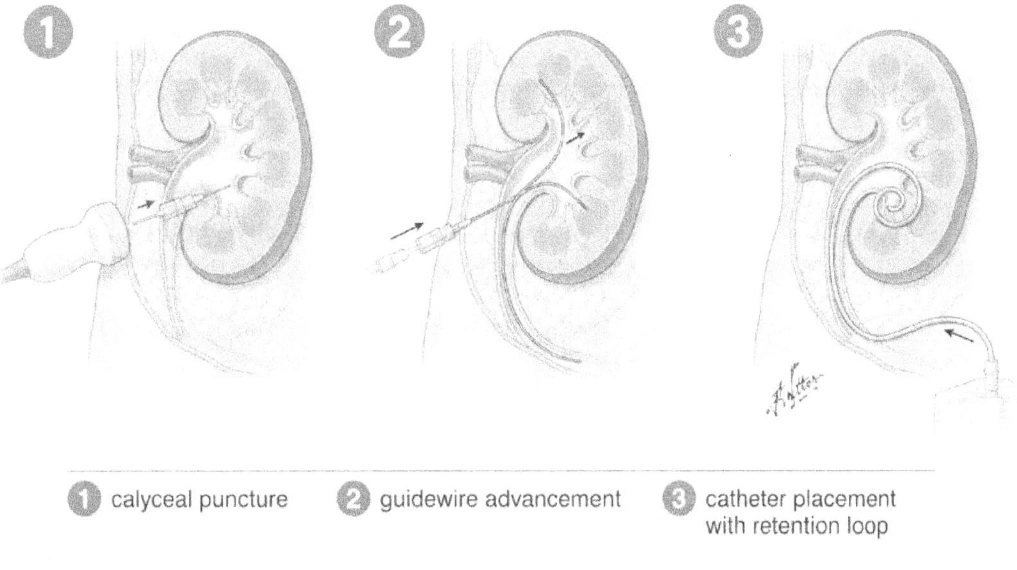

Autosomal Recessive Polycystic Kidney Disease and Other Cystic Syndromes

Autosomal recessive polycystic kidney disease, a distinct and considerably rarer entity typically presenting in infancy or childhood with markedly enlarged, diffusely echogenic or, on MRI, diffusely abnormal-signal kidneys containing innumerable tiny cysts too small to be individually resolved, differs sharply from the adult-onset autosomal dominant form both in its inheritance pattern and its characteristic association with congenital hepatic fibrosis and biliary ductal plate malformation, extrahepatic manifestations that should be specifically assessed when this pediatric-onset entity is suspected or confirmed. Medullary sponge kidney, a comparatively benign entity characterized by cystic dilation of the medullary and papillary collecting ducts producing a characteristic striated or brush-like nephrogram pattern on excretory phase imaging together with a predisposition to medullary nephrocalcinosis and stone formation, and tuberous sclerosis complex, associated with multiple bilateral angiomyolipomas as discussed in the preceding chapter together with renal cysts, round out the major renal cystic disease syndromes relevant to body MRI interpretation, each carrying a distinct genetic basis, clinical trajectory, and extrarenal manifestation pattern worth recognizing beyond the renal cystic appearance alone.

CAUTION: An infected, obstructed collecting system is a urologic emergency requiring urgent decompression, typically with percutaneous nephrostomy or ureteral stenting, regardless of the specific cause of obstruction; identification of this combination should be communicated to the clinical team without delay.

Clinical Case Presentations

Case 1. A 29-year-old woman with fever and flank pain undergoes MRI demonstrating a wedge-shaped area of reduced enhancement in the right kidney with adjacent perinephric fat stranding, without a discrete fluid collection. The radiologist categorizes the findings as uncomplicated acute pyelonephritis and recommends continued antibiotic therapy with clinical follow-up rather than intervention, appropriately distinguishing this pattern from the discrete, rim-enhancing collection that would instead warrant drainage.

Case 2. A 68-year-old man with painless gross hematuria undergoes MRI demonstrating a 1.8-centimeter soft tissue filling defect within the right renal pelvis demonstrating clear postcontrast enhancement on early phase imaging, distinct from the surrounding contrast-opacified collecting system on excretory phase imaging. Recognizing the confirmed enhancement as diagnostic of urothelial tumor rather than stone or clot, the radiologist recommends urologic referral for ureteroscopic evaluation and biopsy, together with dedicated evaluation of the bladder and contralateral upper tract given the field-change risk emphasized in this chapter.

Case 3. A 45-year-old man with acute left flank pain and fever undergoes MRI demonstrating moderate left hydronephrosis with a 6-millimeter non-enhancing filling defect at the ureterovesical junction and no discrete abscess, but with the collecting system appearing tensely dilated and the patient febrile and clinically unwell. Recognizing the combination of obstruction and infection as a urologic emergency regardless of the benign, stone-related cause of the obstruction itself, the radiologist urgently communicates the findings to the clinical team, and the patient undergoes emergent percutaneous nephrostomy placement for source control before definitive stone management is pursued once the infection resolves.

Case 4. A 34-year-old woman with a family history of polycystic kidney disease and known hypertension undergoes surveillance MRI demonstrating bilaterally enlarged kidneys with innumerable cysts of varying size replacing the normal parenchyma, together with several hepatic cysts. The radiologist performs total kidney volume measurement to support prognostic risk stratification and specifically documents the absence of any intracranial finding on the limited sequences available, recommending dedicated intracranial vascular imaging given her family history to screen for the aneurysm risk associated with her underlying autosomal dominant polycystic kidney disease.

Case 5. A 4-year-old girl with recurrent urinary tract infections undergoes MRI demonstrating a duplicated left collecting system with hydronephrosis of the upper pole moiety and an associated ureterocele at the bladder base, with the lower pole moiety appearing grossly normal without hydronephrosis. Applying the Weigert-Meyer rule, the radiologist correctly attributes the hydronephrosis and ureterocele specifically to the upper pole moiety in the report, providing the pediatric urology team with the moiety-specific detail needed for appropriate surgical planning rather than a general description of duplication and hydronephrosis alone.

Case 6. A 58-year-old man with poorly controlled diabetes and a known long-standing left staghorn calculus presents with chronic flank pain and low-grade fevers, and MRI demonstrates a markedly enlarged, nonfunctioning left kidney with multiple dilated, debris-filled calyces in a bear-paw configuration surrounding the known central calculus, with mild extension of inflammatory change into the perinephric fat. Recognizing this combination as characteristic of xanthogranulomatous pyelonephritis rather than an infiltrative renal neoplasm, the radiologist appropriately frames the differential in the report and recommends urology referral for likely nephrectomy given the extensive parenchymal destruction, correctly anticipating the surgical pathology confirmation of this specific chronic inflammatory entity rather than raising undue concern for malignancy.

Case 7. A 61-year-old woman with poorly controlled diabetes presents critically ill with septic shock and left flank pain, and MRI demonstrates extensive signal void within the left renal parenchyma and collecting system consistent with gas, together with extension into the perinephric space. Recognizing this as emphysematous pyelonephritis, the radiologist urgently communicates the findings, and given the patient's hemodynamic stabilization following aggressive resuscitation and the absence of extensive parenchymal destruction on the current examination, the urology team elects percutaneous drainage with intensive antibiotic and glycemic management rather than emergent nephrectomy, achieving renal preservation with resolution confirmed on follow-up imaging.

THE SIGNAL-TO-CATEGORY DECISION SYSTEM — Renal Parenchymal and Collecting System Triage Arc

The Signal Pattern: This chapter's patterns span the renal parenchymal and collecting system risk spectrum, from a perfusion abnormality whose progression to a drainable abscess must be actively excluded, to a collecting system filling defect whose enhancement must be confirmed before a benign stone or clot label is applied.

Category Signature: Renal perfusion abnormalities are categorized as uncomplicated pyelonephritis or drainable abscess based on the presence of a discrete, rim-enhancing collection; collecting system filling defects are categorized as tumor or stone/clot based on confirmed enhancement.

The Decision: Category assignment in this chapter ranges from antibiotics alone to urgent percutaneous drainage, and from benign observation to urologic oncology referral, with every category assigned only after the specific confirmatory feature, a discrete fluid collection or true enhancement, has been explicitly verified.

The Trap Logic: Both patterns in this chapter share a common trap: an early or incompletely evolved finding, an immature abscess or an equivocally enhancing filling defect, that resists confident single-examination categorization and requires either close clinical correlation or interval imaging to resolve.

Pattern Anchor: When single-examination categorization is genuinely equivocal in this chapter, interval change, whether clinical response to antibiotics or imaging persistence versus resolution, is the most reliable secondary discriminator.

Summary and Key Concepts

Loss of corticomedullary differentiation is a nonspecific marker of diffuse renal parenchymal disease; asymmetric involvement should prompt a search for a unilateral, potentially correctable cause such as renal artery stenosis.

Acute pyelonephritis shows wedge-shaped perfusion defects without a discrete collection; a rim-enhancing, non-enhancing-center fluid collection defines abscess and generally requires drainage in addition to antibiotics.

A collecting system filling defect demonstrating true postcontrast enhancement favors urothelial tumor; a non-enhancing defect favors stone or clot, with interval imaging resolving genuinely equivocal cases.

Upper tract urothelial carcinoma carries a field-change risk requiring complete urothelial evaluation, particularly of the bladder, once identified.

An infected, obstructed collecting system is a urologic emergency requiring urgent decompression regardless of the underlying cause of obstruction.

A crossing vessel at the ureteropelvic junction carries direct surgical planning relevance for pyeloplasty; duplicated collecting system findings should be attributed to the specific moiety per the Weigert-Meyer rule.

Autosomal dominant polycystic kidney disease total kidney volume is a validated prognostic biomarker; intracranial aneurysm screening is relevant in patients with a family history of aneurysm rupture.

CHAPTER 14: PROSTATE MRI AND THE PI-RADS FRAMEWORK

Learning Objectives

1. Describe prostate zonal anatomy and its relevance to lesion localization and biopsy planning.
2. Apply the PI-RADS framework to assign a structured suspicion category to a prostate lesion.
3. Recognize the imaging features of clinically significant prostate cancer in the peripheral and transition zones.
4. Apply extraprostatic extension and seminal vesicle invasion assessment relevant to staging and surgical planning.
5. Recognize benign prostatic hyperplasia and prostatitis and distinguish them from clinically significant cancer.

Clinical Overview

Multiparametric prostate MRI has transformed prostate cancer diagnosis over the past decade, shifting the diagnostic pathway from a systematic, essentially blind biopsy sampling approach toward a targeted, image-guided strategy that substantially improves detection of clinically significant cancer while reducing overdiagnosis of the low-grade, indolent disease that need not be treated, and the PI-RADS framework discussed throughout this chapter is the structured reporting system that has made this transformation reproducible and actionable across the radiology community. This chapter proceeds from prostate zonal anatomy, through the PI-RADS framework itself, peripheral and transition zone cancer characterization, extraprostatic extension and staging, and closes with benign prostatic hyperplasia and prostatitis as the major benign mimics of clinically significant disease.

Two instances of the Signal-to-Category Decision System are applied in this chapter, the first to PI-RADS category assignment itself, and the second to the transition zone cancer-versus-benign prostatic hyperplasia nodule distinction, one of the more challenging discriminations in prostate imaging given the zone's inherent heterogeneity.

Prostate Zonal Anatomy and Multiparametric Technique

KEY POINT: Endorectal coil use has declined substantially in contemporary prostate MRI practice as modern surface coil array technology and higher field-strength magnets have narrowed the image quality gap, though an endorectal coil may still be considered for a technically challenging examination or a lower field-strength scanner where the additional signal-to-noise benefit remains clinically meaningful.

Zonal Anatomy: Peripheral, Transition, and Central Zones

The prostate is divided into the peripheral zone, comprising the majority of the gland's posterior and lateral aspect and the site of origin for the substantial majority of clinically significant prostate cancers, the transition zone, surrounding the urethra and the site of origin for benign prostatic hyperplasia as well as a meaningful minority of prostate cancers, and the central zone, a comparatively small region surrounding the ejaculatory ducts that is an uncommon site of primary cancer but can be secondarily involved by seminal vesicle invasion, an anatomic framework introduced by McNeal that remains the foundation for both PI-RADS lesion localization and biopsy and treatment planning throughout this chapter. This zonal framework directly informs the differential diagnosis and imaging interpretation strategy for any given prostate lesion, since a peripheral zone lesion is approached with the cancer-focused interpretive framework discussed in the following section, while a transition zone lesion must be interpreted against the backdrop of the benign prostatic hyperplasia nodularity that is nearly universal in this zone in older men, a distinction that anchors this chapter's second Rhythm Layer instance.

Multiparametric Sequence Protocol and Technical Requirements

Multiparametric prostate MRI, as introduced in the protocol design chapter of this book, requires high-resolution T2-weighted imaging in multiple planes for anatomic and zonal detail, diffusion-weighted imaging with a high b-value acquisition and corresponding apparent diffusion coefficient map as the single most important sequence for lesion detection and characterization, and dynamic contrast-enhanced imaging as a supportive, dominant-sequence-adjacent technique rather than a primary determinant of suspicion category under current PI-RADS criteria. Patient preparation, including a period of ejaculatory abstinence to reduce seminal vesicle distension and, in some protocols, a preceding bowel preparation to reduce rectal gas and peristalsis artifact that can degrade diffusion-weighted image quality, meaningfully affects diagnostic image quality, and technical inadequacy from motion, susceptibility artifact related to rectal gas, or suboptimal diffusion-weighted image quality should be explicitly acknowledged in the report when present, since a technically limited examination carries a correspondingly limited negative predictive value that the referring urologist should understand before relying on a reassuring interpretation to defer biopsy.

Epidemiology of Prostate Cancer and Screening Considerations

Prostate cancer is among the most commonly diagnosed malignancies in men, though its clinical behavior spans an unusually wide spectrum from indolent, low-grade disease that may never require treatment to aggressive, high-grade disease with substantial metastatic potential, a biologic heterogeneity that has historically complicated screening strategy given the risk of overdiagnosing and overtreating indolent disease inherent to serum prostate-specific antigen-based screening alone. The incorporation of multiparametric MRI into the diagnostic pathway, generally performed after an elevated prostate-specific antigen result but before biopsy, has meaningfully improved this risk-benefit calculus by allowing a substantial proportion of men with a low-suspicion examination to safely defer biopsy, reducing both the number of biopsies performed and the detection of clinically insignificant disease that a purely prostate-specific antigen-triggered systematic biopsy approach would otherwise identify, representing one of the more significant recent advances in prostate cancer diagnostic strategy.

Anatomic Boundaries and Landmark Structures Relevant to Reporting

Beyond the three glandular zones discussed above, several additional anatomic structures carry direct relevance to prostate MRI reporting: the neurovascular bundles, coursing along the posterolateral prostate margin and responsible for erectile function, whose proximity to a peripheral zone lesion should be specifically documented given direct implications for nerve-sparing surgical planning, the anterior fibromuscular stroma, a non-glandular band along the anterior prostate surface that is an uncommon but recognized site of cancer origin discussed further below, and the prostate apex and base, whose precise involvement by a lesion should be documented using the standardized twelve-sector or thirty-nine-sector PI-RADS sector map framework rather than a general anatomic description, ensuring the biopsy team can precisely localize the same lesion identified on imaging during the subsequent targeted procedure.

Interobserver Variability and Quality Assurance in Prostate MRI Interpretation

PI-RADS category assignment, despite its structured framework, retains a meaningful degree of interobserver variability, particularly at the category 3-versus-4 boundary where the distinction can hinge on subtle differences in apparent diffusion coefficient signal interpretation or lesion size measurement near a threshold value, and this variability has driven increasing emphasis on dedicated reader training, volume-based experience thresholds, and structured quality assurance programs at institutions performing prostate MRI, reflecting an accumulating body of evidence that reader experience meaningfully affects both cancer detection rate and the appropriate, judicious use of the category 3 designation rather than its overuse as a default categorization for genuine diagnostic uncertainty. Institutional and national quality assurance initiatives, including standardized reporting templates, structured sector map documentation, and periodic outcome correlation between assigned PI-RADS category and eventual biopsy pathology, are increasingly recognized as essential components of a mature prostate MRI program rather than optional adjuncts, given the direct clinical consequences, missed clinically significant cancer from undercalling or unnecessary biopsy from overcalling, that flow directly from category assignment accuracy.

The PI-RADS Framework

PI-RADS Category Assignment: Dominant Sequence by Zone

The PI-RADS framework assigns a five-point suspicion category to each identified lesion based on a zone-specific dominant sequence: in the peripheral zone, diffusion-weighted imaging and its corresponding apparent diffusion coefficient map serve as the dominant sequence, with T2-weighted imaging playing a supportive role, while in the transition zone, T2-weighted imaging serves as the dominant sequence given the greater diagnostic value of morphologic assessment in this zone's structurally heterogeneous, hyperplastic background, with diffusion-weighted imaging playing a supportive role, an inverted dominant-sequence assignment between the two zones that reflects each zone's distinct underlying tissue architecture and the resulting differential diagnostic value of each sequence type. Category 1 and 2 findings are considered very low and low probability of clinically significant cancer respectively, category 3 represents genuine indeterminate probability, category 4 represents high probability, and category 5 represents very high probability, with the specific descriptive criteria for each category, size and morphology thresholds for the dominant sequence findings, defined in detail within the PI-RADS technical specification that guides consistent category assignment across readers and institutions.

Dynamic Contrast Enhancement and Category Modification

Dynamic contrast-enhanced imaging's primary role under current PI-RADS criteria is to potentially upgrade a peripheral zone category 3 lesion to category 4 when focal, early, and corresponding enhancement is present at the same location as the equivocal diffusion-weighted finding, a specific and limited modifying role rather than an independent category-determining sequence, reflecting the framework's emphasis on diffusion-weighted imaging as the primary peripheral zone determinant with dynamic contrast enhancement functioning as a corroborating, category-nudging adjunct only in this specific intermediate-category scenario. This comparatively limited role for dynamic contrast enhancement represents an evolution from earlier prostate MRI reporting approaches that weighted contrast enhancement more heavily, reflecting accumulated evidence that diffusion-weighted imaging alone carries superior standalone diagnostic performance for clinically significant cancer detection, though dynamic contrast-enhanced imaging remains part of the standard multiparametric protocol given its category 3-to-4 modifying value and its contribution to characterizing lesions in a technically limited diffusion-weighted acquisition.

THE SIGNAL-TO-CATEGORY DECISION SYSTEM — PI-RADS Category Assignment

---

The Signal Pattern: A prostate lesion is identified, and the reader must first establish its zone of origin before assessing the dominant-sequence finding appropriate to that zone.

Category Signature: In the peripheral zone, a lesion is categorized primarily by its diffusion-weighted imaging and apparent diffusion coefficient appearance, ranging from category 1, normal, through category 5, a markedly hypointense apparent diffusion coefficient focus with corresponding high b-value hyperintensity measuring 1.5 centimeters or greater or demonstrating definite extraprostatic extension; in the transition zone, a lesion is categorized primarily by its T2-weighted morphology, ranging from category 1, a normal, encapsulated hyperplastic nodule, through category 5, a lenticular or non-circumscribed, markedly hypointense mass measuring 1.5 centimeters or greater.

The Decision: Category 1 and 2 lesions generally do not warrant targeted biopsy; category 3 lesions warrant clinical correlation, often with serum prostate-specific antigen density, before a biopsy decision is finalized, with dynamic contrast enhancement potentially upgrading a peripheral zone category 3 lesion as discussed above; category 4 and 5 lesions warrant targeted biopsy given their substantial probability of clinically significant cancer.

Trap Logic: A lesion straddling the peripheral and transition zone boundary, or one whose zone of origin is genuinely ambiguous given distortion from an adjacent large hyperplastic nodule, can be miscategorized if the wrong zone-specific dominant sequence framework is applied; the discriminating step is careful, deliberate zonal localization on high-resolution T2-weighted imaging in multiple planes before applying either zone's category criteria, since applying the peripheral zone's diffusion-dominant framework to a genuinely transition zone lesion, or the reverse, can produce a meaningfully different and potentially inaccurate category assignment.

Pattern Anchor: Confirm the lesion's zone of origin before applying category criteria; the dominant sequence differs by zone, and misapplying the wrong zone's framework produces an inaccurate category.

PI-RADS Structured Reporting and Sector Map Documentation

A complete PI-RADS report documents each identified lesion's location using the standardized sector map, its size in at least two dimensions, its assigned category with the specific dominant and supportive sequence findings supporting that assignment, and, when relevant, extraprostatic extension or seminal vesicle invasion findings discussed later in this chapter, a level of structured detail considerably more granular than a general narrative description of prostate findings and one that directly supports both the biopsy team's precise targeting and the surgical team's operative planning when treatment is ultimately pursued. Overall gland assessment, including prostate volume calculation and a general description of background transition zone hyperplastic change, is typically included alongside the individual lesion-specific findings, providing the referring clinician with both the overall gland context, relevant to symptom correlation and prostate-specific antigen density calculation, and the specific, actionable lesion-level detail that drives the biopsy and treatment planning decision.

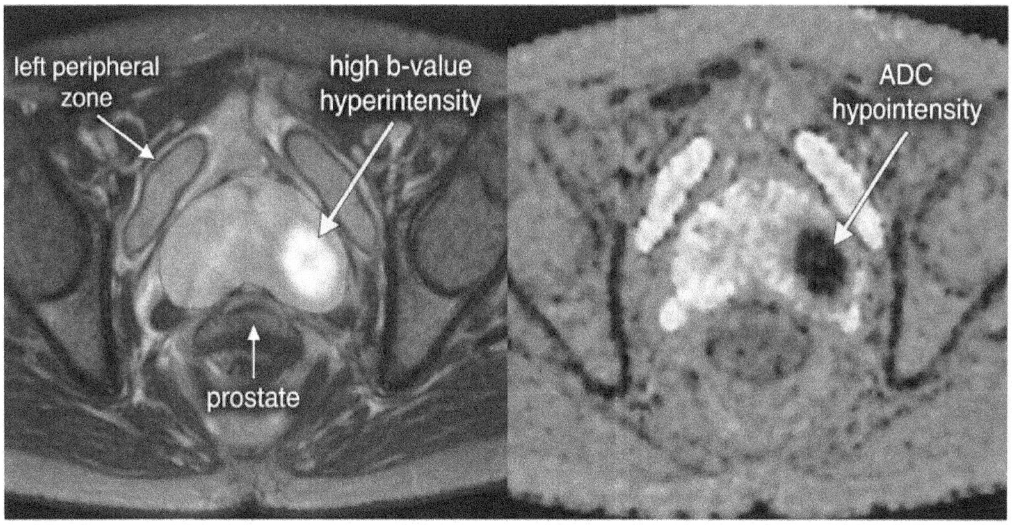

Figure 14.1: PI-RADS Category 5 Peripheral Zone Lesion.

Active Surveillance and the Role of MRI in Monitoring

Active surveillance, involving serial monitoring rather than immediate treatment, has become an increasingly accepted management strategy for men with lower-risk, biopsy-confirmed prostate cancer, reflecting the recognition that many such cancers carry a sufficiently indolent natural history that immediate treatment, with its associated risk of urinary and sexual side effects, may not offer a meaningful survival benefit over careful monitoring with treatment reserved for evidence of progression, and multiparametric MRI has assumed a central role in this monitoring strategy, both at surveillance entry to confirm the absence of a higher-suspicion lesion that may have been missed by the original systematic biopsy sampling, and at surveillance intervals to detect interval change in a previously identified lesion. Interval increase in PI-RADS category, lesion size, or the development of a new lesion on surveillance MRI generally prompts repeat targeted biopsy to reassess for grade progression, while a stable examination supports continued surveillance without repeat biopsy in some protocols, reflecting an evolving, imaging-integrated approach to active surveillance that reduces the biopsy burden relative to protocols relying on scheduled biopsy alone regardless of interval imaging findings.

Peripheral and Transition Zone Cancer Characterization

Peripheral Zone Cancer: Morphology and Grading Correlation

Clinically significant peripheral zone cancer typically demonstrates a focal, round or lenticular area of restricted diffusion with corresponding low T2 signal, and the degree of diffusion restriction correlates, albeit imperfectly, with the Gleason grade group that will ultimately be established on biopsy, with more markedly restricted diffusion generally, though not invariably, corresponding to higher-grade disease, a correlation that contributes to, without independently determining, the pretest probability assessment the urologist applies alongside the formal PI-RADS category when counseling a patient about biopsy. Low-grade, low-volume peripheral zone cancer can present with subtle or absent imaging findings, an important limitation underlying the framework's design intent of prioritizing detection of clinically significant, intermediate-to-high-grade disease over exhaustive detection of every focus of cancer regardless of grade, since indolent, low-grade disease, sometimes termed clinically insignificant cancer given its minimal metastatic potential, need not necessarily be detected or treated, and a normal or low-category multiparametric examination should not be interpreted as excluding all prostate cancer, only as substantially lowering the probability of the clinically significant disease this framework is specifically designed to detect.

Transition Zone Cancer Versus Benign Prostatic Hyperplasia Nodule

Transition zone cancer typically presents as a lenticular or non-circumscribed, homogeneously markedly hypointense mass on T2-weighted imaging with corresponding diffusion restriction, an appearance termed the erased charcoal sign given its smudged, non-encapsulated margin, in contrast to the well-circumscribed, encapsulated, and often heterogeneous appearance of a benign hyperplastic nodule, which frequently demonstrates a mixed stromal and glandular composition producing variable T2 signal intensity within a single nodule and a discrete, encapsulating pseudocapsule that a transition zone cancer characteristically lacks. This morphologic distinction, well-circumscribed and encapsulated favoring benign hyperplasia versus non-circumscribed and homogeneously hypointense favoring cancer, is the essential interpretive skill for transition zone lesion characterization, and its reliable application requires deliberate attention to lesion margin and internal heterogeneity rather than size or overall T2 signal intensity alone, since a large benign hyperplastic nodule can demonstrate substantial T2 hypointensity in its stromal-predominant component that superficially resembles cancer if margin and encapsulation are not specifically assessed.

THE SIGNAL-TO-CATEGORY DECISION SYSTEM — Transition Zone Cancer versus Benign Prostatic Hyperplasia Nodule

The Signal Pattern: A transition zone lesion with reduced T2 signal is identified, and the reader must determine whether its morphology favors benign hyperplastic nodularity or transition zone cancer before assigning a PI-RADS category.

Category Signature: A well-circumscribed, encapsulated lesion, particularly one demonstrating heterogeneous internal signal reflecting mixed stromal and glandular composition, is categorized as favoring benign hyperplastic nodule; a lenticular or non-circumscribed lesion with homogeneous, markedly reduced T2 signal lacking a discrete capsule is categorized as favoring cancer.

The Decision: A lesion favoring benign hyperplasia is generally assigned a lower PI-RADS category without targeted biopsy in the absence of other concerning features; a lesion favoring cancer with a non-circumscribed, homogeneously hypointense morphology is assigned a higher category and proceeds to targeted biopsy.

Trap Logic: A large, stromal-predominant benign hyperplastic nodule can demonstrate substantial homogeneous T2 hypointensity that superficially resembles the cancer pattern if margin and encapsulation are not specifically and deliberately assessed; the discriminating step is systematically evaluating lesion margin and the presence or absence of a discrete encapsulating pseudocapsule on high-resolution T2-weighted imaging before relying on signal intensity alone.

Pattern Anchor: Margin and encapsulation, not signal intensity alone, distinguish benign hyperplastic nodule from transition zone cancer; a stromal-predominant nodule can mimic cancer's hypointensity without deliberate margin assessment.

Anterior Fibromuscular Stroma and Rare Sites of Origin

Cancer arising from or extending into the anterior fibromuscular stroma, an uncommon but recognized site given this structure's predominantly non-glandular, fibromuscular composition, presents a distinct diagnostic challenge given the region's inherently low baseline signal on both T2-weighted and diffusion-weighted imaging, which can obscure a tumor's contrast against this already hypointense background more than in the more conventionally assessed peripheral or transition zone, requiring the reader to specifically and deliberately assess this anterior region rather than relying on the same signal contrast expectations applied elsewhere in the gland. A transition zone or anterior fibromuscular stroma cancer of sufficient size can produce a bulging anterior gland contour or capsular abnormality analogous to the extraprostatic extension signs discussed later in this chapter, and recognizing this specific anterior location and its distinct interpretive challenges is particularly relevant given that anterior tumors are disproportionately more likely to be missed by a standard systematic biopsy template, which historically sampled the posterior peripheral zone more comprehensively than the anterior gland, underscoring one of the specific detection advantages multiparametric MRI-targeted biopsy offers over systematic sampling alone.

Multifocal and Bilateral Disease

Prostate cancer not infrequently presents as multiple, spatially distinct foci within the same gland, a pattern with direct relevance to treatment planning, particularly for focal therapy approaches that treat only a targeted portion of the gland rather than the entire prostate, since unrecognized multifocality can result in undertreatment of a clinically significant focus outside the primary treatment zone, making complete, systematic documentation of every identified lesion, not solely the single highest-category index lesion, an essential component of a comprehensive prostate MRI report when focal therapy is being considered as a treatment option. When multiple lesions of differing PI-RADS category are identified, the highest-category lesion, generally termed the index lesion, is typically the primary driver of the biopsy and treatment planning decision given its correlation with the tumor most likely to determine overall prognosis, though secondary lesions still warrant biopsy consideration and documentation, particularly when a focal or partial-gland treatment approach that would need to account for their location is under consideration.

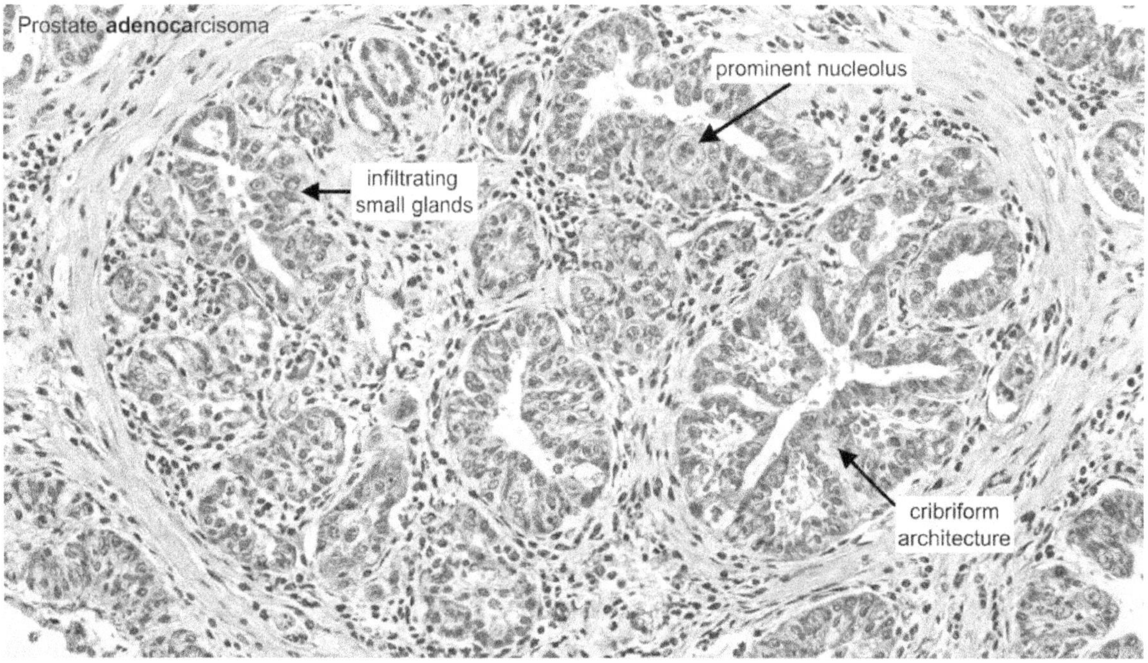

Extraprostatic Extension and Staging

Assessing Extraprostatic Extension

Extraprostatic extension, tumor extension beyond the prostatic capsule into the periprostatic fat, is assessed through a combination of direct and indirect signs, including a bulging or irregular capsular contour, capsular disruption with direct tumoral extension into periprostatic fat, obliteration of the normally visible rectoprostatic angle, and, most specifically, measurable tumor-capsule contact length, with a longer length of capsular contact correlating with a substantially elevated probability of true extraprostatic extension even in the absence of a frank, unambiguous capsular breach. This assessment carries direct treatment planning relevance, since confirmed or highly suspected extraprostatic extension generally favors a non-nerve-sparing or wide-margin surgical approach when radical prostatectomy is pursued, given the elevated positive margin risk a nerve-sparing approach would carry in this setting, or may favor a primary radiation-based treatment approach over surgery altogether depending on the extent and location of extension, making precise, side-specific documentation of extraprostatic extension, including its location and estimated extent, essential information for the treating urologist or radiation oncologist.

Seminal Vesicle Invasion and Nodal Assessment

Seminal vesicle invasion, most reliably identified as loss of the normal seminal vesicle's tubular, feathery internal architecture with replacement by solid, low T2 signal tumor tissue, together with direct tumoral extension from the prostate base along the ejaculatory duct complex into the seminal vesicle, represents locally advanced disease carrying a substantially worse prognosis than organ-confined cancer and, similar to extraprostatic extension, meaningfully influences the surgical approach and the appropriateness of surgery as a primary treatment modality at all in more extensive cases. Regional lymph node assessment in prostate cancer staging focuses on the obturator, internal iliac, and external iliac nodal stations, using morphologic criteria, size together with rounded configuration and loss of the normal fatty hilum, similar to the criteria applied to lymphadenopathy elsewhere in this book, though conventional cross-sectional imaging carries recognized limitations in detecting microscopic nodal metastatic disease, a limitation that has driven increasing use of dedicated molecular imaging techniques for higher-risk disease, a topic addressed further in the whole-body oncologic imaging chapter later in this book.

Post-Treatment Imaging: Recurrence After Prostatectomy and Radiation

Following radical prostatectomy, local recurrence presents as a soft tissue nodule at the vesicourethral anastomosis or within the prostatectomy bed demonstrating restricted diffusion and, on dynamic contrast-enhanced imaging, early, focal enhancement against the expected absence of any residual normal prostate tissue in this surgically altered anatomy, a comparatively more straightforward interpretive scenario than post-radiation recurrence given the complete absence of background glandular tissue that could otherwise confound the differential. Following radiation therapy, by contrast, the entire gland typically demonstrates diffusely decreased T2 signal and altered background diffusion characteristics from radiation-induced fibrosis, complicating recurrence detection relative to the post-prostatectomy setting, and a focal area of recurrent restricted diffusion and early enhancement within this diffusely altered background, particularly correlating with a site of prior known disease or a rising serum prostate-specific antigen after an initial post-treatment nadir, is the key pattern the reader should specifically seek against this more challenging, diffusely abnormal post-radiation background.

Special Populations: BRCA and Hereditary Prostate Cancer Risk

Germline BRCA2 mutation, and to a lesser extent BRCA1 mutation, carries a meaningfully elevated prostate cancer risk together with an association with higher-grade, more aggressive disease at diagnosis relative to sporadic prostate cancer, an association that has prompted some professional guidelines to recommend earlier and more frequent screening in known BRCA mutation carriers than the general population screening interval, and recognizing a family history suggestive of hereditary breast, ovarian, or prostate cancer syndrome in a patient undergoing prostate MRI provides relevant context that can appropriately heighten the reader's vigilance for a subtle but clinically significant lesion, particularly given this population's association with more aggressive disease biology. This hereditary risk context, while not directly changing the mechanics of PI-RADS category assignment itself, appropriately informs the broader clinical risk stratification the referring urologist applies alongside the imaging findings when counseling a BRCA-positive patient about screening frequency and the threshold for biopsy of an intermediate-category finding.

Figure 14.3

Figure 14.3: Prostate Zonal Anatomy and Neurovascular Bundle Relationships

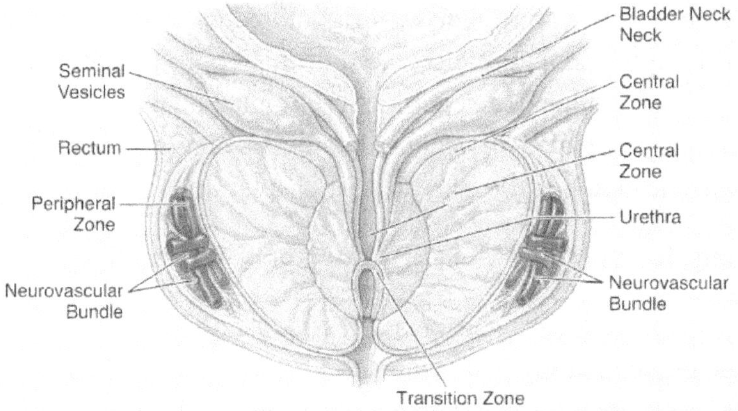

Benign Prostatic Hyperplasia and Prostatitis

Benign Prostatic Hyperplasia: Imaging Pattern and Clinical Correlation

Benign prostatic hyperplasia, an essentially universal finding in aging men reflecting progressive transition zone glandular and stromal proliferation, produces the heterogeneous, nodular, encapsulated transition zone appearance discussed above and, when sufficiently large, can produce significant lower urinary tract symptoms and bladder outlet obstruction addressed further in the following chapter's bladder discussion, though the correlation between prostate size and symptom severity is genuinely imperfect, such that imaging-based gland volume measurement, while useful for surgical planning when intervention is indicated, should not be over-interpreted as a direct proxy for symptom burden in isolation from the patient's clinical presentation. Prostate volume, generally calculated using an ellipsoid formula from three orthogonal diameter measurements, is also a component of prostate-specific antigen density calculation, dividing serum prostate-specific antigen by prostate volume to normalize for the expected antigen elevation from benign hyperplastic tissue alone, a calculation with direct relevance to the category 3 biopsy decision discussed earlier in this chapter, since a lower prostate-specific antigen density in a patient with a large gland reduces the probability that an elevated absolute prostate-specific antigen reflects clinically significant cancer rather than benign hyperplasia alone.

Prostatitis and Its Imaging Mimicry of Cancer

Acute and chronic prostatitis can produce peripheral zone signal abnormality with restricted diffusion that closely mimics the appearance of clinically significant cancer, an important and well-recognized diagnostic pitfall given prostatitis's relative commonality, particularly in a younger patient or one with a compatible clinical history of recent instrumentation, infection, or pelvic pain syndrome, and this mimicry underscores why clinical correlation, including recent symptoms, prior biopsy or instrumentation history, and, when genuinely ambiguous, a period of anti-inflammatory or antibiotic treatment with interval follow-up imaging, contributes meaningfully to accurate interpretation beyond the imaging findings considered in complete clinical isolation. Diffuse or geographic, ill-defined peripheral zone signal abnormality without a discrete, focal, round or lenticular lesion morphology favors a diffuse inflammatory process such as prostatitis over the more focal, discrete morphology typical of clinically significant cancer, though this distinction is imperfect and a genuinely indeterminate or clinically concerning finding, particularly with an elevated or rising serum prostate-specific antigen, should not be dismissed as inflammatory without appropriate clinical correlation and, when warranted, biopsy.

Prostate Biopsy Complications and Post-Biopsy Hemorrhage

Post-biopsy hemorrhage within the prostate gland and, less commonly, the seminal vesicles is a near-universal finding on MRI performed within several weeks of a prostate biopsy, appearing as elevated T1 signal that can obscure or, more concerningly, mimic tumor signal on subsequent imaging if the recent biopsy history is not known or specifically accounted for, such that current guidelines generally recommend a waiting interval, commonly around four to six weeks though institutional protocols vary, between biopsy and subsequent MRI, or between MRI and a prior biopsy when imaging is obtained specifically to assess for recurrence or to plan a repeat targeted procedure, to allow hemorrhage to sufficiently resolve and avoid this specific interpretive confound. Precontrast T1-weighted imaging, obtained as a standard component of the multiparametric protocol, is essential for recognizing post-biopsy hemorrhage as the explanation for an area of signal abnormality that might otherwise be misinterpreted on postcontrast or diffusion-weighted sequences alone, underscoring the importance of reviewing the complete multiparametric sequence set together rather than any single sequence in isolation, particularly in a patient with a known recent biopsy history that the requisition or clinical history should specifically flag for the interpreting radiologist.

PI-RADS Category	Suspicion Level	Typical Management
1	Very low	No biopsy
2	Low	No biopsy
3	Intermediate	Clinical correlation, PSA density; biopsy per shared decision
4	High	Targeted biopsy
5	Very high	Targeted biopsy

Focal Therapy Planning and MRI-Guided Ablation

Focal therapy, treating only the identified index lesion and a surrounding margin of tissue rather than the entire gland, has emerged as an intermediate treatment option between active surveillance and definitive whole-gland therapy for carefully selected patients with unifocal, lower-to-intermediate risk disease, and MRI plays an essential planning role in this approach by precisely delineating the lesion's size, location, and margin relative to critical structures including the neurovascular bundles and urethra, information that directly determines the ablation zone geometry for the various energy modalities used in focal therapy, including cryoablation, high-intensity focused ultrasound, and irreversible electroporation. Post-ablation MRI, generally obtained at defined intervals following focal therapy, assesses treatment zone coverage and screens for residual or recurrent disease at the ablation margin or elsewhere in the untreated gland, applying the same restricted diffusion and enhancement principles discussed throughout this chapter to this specific post-treatment surveillance context, with the complete absence of expected treatment-zone signal change or, conversely, any new or persistent suspicious signal within or adjacent to the treated zone warranting further evaluation.

Figure 14.4: MRI-Ultrasound Fusion Targeted Prostate Biopsy Technique

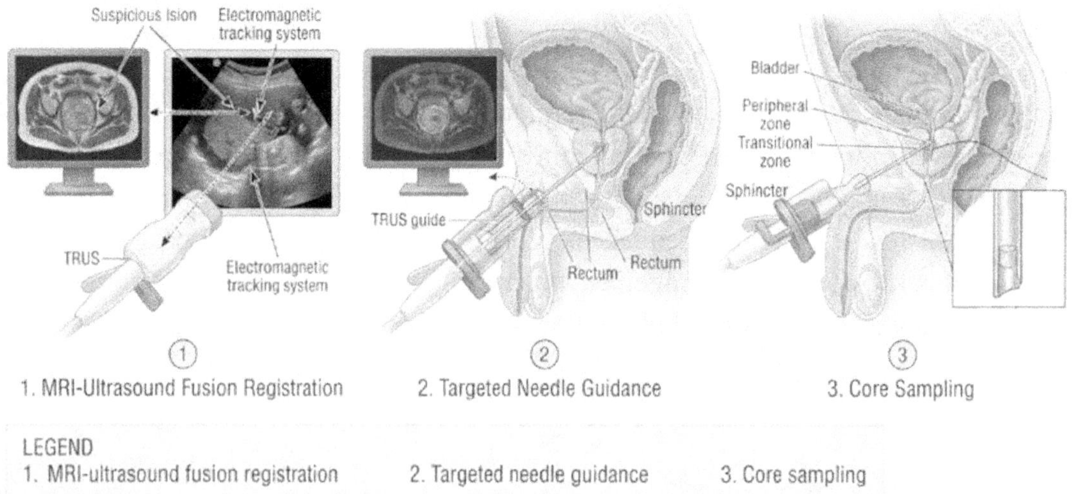

Clinical Case Presentations

Case 1. A 64-year-old man with an elevated prostate-specific antigen of 6.8 undergoes multiparametric MRI demonstrating a 1.6-centimeter round focus of marked apparent diffusion coefficient hypointensity with corresponding high b-value hyperintensity in the right peripheral zone, without extraprostatic extension. The radiologist categorizes the lesion as PI-RADS category 5 and recommends targeted biopsy, and MRI-ultrasound fusion biopsy confirms Gleason grade group 3 adenocarcinoma, directly guiding the patient's subsequent treatment planning discussion.

Case 2. A 71-year-old man with a markedly enlarged prostate and moderate lower urinary tract symptoms undergoes MRI demonstrating a large, heterogeneous, well-circumscribed transition zone nodule with a discrete encapsulating pseudocapsule and mixed stromal and glandular internal signal. Recognizing the encapsulated, heterogeneous morphology as characteristic of benign prostatic hyperplasia rather than transition zone cancer, the radiologist categorizes the finding as PI-RADS category 2 and calculates prostate-specific antigen density using the measured gland volume, providing the urologist with reassuring context for the patient's modestly elevated absolute prostate-specific antigen.

Case 3. A 58-year-old man undergoes MRI demonstrating a 2.2-centimeter peripheral zone lesion at the prostate base with a broad area of capsular contact, mild capsular bulging, and partial obliteration of the ipsilateral rectoprostatic angle, together with loss of the normal feathery architecture of the adjacent seminal vesicle. The radiologist categorizes the lesion as PI-RADS category 5 with confirmed extraprostatic extension and seminal vesicle invasion, explicitly documenting the specific location and extent of extension to support the urologic and radiation oncology teams' joint discussion of treatment approach given this locally advanced staging.

Case 4. A 55-year-old man with a recent history of prostatitis treated with antibiotics undergoes MRI demonstrating diffuse, ill-defined, geographic signal abnormality with mild diffusion restriction throughout the peripheral zone bilaterally, without a discrete focal lesion. Recognizing this pattern as favoring diffuse inflammatory change over focal clinically significant cancer, the radiologist recommends clinical correlation and interval follow-up imaging rather than immediate biopsy, appropriately applying the mimicry awareness this chapter's framework specifically emphasizes rather than assigning a high suspicion category to a diffuse, non-focal finding.

Case 5. A 60-year-old man on active surveillance for low-grade prostate cancer diagnosed three years earlier undergoes routine surveillance MRI demonstrating interval increase in the size of his previously known peripheral zone lesion, now measuring 1.4 centimeters with more pronounced diffusion restriction than on the baseline examination, with the category increasing from 3 to 4. Given this interval progression, the radiologist recommends repeat targeted biopsy to reassess for grade progression rather than continued surveillance without biopsy, appropriately applying the imaging-integrated active surveillance monitoring approach this chapter's framework describes, and the repeat biopsy confirms upgrade to a higher Gleason grade group, prompting the patient and his care team to transition from surveillance to active treatment.

Case 6. A 62-year-old man with unifocal, intermediate-risk prostate cancer confirmed on targeted biopsy of a well-defined 1.2-centimeter peripheral zone lesion elects focal cryoablation rather than whole-gland treatment. Preoperative MRI precisely delineates the lesion's margin relative to the adjacent neurovascular bundle to guide ablation zone planning, and follow-up MRI at six months demonstrates the expected treatment-zone signal change without any new or persistent suspicious focus within or adjacent to the ablation zone, supporting continued surveillance of the treated and untreated gland per the focal therapy monitoring protocol described in this chapter.

THE SIGNAL-TO-CATEGORY DECISION SYSTEM — Prostate Lesion Triage Arc

---

The Signal Pattern: This chapter's patterns span the full prostate risk spectrum, from a peripheral zone lesion whose diffusion-weighted appearance anchors PI-RADS category assignment, to a transition zone lesion whose margin and encapsulation must be assessed before a benign hyperplastic nodule label is applied.

Category Signature: Peripheral zone lesions are categorized 1 through 5 based on diffusion-weighted and apparent diffusion coefficient findings; transition zone lesions are categorized based on T2-weighted morphology, margin, and encapsulation.

The Decision: Category assignment in this chapter ranges from no biopsy for a low category to targeted biopsy and, when extraprostatic extension or seminal vesicle invasion is confirmed, complex multidisciplinary treatment planning, with every category assigned only after applying the correct zone-specific dominant sequence framework.

The Trap Logic: Both patterns in this chapter share a common trap: a benign mimic, prostatitis or a stromal-predominant hyperplastic nodule, that superficially resembles the cancer-defining pattern without the specific discriminating morphologic feature this chapter's framework requires.

Pattern Anchor: Confirm zone of origin and the zone-specific dominant sequence finding before assigning a PI-RADS category; benign mimics are common in both zones and require deliberate morphologic scrutiny to exclude.

Summary and Key Concepts

Prostate zonal anatomy, peripheral, transition, and central, determines the appropriate PI-RADS dominant sequence: diffusion-weighted imaging in the peripheral zone, T2-weighted imaging in the transition zone.

PI-RADS categories 1 through 5 stratify the probability of clinically significant cancer; dynamic contrast enhancement plays a limited role, potentially upgrading a peripheral zone category 3 lesion to category 4.

Transition zone cancer demonstrates a non-circumscribed, homogeneously hypointense erased charcoal sign, distinguishing it from the encapsulated, heterogeneous appearance of a benign hyperplastic nodule.

Extraprostatic extension is assessed through capsular contour, capsular disruption, rectoprostatic angle obliteration, and tumor-capsule contact length; each carries direct surgical and treatment planning implications.

Seminal vesicle invasion presents as loss of the normal feathery internal architecture with tumoral replacement and represents locally advanced disease.

Prostatitis can closely mimic clinically significant cancer on diffusion-weighted imaging; diffuse, ill-defined signal abnormality favors inflammation over the focal, discrete morphology typical of cancer.

Prostate-specific antigen density, calculated from MRI-derived gland volume, contributes to the biopsy decision for a PI-RADS category 3 lesion.

CHAPTER 15: BLADDER AND MALE PELVIC IMAGING

Learning Objectives

1. Apply the VI-RADS framework to stratify bladder lesions by the probability of muscle invasion.
2. Recognize bladder urothelial carcinoma and distinguish it from benign mimics including trabeculation and blood clot.
3. Recognize testicular and scrotal masses relevant to body MRI referral and distinguish intratesticular from extratesticular lesions.
4. Characterize penile and urethral pathology relevant to body MRI interpretation.
5. Recognize benign prostatic hyperplasia-related bladder outlet obstruction and its structural sequelae.

Clinical Overview

This chapter closes Part IV of this book with the bladder and the remaining male pelvic structures not addressed in the preceding prostate-focused chapter, completing the genitourinary coverage before the book turns to the female pelvis. Bladder cancer staging, in particular, has undergone a transformation paralleling the PI-RADS-driven evolution of prostate imaging discussed in the preceding chapter, with the VI-RADS framework now providing a comparably structured, reproducible approach to the single most consequential bladder imaging question, whether a lesion invades the muscularis propria. This chapter proceeds from the VI-RADS framework and bladder urothelial carcinoma, through testicular and scrotal imaging, penile and urethral pathology, and closes with bladder outlet obstruction and its structural sequelae.

Two instances of the Signal-to-Category Decision System are applied in this chapter, the first to VI-RADS category assignment itself, and the second to the intratesticular-versus-extratesticular triage that is the foundational first step in any scrotal mass characterization.

The VI-RADS Framework and Bladder Urothelial Carcinoma

Epidemiology of Bladder Cancer and Risk Factors

Bladder cancer demonstrates a marked male predominance, occurring several times more frequently in men than women, and shares its dominant risk factor, cigarette smoking, with the urothelial malignancies discussed throughout the preceding two chapters, with smoking accounting for a substantial proportion of cases across most epidemiologic series, together with occupational exposure to aromatic amines in industries including dye, rubber, and textile manufacturing, and, in endemic regions, chronic Schistosoma haematobium infection, which carries a specific and well-established association with the squamous cell carcinoma subtype discussed later in this chapter rather than the more common urothelial carcinoma seen in non-endemic populations. Hematuria, whether gross or microscopic, remains the dominant presenting symptom prompting the imaging evaluation discussed throughout this chapter, and current guidelines generally recommend cross-sectional urographic imaging as part of the standard hematuria workup in an appropriately risk-stratified adult patient, a workup pathway that, together with cystoscopy, forms the complementary anatomic and direct-visualization evaluation strategy for this common clinical presentation.

MRI Technique Considerations for Bladder and Male Pelvic Imaging

A dedicated bladder MRI protocol, as introduced in this chapter's discussion of adequate distension, benefits from patient instructions regarding bladder filling timed to the examination, high-resolution T2-weighted imaging in multiple planes analogous to the multiplanar emphasis in the prostate protocol discussed in the preceding chapter, and diffusion-weighted imaging with attention to minimizing distortion artifact, which can be particularly pronounced in the pelvis given the interfaces between bladder, bowel gas, and pelvic sidewall soft tissue discussed in the artifact recognition chapter earlier in this book. When testicular or penile imaging is performed, dedicated small field-of-view, high-resolution surface coil technique, analogous in principle to the dedicated coil considerations discussed for prostate imaging, substantially improves the spatial resolution needed to characterize these comparatively small structures, and taping the penis to the abdominal wall in a stretched position for penile MRI, a specific positioning technique with direct relevance to Peyronie disease and penile carcinoma staging, improves both patient comfort and diagnostic image quality relative to imaging the organ in its resting, non-stretched position.

Bladder Wall Anatomy and the Muscle Invasion Question

The bladder wall comprises the mucosa and lamina propria, together constituting the submucosa relevant to non-muscle-invasive staging, and the muscularis propria, the detrusor muscle whose invasion by tumor represents the single most important staging threshold in bladder cancer, since muscle-invasive disease generally requires radical cystectomy or definitive chemoradiation, while non-muscle-invasive disease is managed with transurethral resection and intravesical therapy, a binary treatment fork that makes the muscle invasion determination the central organizing question of this chapter's bladder discussion, analogous in its outsized clinical weight to the Bosniak category assignment task in the renal chapter earlier in this book. Adequate bladder distension, generally achieved through a combination of oral hydration, intravenous fluid administration, or a period of examination timing coordinated with the patient's natural bladder filling, is an essential technical prerequisite for confident bladder wall assessment, since an underdistended bladder produces wall thickening and folding that can obscure a lesion or mimic wall invasion, a technical consideration analogous to the excretory phase distension requirement discussed in the preceding renal chapter.

VI-RADS Category Criteria

The VI-RADS framework assigns a five-point category based primarily on T2-weighted morphology and diffusion-weighted imaging, evaluating the integrity of the low-signal muscularis propria layer deep to the lesion: category 1 and 2 findings demonstrate a lesion confined to the mucosa or lamina propria with an intact, uninterrupted muscularis propria layer beneath, favoring non-muscle-invasive disease, category

3 represents genuine indeterminate probability of muscle invasion, and category 4 and 5 findings demonstrate disruption or discontinuity of the muscularis propria layer with tumor signal extending through it, favoring muscle-invasive disease, with category 5 reserved for lesions demonstrating extravesical extension beyond the bladder wall entirely. As with PI-RADS in the preceding chapter, diffusion-weighted imaging and its apparent diffusion coefficient map serve as a key contributing sequence, with a stalk-like configuration on diffusion-weighted imaging, in which the lesion demonstrates a discrete, non-invasive base connecting to an otherwise intact muscularis propria layer, favoring the lower, non-invasive categories, while a broad-based or sessile morphology with diffusion signal extending into and disrupting the muscularis layer favors the higher, invasive categories.

Figure 15.1: VI-RADS Category 4 Bladder Lesion with Muscularis Invasion

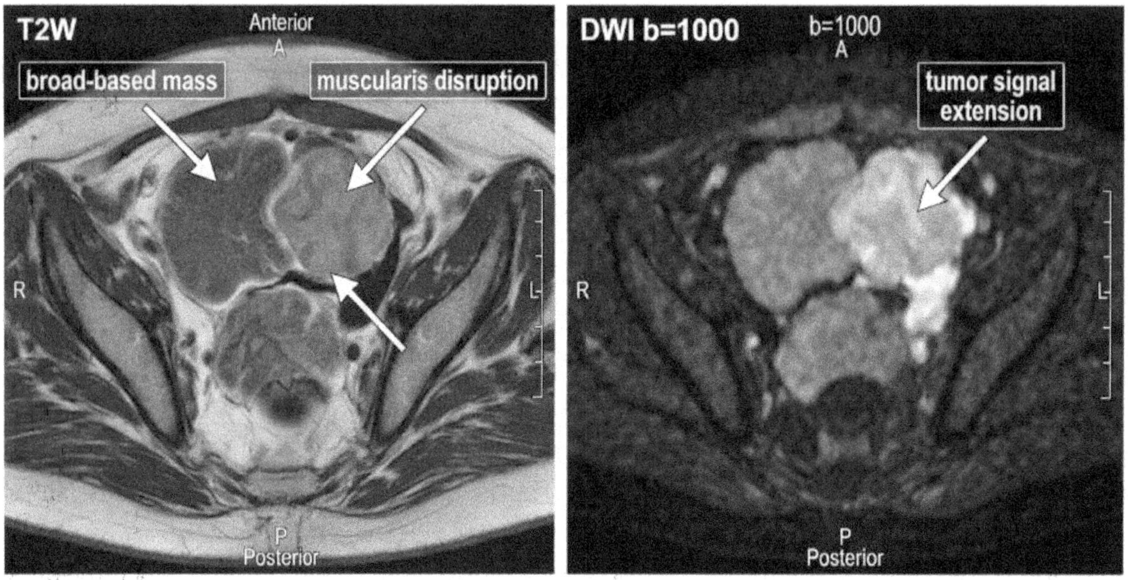

THE SIGNAL-TO-CATEGORY DECISION SYSTEM — VI-RADS Category Assignment

The Signal Pattern: A bladder lesion is identified on a technically adequate, well-distended examination, and the reader must assess the integrity of the muscularis propria layer immediately deep to the lesion on both T2-weighted and diffusion-weighted imaging.

Category Signature: A lesion with a stalk-like configuration and an intact, continuous low-signal muscularis propria layer is categorized as VI-RADS 1 or 2; a lesion with morphology or signal that is genuinely ambiguous for muscularis integrity is categorized as VI-RADS 3; a lesion with clear disruption of the muscularis propria layer by tumor signal is categorized as VI-RADS 4, and extravesical extension defines VI-RADS 5.

The Decision: VI-RADS 1 through 3 lesions proceed to transurethral resection, which remains both diagnostic and, for non-muscle-invasive disease, therapeutic, with the resection pathology providing the definitive muscle invasion determination; VI-RADS 4 and 5 lesions strongly suggest muscle-invasive disease and support upfront planning for radical cystectomy or definitive chemoradiation discussion even before the confirmatory resection pathology is available.

Trap Logic: Prior transurethral resection, intravesical therapy, or biopsy can produce inflammatory or fibrotic change in the bladder wall that mimics muscle invasion on subsequent imaging, a pitfall directly analogous to the post-biopsy hemorrhage confound discussed for the prostate in the preceding chapter; the discriminating step is obtaining VI-RADS imaging before any resection or biopsy whenever feasible, and, when post-treatment imaging is unavoidable, explicitly accounting for the recent intervention history when characterizing wall signal abnormality.

Pattern Anchor: Assess muscularis propria integrity, not lesion size or number, as the primary category-determining feature; obtain VI-RADS imaging before biopsy or resection whenever possible to avoid treatment-related mimicry.

Non-Muscle-Invasive Disease Risk Stratification and Surveillance

Non-muscle-invasive bladder cancer, comprising the majority of newly diagnosed cases, is further risk-stratified following transurethral resection using pathologic grade, tumor size and multifocality, and the presence of concurrent carcinoma in situ, a flat, high-grade lesion that can be genuinely difficult to detect on MRI given its lack of a discrete mass-like morphology, into low, intermediate, and high-risk categories that determine the intensity of subsequent intravesical therapy and surveillance cystoscopy, with high-risk non-muscle-invasive disease carrying a substantial risk of both recurrence and progression to muscle-invasive disease that warrants considerably closer surveillance than low-risk disease. MRI's role in this surveillance context remains generally secondary to cystoscopy, which retains superior sensitivity for the flat, subtle lesions including carcinoma in situ that VI-RADS imaging can miss, echoing the same bladder field-change surveillance principle discussed for the upper tract urothelial carcinoma follow-up protocol in the preceding chapter, though MRI can contribute meaningfully when a cystoscopically identified abnormality requires staging clarification or when upper tract evaluation is being performed concurrently for the same field-change risk.

Non-Urothelial Bladder Malignancies

While urothelial carcinoma accounts for the substantial majority of bladder malignancies in most populations, squamous cell carcinoma, associated with chronic bladder irritation from a long-standing indwelling catheter, chronic infection, or, in endemic regions, schistosomiasis, and adenocarcinoma, which can arise from the native bladder mucosa or, in a distinctive pattern, from a urachal remnant along the dome of the bladder extending toward the umbilicus, together comprise the minority non-urothelial bladder malignancy differential worth recognizing when a bladder mass demonstrates an atypical location or a relevant risk factor history inconsistent with typical urothelial carcinoma. Urachal adenocarcinoma specifically presents as a mass centered along the urachal remnant at the bladder dome, often with associated calcification, and its distinctive location, at the dome rather than the more typical urothelial carcinoma distribution throughout the bladder, together with a relevant history, should prompt consideration of this specific, comparatively rare non-urothelial entity rather than assuming urothelial carcinoma by default for every bladder mass encountered.

Bladder Urothelial Carcinoma: Epidemiology and Benign Mimics

Bladder urothelial carcinoma shares its major risk factors, cigarette smoking foremost among them, with the upper tract urothelial carcinoma discussed in the preceding chapter, reflecting the shared field-change carcinogenic exposure across the entire urothelium, and a diagnosis of bladder urothelial carcinoma should similarly prompt attention to the upper tracts for synchronous disease, just as the reverse evaluation sequence was emphasized in the preceding chapter. Benign mimics of bladder cancer on imaging include bladder wall trabeculation from chronic outlet obstruction, discussed later in this chapter, which produces a nodular, irregular luminal contour that can be mistaken for a mass if not correlated with the diffuse, symmetric distribution typical of trabeculation versus the focal, asymmetric morphology typical of tumor, and blood clot, which, like the ureteral clot discussed in the preceding chapter, demonstrates no true enhancement and can be distinguished from tumor by this feature together with its tendency to change position or resolve on interval or repositioned imaging given its non-fixed, mobile nature within the bladder lumen.

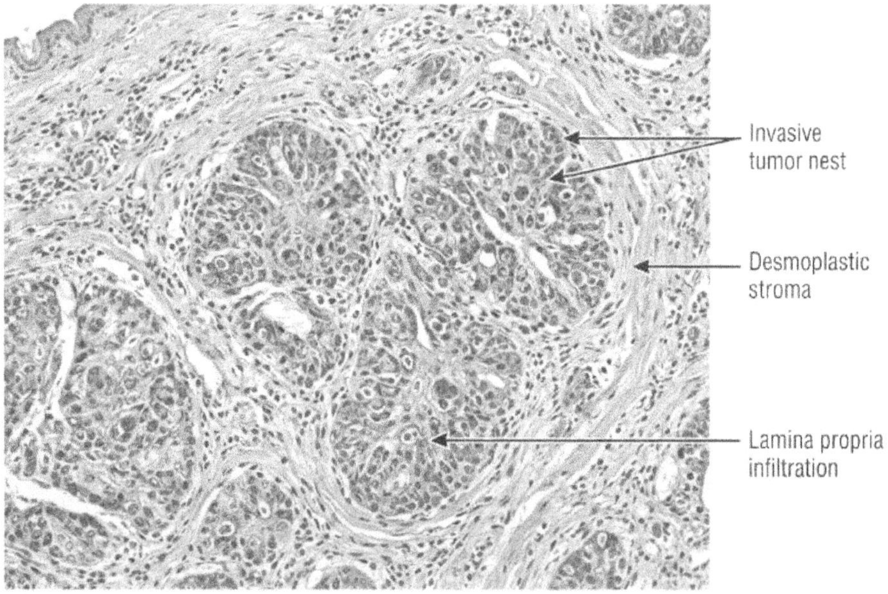

Figure 15.2 Histopathology of HE sided photomicrograph 20x)

Testicular and Scrotal Imaging

Epididymitis, Orchitis, and Testicular Torsion

Acute epididymitis and orchitis, most often related to ascending bacterial infection or, in a sexually active younger man, a sexually transmitted pathogen, present with epididymal or testicular enlargement, edema, and hyperemia that on MRI corresponds to T2 hyperintensity and increased postcontrast enhancement relative to the contralateral side, findings that, while more commonly assessed with ultrasound as the first-line modality given its real-time capability and lower cost, translate directly to MRI when this modality is used, most often as a problem-solving tool for a clinically ambiguous presentation or when ultrasound is technically limited. Testicular torsion, a true surgical emergency in which the spermatic cord twists and compromises testicular blood flow, is likewise primarily assessed with ultrasound given the time-critical nature of the diagnosis and the several-hour window before irreversible testicular infarction occurs, and while MRI can demonstrate the whirlpool sign of a twisted spermatic cord together with reduced or absent testicular enhancement in confirmed torsion, its comparatively longer acquisition time makes it an inappropriate first-line choice for this specific time-critical emergency, reserved instead for the rare scenario where ultrasound is entirely unavailable or has produced a genuinely indeterminate result requiring urgent clarification.

Testicular Microlithiasis and Incidental Findings

Testicular microlithiasis, characterized by numerous tiny calcific foci scattered throughout the testicular parenchyma, most reliably identified on ultrasound given calcification's subtle MRI signal characteristics analogous to the calcification detection limitations discussed for other organs throughout this book, is generally an incidental, benign finding, though its historical association with an elevated germ cell tumor risk, now understood to be modest and most relevant when additional risk factors such as cryptorchidism history or a contralateral testicular tumor are also present, has generated ongoing debate about the appropriate surveillance intensity for an otherwise asymptomatic patient with isolated microlithiasis and no other risk factors, with most current guidelines favoring patient self-examination education over routine imaging surveillance in this specific low-additional-risk scenario. Cryptorchidism, an undescended testis most often identified and addressed in infancy, carries an independently elevated germ cell tumor risk that persists even after surgical orchiopexy repositions the testis into the scrotum, such that a history of cryptorchidism, whether or not previously corrected, provides relevant risk context that should heighten suspicion for a subtle intratesticular finding in this specific population relative to a patient without this history.

The Role of MRI in Scrotal Imaging

Ultrasound remains the primary, first-line imaging modality for scrotal pathology given its excellent spatial resolution, real-time capability, and low cost, and MRI is generally reserved as a problem-solving tool for cases where ultrasound findings are genuinely indeterminate, most often to further characterize an equivocal testicular lesion, to assess local extent and staging once testicular malignancy is confirmed or strongly suspected, or to further evaluate a complex extratesticular finding, such that the radiologist approaching a scrotal MRI should understand this problem-solving, second-line role rather than treating scrotal MRI as a routine first-line examination. Intratesticular-versus-extratesticular localization is the first and most fundamental branch point in scrotal mass characterization, directly analogous in its foundational, upstream diagnostic importance to the cystic-versus-solid triage in renal imaging and the zonal localization task in prostate imaging discussed in preceding chapters, since intratesticular masses carry a substantially higher malignant probability, particularly in an adult, than the predominantly benign extratesticular mass differential.

Epidemiology and Risk Factors for Testicular Germ Cell Tumors

Testicular germ cell tumors demonstrate a peak incidence in young to middle-aged adult men, making them among the most common solid malignancies in this specific age demographic despite their overall rarity relative to malignancy incidence across the full adult population, and beyond the cryptorchidism risk discussed later in this chapter, additional recognized risk factors include a personal history of a contralateral testicular tumor, which carries a substantially elevated risk of a second, metachronous primary in the remaining testis warranting heightened surveillance vigilance, a family history of testicular cancer in a first-degree relative, and certain disorders of sex development. Testicular germ cell tumors carry an excellent overall prognosis with contemporary multimodal treatment, including surgery, chemotherapy, and, for seminoma, radiation therapy, even in the setting of metastatic disease at diagnosis, a favorable prognosis that, together with the tumor's characteristic serum marker profile discussed below, distinguishes it from most other solid malignancies discussed throughout this book and appropriately shapes both the urgency and the specific staging protocol applied once the diagnosis is confirmed.

Testicular Germ Cell Tumors

Testicular germ cell tumors, the most common testicular malignancy in young to middle-aged men, present as an intratesticular mass demonstrating variable signal characteristics depending on the specific histologic subtype, with seminoma typically presenting as a homogeneous, moderately hypointense mass on T2-weighted imaging with fibrovascular septa producing a lobulated internal architecture, and the non-seminomatous germ cell tumors, including embryonal carcinoma, yolk sac tumor, choriocarcinoma, and teratoma, typically presenting as a more heterogeneous mass reflecting the mixed and often hemorrhagic, necrotic, or cystic internal composition characteristic of this histologically diverse tumor group. Any solid intratesticular mass in an adult should be considered malignant until proven otherwise, given the low prevalence of a solid benign intratesticular neoplasm in this population, and this default-malignant approach, together with prompt correlation with serum tumor markers including alpha-fetoprotein, beta-human chorionic gonadotropin, and lactate dehydrogenase, which carry both diagnostic and, once malignancy is confirmed, staging and treatment-response monitoring value specific to the germ cell tumor differential, generally drives the radical orchiectomy pathway that remains the standard diagnostic and initial treatment approach for a suspicious solid intratesticular mass rather than percutaneous biopsy, which carries a recognized risk of tumor seeding along the biopsy tract in this specific anatomic context.

THE SIGNAL-TO-CATEGORY DECISION SYSTEM — Intratesticular versus Extratesticular Scrotal Mass Triage

The Signal Pattern: A scrotal mass is identified, and the reader must first establish whether it arises from within the testicular parenchyma itself or from an extratesticular structure before applying the appropriate differential diagnosis.

Category Signature: A mass clearly surrounded by and distinct from normal testicular parenchyma, with the testis itself identifiable as a separate structure, is categorized as extratesticular; a mass replacing or distorting the normal testicular parenchymal architecture, with no discernible normal testis separate from the mass, is categorized as intratesticular.

The Decision: An extratesticular mass is generally approached with a predominantly benign differential, including epididymal cyst, spermatocele, and varicocele, with malignancy a distinctly uncommon consideration reserved for a mass with specifically concerning features; an intratesticular solid mass in an adult is treated as malignant until proven otherwise and proceeds to radical orchiectomy rather than biopsy.

Trap Logic: A large extratesticular mass can compress and distort the adjacent testis sufficiently to create diagnostic ambiguity about its precise origin, and conversely, a testicular tumor that has extended through the tunica albuginea can create an extratesticular component that obscures its true intratesticular origin; the discriminating step is deliberate identification of the tunica albuginea, the testis's fibrous capsule, on multiplanar imaging to confirm whether the mass originates from within or outside this specific anatomic boundary.

Pattern Anchor: Confirm the mass's relationship to the tunica albuginea before assigning intratesticular versus extratesticular category; an intratesticular solid mass in an adult defaults to malignant and proceeds to orchiectomy, not biopsy.

Extratesticular Masses and Benign Findings

Epididymal cyst and spermatocele, both common, entirely benign extratesticular findings arising from the epididymis, demonstrate simple or, for spermatocele given its proteinaceous, sperm-containing fluid content, mildly complex fluid signal without solid enhancing components, and require no further workup once confidently characterized as such. Varicocele, dilation of the pampiniform venous plexus most commonly on the left side given the left testicular vein's more vertical, higher-resistance drainage into the left renal vein compared to the right testicular vein's more oblique, lower-resistance direct drainage into the inferior vena cava, presents as a serpiginous, tubular structure demonstrating flow-related signal characteristics, and a new, isolated right-sided varicocele, or a left varicocele that fails to decompress in the supine position, should prompt a search for a retroperitoneal process obstructing venous outflow, echoing the renal vein and inferior vena cava tumor thrombus considerations discussed in the preceding renal chapter, rather than being attributed to simple idiopathic varicocele without this specific evaluation.

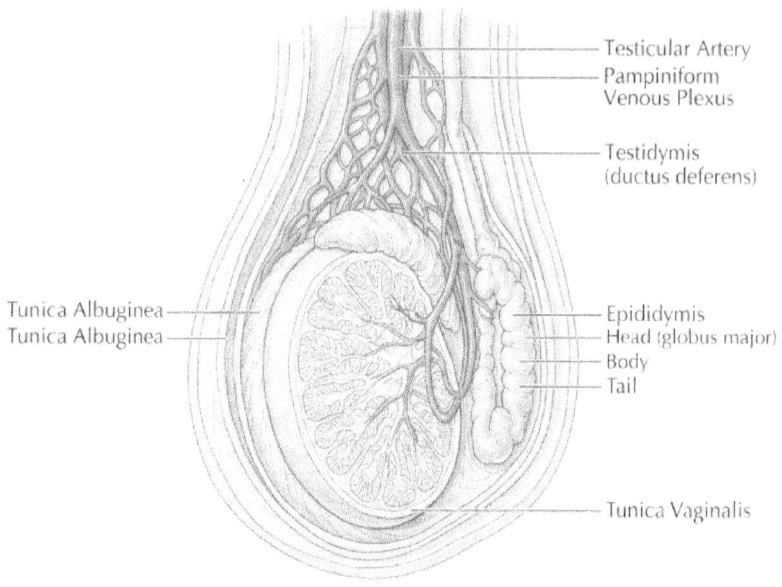

Penile and Urethral Pathology

Penile Anatomy and Peyronie Disease

The penis comprises the paired corpora cavernosa, the primary erectile bodies, and the corpus spongiosum, surrounding the urethra and terminating in the glans, each surrounded by the tunica albuginea, and MRI of the penis, while an uncommon indication relative to the other structures discussed in this chapter, is most often performed for Peyronie disease, a fibrotic condition of the tunica albuginea producing a palpable plaque and, clinically, penile curvature during erection, or for staging of the comparatively rare penile carcinoma. Peyronie disease plaque demonstrates low T2 signal reflecting its dense fibrous composition, with MRI contributing plaque localization and size characterization relevant to surgical planning when intervention, whether plaque incision and grafting or a penile prosthesis procedure, is being considered for a patient with functionally significant curvature or erectile dysfunction not adequately addressed by medical therapy alone.

Priapism and Vascular Penile Pathology

Priapism, a prolonged, often painful erection unrelated to sexual stimulation, is classified as ischemic, a compartment syndrome-like emergency related to impaired venous outflow that requires urgent decompression to prevent irreversible corporal smooth muscle damage and subsequent erectile dysfunction, or non-ischemic, generally related to a traumatic arterial-cavernosal fistula and carrying a considerably lower urgency given preserved arterial inflow and venous outflow, a distinction traditionally made with cavernosal blood gas sampling but for which MRI, demonstrating diffusion restriction and reduced or absent enhancement within the corpora cavernosa in ischemic priapism versus preserved enhancement and, often, a visible high-flow fistula in non-ischemic priapism, can provide valuable confirmatory or clarifying information particularly when initial clinical and laboratory assessment is ambiguous. This ischemic-versus-non-ischemic distinction carries direct and urgent management implications analogous to several other binary triage decisions addressed throughout this book, since ischemic priapism requires emergent corporal aspiration and irrigation, with surgical shunt procedures reserved for refractory cases, while non-ischemic priapism can generally be managed conservatively or with selective arterial embolization on a considerably less urgent timeline, making accurate, prompt distinction between these two entities clinically consequential.

Penile Carcinoma and Urethral Pathology

Penile carcinoma, most commonly squamous cell carcinoma and strongly associated with human papillomavirus infection and, in uncircumcised men, phimosis and chronic inflammatory conditions of the foreskin, presents as a mass or infiltrative thickening most often involving the glans, with MRI staging focused on assessing the depth of invasion into the corpus spongiosum and, more consequentially for prognosis and surgical planning, the corpora cavernosa, since invasion of the cavernosal bodies generally necessitates a more extensive partial or total penectomy than disease confined to the glans or corpus spongiosum alone, making this specific depth assessment the central staging task analogous to the muscle invasion determination in bladder cancer discussed earlier in this chapter. Urethral pathology, including urethral stricture, most reliably characterized with dedicated retrograde or voiding urethrography rather than MRI as the primary technique, and the considerably rarer primary urethral carcinoma, which MRI can help stage by assessing local extent and corpal body invasion analogous to the penile carcinoma staging task, round out the male pelvic pathology relevant to this chapter, each representing a comparatively uncommon but clinically significant indication for body MRI referral in this specific anatomic region.

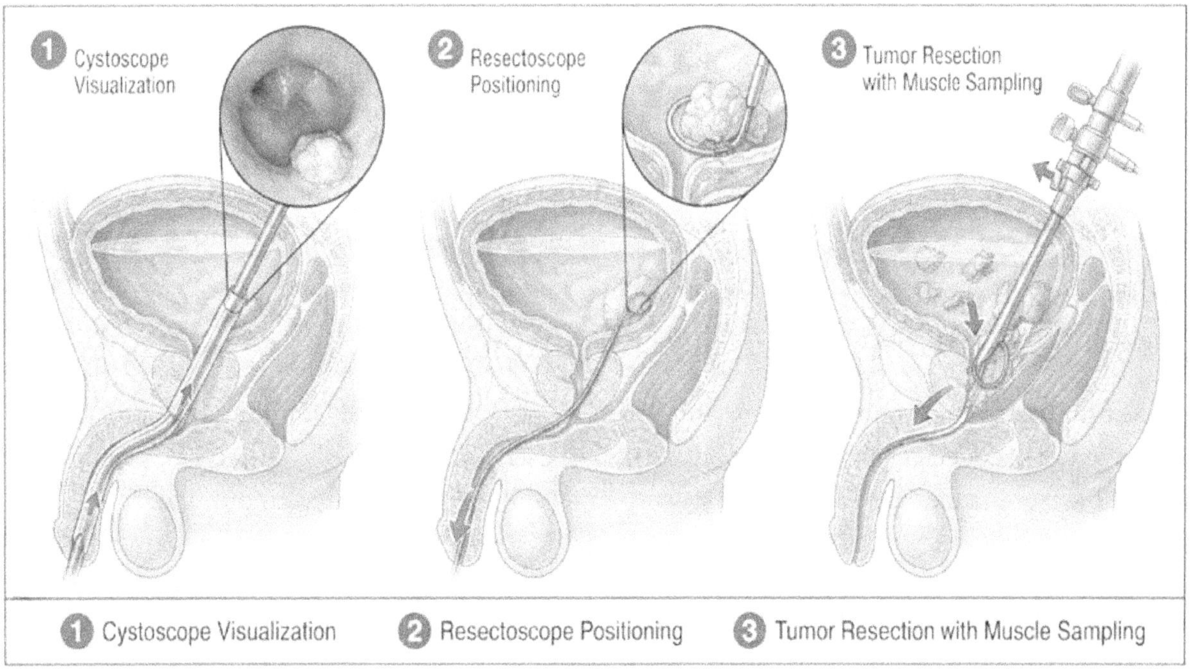

Figure 15.4: Transurethral Resection of Bladder Tumor Technique

Bladder Outlet Obstruction and Structural Sequelae

Post-Cystectomy and Urinary Diversion Imaging

Following radical cystectomy for muscle-invasive bladder cancer, urinary diversion, most commonly an ileal conduit directing urine to a cutaneous stoma or, in select patients, an orthotopic neobladder constructed from a segment of bowel and anastomosed directly to the urethra to preserve a more physiologic voiding pattern, creates a substantially altered pelvic anatomy that the radiologist should recognize and correctly interpret on any subsequent surveillance or symptom-driven imaging, avoiding the misinterpretation of expected postsurgical anatomy, bowel used for diversion construction, as a pathologic finding. Surveillance imaging following cystectomy focuses on detecting local pelvic recurrence at the cystectomy bed and urethral remnant when present, upper tract complications including stricture at the ureteroenteric anastomosis producing hydronephrosis, and distant metastatic disease, with the specific surveillance interval and imaging protocol generally determined by the original tumor stage and any adjuvant therapy received, a comprehensive post-treatment surveillance framework the radiologist should understand when interpreting imaging in this specific postsurgical population.

Bladder Trabeculation and Diverticula

Chronic bladder outlet obstruction, most commonly related to benign prostatic hyperplasia discussed in the preceding chapter, produces detrusor muscle hypertrophy and a resulting trabeculated, nodular luminal contour as the thickened muscle bundles become visible against the bladder lumen, a diffuse, symmetric pattern that, as discussed earlier in this chapter, should be distinguished from the focal, asymmetric morphology of a mass. Bladder diverticula, outpouchings of mucosa herniating through a weakened area of the detrusor muscle, most often between hypertrophied trabecular muscle bundles, are a recognized long-term consequence of chronic outlet obstruction and carry their own specific complication risks, including urinary stasis predisposing to infection and stone formation, and, less commonly but importantly, an elevated risk of urothelial carcinoma developing specifically within the diverticulum, where the absence of a normal muscularis propria layer, the diverticulum being a mucosa-lined outpouching without the muscular wall of the native bladder, means that a tumor arising within a diverticulum has no muscle layer to invade before reaching the perivesical fat directly, an important anatomic consideration that alters the usual VI-RADS muscle-invasion framework for a diverticular lesion specifically.

Cystitis and Inflammatory Bladder Conditions

Acute cystitis, most often related to ascending bacterial infection and considerably more common in women given the shared anatomic susceptibility discussed for pyelonephritis in the preceding chapter, produces diffuse bladder wall thickening and mucosal enhancement without the focal, mass-like morphology of a tumor, and this diffuse, symmetric pattern, together with a compatible clinical presentation of dysuria and urinary frequency, should favor cystitis over a neoplastic process, though a focal or asymmetric area of thickening within an otherwise diffusely inflamed bladder still warrants the same VI-RADS-informed scrutiny applied to any other bladder wall abnormality. Radiation cystitis, a recognized late complication of pelvic radiation therapy administered for prostate, bladder, gynecologic, or rectal malignancy, produces a similarly diffuse pattern of bladder wall thickening and, in more severe cases, hemorrhagic cystitis with intraluminal blood products, and correlating imaging findings with the patient's specific radiation treatment history and time course is essential to correctly attributing bladder wall changes to this specific radiation-related etiology rather than pursuing an unnecessary evaluation for tumor recurrence in a patient with a known and expected pattern of radiation-related bladder injury.

Neurogenic Bladder and Special Populations

Neurogenic bladder, arising from a variety of neurologic conditions affecting bladder innervation, including spinal cord injury, multiple sclerosis, and spina bifida, produces a spectrum of bladder wall and functional abnormalities ranging from a similarly trabeculated, thick-walled pattern to a small-capacity, poorly compliant bladder, depending on the specific pattern of neurologic injury, and this population carries an elevated long-term bladder cancer risk, particularly with chronic indwelling catheter use, that should inform a heightened index of suspicion for a new bladder mass in this specific clinical context. In the pediatric population, posterior urethral valves, an obstructing congenital anomaly in male infants, produce a similar downstream pattern of bladder wall thickening and trabeculation together with bilateral hydronephrosis and, in more severe cases, renal parenchymal dysplasia from the sustained back-pressure effect on the developing kidneys, underscoring the importance of prompt postnatal diagnosis and decompression to preserve long-term renal function in this specific and time-sensitive pediatric obstructive uropathy.

VI-RADS Category	Muscularis Propria Status	Typical Management
1-2	Intact, continuous layer	Transurethral resection (diagnostic and therapeutic)
3	Indeterminate	Transurethral resection with close attention to deep margin
4	Disrupted by tumor	Resection plus upfront staging for likely cystectomy/chemoradiation
5	Extravesical extension	Staging workup, multidisciplinary treatment planning

CAUTION: Prior transurethral resection or intravesical therapy produces inflammatory and fibrotic change that can mimic muscle invasion on subsequent imaging; obtain VI-RADS imaging before biopsy or resection whenever clinically feasible.

Clinical Case Presentations

Special Populations: Pregnancy and Pediatric Bladder Considerations

In pregnancy, bladder and pelvic MRI without gadolinium contrast is occasionally required for a suspected mass or complex presentation not adequately characterized by ultrasound, and the gravid uterus produces predictable bladder displacement and compression that should be accounted for when characterizing bladder wall thickness and contour, since physiologic compression from the enlarging uterus can produce an asymmetric bladder contour that should not be mistaken for a mass or focal wall abnormality without correlation to the expected anatomic distortion at the patient's specific gestational age. In the pediatric population, posterior urethral valves and other congenital anomalies discussed in the preceding chapter's hydronephrosis section frequently produce secondary bladder wall changes, including trabeculation and, in severe cases, a thick-walled, poorly compliant bladder pattern similar to the neurogenic bladder pattern discussed above, and recognizing this congenital obstructive etiology as the underlying cause of pediatric bladder wall thickening, rather than an acquired process more typical of the adult differential emphasized throughout this chapter, is essential to correctly directing the pediatric urology evaluation toward the appropriate age-specific differential.

KEY POINT: Physiologic bladder compression and asymmetry from the gravid uterus in pregnancy should not be mistaken for a mass or focal wall abnormality; correlate any apparent asymmetry with the expected anatomic distortion at the patient's specific gestational age.

Case 1. A 67-year-old man with gross hematuria undergoes bladder MRI demonstrating a 2.5-centimeter papillary mass with a discrete stalk and an intact, continuous muscularis propria layer beneath it. The radiologist categorizes the lesion as VI-RADS 2 and communicates the low probability of muscle invasion to the urology team, who proceed with transurethral resection, confirmed on pathology as non-muscle-invasive papillary urothelial carcinoma consistent with the imaging prediction.

Case 2. A 58-year-old woman with gross hematuria undergoes MRI demonstrating a broad-based, sessile bladder mass with clear disruption of the underlying muscularis propria layer by tumor signal extending toward the perivesical fat. The radiologist categorizes the lesion as VI-RADS 5 given the apparent extravesical extension and recommends staging workup and multidisciplinary discussion for likely radical cystectomy or definitive chemoradiation, providing the urology team with actionable pretreatment staging information before the confirmatory resection is performed.

Case 3. A 26-year-old man presents with a painless testicular mass, and MRI demonstrates a solid intratesticular mass replacing a portion of the normal testicular parenchyma, with the tunica albuginea intact and the mass confirmed as arising from within the testis rather than compressing it from outside. Recognizing this solid intratesticular mass as malignant until proven otherwise, the radiologist recommends radical orchiectomy rather than biopsy, and serum tumor markers together with the surgical pathology confirm mixed germ cell tumor, directing the patient's subsequent oncologic staging and treatment.

Case 4. A 71-year-old man with long-standing benign prostatic hyperplasia and chronic urinary retention undergoes MRI demonstrating marked bladder wall trabeculation with a large bladder diverticulum arising between hypertrophied trabecular bundles, and a small enhancing soft tissue nodule within the diverticulum wall itself. Recognizing that the diverticulum lacks a muscularis propria layer, the radiologist explicitly notes that any tumor within this diverticulum has direct access to the perivesical fat without an intervening muscle layer to invade, providing this important anatomic caveat to the urology team as they plan biopsy and staging for this diverticular lesion.

Case 5. A 38-year-old man presents with a prolonged, painful erection lasting six hours without recent trauma, and MRI demonstrates diffusion restriction and absent enhancement within both corpora cavernosa. Recognizing this as ischemic priapism, the radiologist urgently communicates the findings, and the patient undergoes emergent corporal aspiration and irrigation, achieving detumescence and avoiding the irreversible corporal smooth muscle damage that delayed treatment of ischemic priapism can produce.

Case 6. A 24-year-old man with a history of orchiopexy for cryptorchidism in infancy presents for routine follow-up, and MRI performed for an unrelated indication incidentally demonstrates numerous tiny calcific foci scattered throughout both testes without a discrete mass. Recognizing this as testicular microlithiasis and noting the patient's cryptorchidism history as an independent risk factor for germ cell tumor, the radiologist recommends patient self-examination education and continued routine follow-up rather than aggressive surveillance imaging, appropriately calibrating the recommendation to this specific combination of findings and history per current guidance.

Case 7. A 74-year-old man with a history of pelvic radiation therapy for prostate cancer two years earlier presents with new gross hematuria, and MRI demonstrates diffuse bladder wall thickening with mucosal enhancement and small foci of intraluminal blood product signal, without a discrete focal mass or muscularis disruption. Correlating the diffuse pattern with the patient's radiation history and time course, the radiologist favors radiation cystitis over tumor recurrence, and cystoscopy with biopsy confirms benign radiation-related changes without evidence of recurrent malignancy, sparing the patient an unnecessarily aggressive re-staging workup.

THE SIGNAL-TO-CATEGORY DECISION SYSTEM — Bladder and Male Pelvic Triage Arc

The Signal Pattern: This chapter's patterns span the bladder and male pelvic risk spectrum, from a bladder lesion whose muscularis propria integrity must be assessed for VI-RADS category assignment, to a scrotal mass whose relationship to the tunica albuginea must be confirmed before intratesticular-versus-extratesticular categorization.

Category Signature: Bladder lesions are categorized VI-RADS 1 through 5 based on muscularis propria integrity; scrotal masses are categorized as intratesticular, defaulting to malignant, or extratesticular, defaulting to benign, based on their relationship to the tunica albuginea.

The Decision: Category assignment in this chapter ranges from transurethral resection alone to radical cystectomy planning, and from benign observation to radical orchiectomy without biopsy, with every category assigned only after the specific confirmatory anatomic relationship, muscularis integrity or tunica albuginea origin, has been explicitly verified.

The Trap Logic: Both patterns in this chapter share a common trap: a technical or anatomic confound, prior treatment mimicking invasion or a large mass distorting adjacent structures, that can obscure the specific anatomic relationship this chapter's framework requires for accurate categorization.

Pattern Anchor: Confirm the specific anatomic relationship, muscularis integrity or tunica albuginea origin, deliberately and explicitly before committing to a final category in this chapter; technical and treatment-related confounds are common and must be actively excluded.

Summary and Key Concepts

VI-RADS stratifies bladder lesions by the probability of muscle invasion using T2-weighted morphology and diffusion-weighted imaging assessment of muscularis propria integrity; obtain imaging before biopsy or resection to avoid treatment-related mimicry.

A stalk-like configuration with intact muscularis propria favors non-invasive disease; a broad-based lesion with muscularis disruption favors invasive disease.

Intratesticular-versus-extratesticular localization is the foundational scrotal mass triage; a solid intratesticular mass in an adult is malignant until proven otherwise and proceeds to orchiectomy, not biopsy.

A new isolated right-sided varicocele or a left varicocele failing to decompress supine should prompt evaluation for a retroperitoneal process obstructing venous outflow.

Peyronie disease plaque demonstrates low T2 signal from dense fibrosis; penile carcinoma staging focuses on depth of invasion into the corpus spongiosum versus the corpora cavernosa.

Bladder diverticula lack a muscularis propria layer, so a tumor within a diverticulum has direct access to perivesical fat without an intervening muscle layer to invade.

Posterior urethral valves in male infants produce bladder trabeculation, bilateral hydronephrosis, and potential renal dysplasia, requiring prompt postnatal diagnosis and decompression.

CHAPTER 16: UTERINE IMAGING

Learning Objectives

1. Describe normal uterine zonal anatomy and its variation across the menstrual cycle and reproductive life stages.
2. Distinguish leiomyoma from leiomyosarcoma using a structured, multi-feature approach.
3. Recognize adenomyosis and distinguish it from leiomyoma.
4. Apply endometrial carcinoma staging principles relevant to myometrial and cervical stromal invasion assessment.
5. Recognize congenital uterine anomalies and their classification.

Clinical Overview

This chapter opens Part V of this book with the uterus, an organ whose MRI evaluation spans a comparatively benign but symptomatically significant differential, leiomyoma and adenomyosis foremost among them, together with endometrial carcinoma, one of the more common gynecologic malignancies, whose staging depends substantially on the same zonal anatomy that governs benign disease characterization. This chapter proceeds from uterine zonal anatomy, through the leiomyoma-versus-sarcoma distinction, adenomyosis, endometrial carcinoma staging, and closes with congenital uterine anomalies.

Two instances of the Signal-to-Category Decision System are applied in this chapter, the first to the leiomyoma-versus-leiomyosarcoma triage that anchors uterine mass characterization, and the second to the myometrial invasion depth assessment that is the central determinant of endometrial carcinoma staging.

Uterine Zonal Anatomy and Imaging Technique

Normal Zonal Anatomy: Endometrium, Junctional Zone, and Myometrium

The uterus demonstrates a characteristic trilaminar zonal appearance on T2-weighted imaging that forms the essential anatomic foundation for nearly every diagnostic task in this chapter: the endometrium, centrally located and demonstrating high T2 signal reflecting its glandular, mucosal composition, with thickness varying substantially across the menstrual cycle from a thin, quiescent postmenstrual endometrium to a thick, secretory-phase endometrium; the junctional zone, a thin, low T2 signal band representing the innermost, compact layer of myometrium, whose thickness and integrity are central to both the adenomyosis diagnosis discussed later in this chapter and endometrial carcinoma myometrial invasion staging; and the outer myometrium, demonstrating intermediate T2 signal and comprising the bulk of the uterine wall. Menstrual cycle timing meaningfully affects the appearance of each of these zones, and when clinically feasible, imaging performed during the early proliferative phase, when the endometrium is thin and the junctional zone is most clearly delineated, provides optimal conditions for the zonal anatomy assessment this chapter's diagnostic framework depends upon, a scheduling consideration worth incorporating into elective uterine MRI protocol planning.

Age-Related and Physiologic Variation

Uterine size and zonal anatomy vary substantially across a woman's reproductive life stages, with the prepubertal uterus demonstrating a comparatively small, tubular configuration without the well-developed zonal differentiation of the mature, estrogenized uterus, the reproductive-age uterus demonstrating the classic trilaminar pattern described above, and the postmenopausal uterus demonstrating progressive involution with a thinned myometrium, an often indistinct junctional zone, and a thin endometrial stripe, such that failure to account for this expected age-related involution risks either under-recognizing a genuinely abnormal finding in a younger patient whose baseline anatomy differs from postmenopausal norms, or over-interpreting the expected postmenopausal thinning as pathologic atrophy requiring further workup. Postmenopausal endometrial thickness carries specific, validated threshold values relevant to endometrial carcinoma risk assessment discussed later in this chapter, with a thin endometrial stripe below a validated threshold, generally cited around four to five millimeters, carrying a low probability of clinically significant endometrial pathology in an asymptomatic postmenopausal woman, though postmenopausal bleeding of any kind warrants endometrial sampling regardless of measured thickness given the direct clinical significance of this specific symptom.

Epidemiology and Common Presenting Symptoms of Uterine Disease

Uterine pathology is among the most common indications for pelvic MRI in women of reproductive age, with abnormal uterine bleeding, pelvic pain and pressure, and infertility together accounting for the majority of clinical presentations prompting the imaging evaluations discussed throughout this chapter, and the specific presenting symptom often meaningfully narrows the relevant differential even before imaging is reviewed, since heavy, regular menstrual bleeding more often points toward leiomyoma or adenomyosis, postmenopausal bleeding demands specific exclusion of endometrial carcinoma as discussed later in this chapter, and recurrent pregnancy loss or infertility raises the congenital anomaly differential addressed at the close of this chapter. Ultrasound remains the first-line imaging modality for most uterine indications given its widespread availability, lower cost, and excellent performance for many common findings, with MRI reserved as a problem-solving tool for cases where ultrasound findings are indeterminate, where a large or complex uterus limits ultrasound's field of view and tissue characterization, or where the specific diagnostic task, such as the leiomyoma-versus-sarcoma distinction or precise endometrial carcinoma staging discussed in this chapter, benefits from MRI's superior soft tissue contrast and larger field of view relative to ultrasound.

MRI Technique Considerations for Uterine Imaging

A dedicated uterine MRI protocol incorporates high-resolution T2-weighted imaging in multiple planes, generally including a plane oriented along the true short axis of the uterine body to optimize zonal anatomy depiction, diffusion-weighted imaging, increasingly standard given its contribution to both the leiomyosarcoma risk assessment and endometrial carcinoma characterization discussed throughout this chapter, and dynamic contrast-enhanced imaging, particularly valuable for the myometrial invasion depth assessment central to endometrial carcinoma staging. Patient preparation, including administration of an antiperistaltic agent to reduce bowel motion artifact and, in some protocols, a period of bladder filling optimization analogous to the bladder distension considerations discussed in the preceding chapter, meaningfully affects image quality for the pelvic MRI examinations discussed throughout this and the following two chapters, and technical factors specific to patient body habitus, including the comparatively greater distance from the surface coil array in a patient with a larger body habitus, should be anticipated and addressed with appropriate coil selection and acquisition parameter adjustment.

Postpartum and Puerperal Uterine Imaging

Postpartum MRI, generally reserved for a complicated puerperal course rather than routine use, most often evaluates for retained products of conception, presenting as heterogeneous, enhancing tissue within the endometrial cavity distinct from the expected postpartum blood products and debris, or postpartum hemorrhage from an underlying vascular abnormality including uterine artery pseudoaneurysm, sharing the same enhancing structure morphology and management urgency as the pseudoaneurysms discussed in the splenic and hepatic contexts earlier in this book, or arteriovenous malformation, a less common but important cause of delayed, sometimes severe postpartum hemorrhage. Distinguishing retained products of conception from a uterine arteriovenous malformation carries direct management implications, since retained products are managed with uterine evacuation, while an arteriovenous malformation, if inadvertently curetted, can produce catastrophic hemorrhage given its abnormal, high-flow vascular architecture, such that a puerperal patient with a vascular-appearing uterine abnormality demonstrating prominent flow voids or a tangle of abnormal vessels on MRI should be specifically flagged for interventional radiology consultation and embolization consideration rather than proceeding directly to curettage without this specific vascular characterization.

Leiomyoma and the Leiomyosarcoma Distinction

Epidemiology of Leiomyoma and Risk Factors

Uterine leiomyoma demonstrates a strikingly high prevalence in women of reproductive age, present in a substantial majority of women by the time of menopause when assessed by careful pathologic examination even though many remain clinically silent and never come to imaging attention, with established risk factors including advancing reproductive age until menopause, obesity, and a family history of leiomyoma, while parity and prolonged combined oral contraceptive use are each associated with a modestly reduced risk, and Black women demonstrate a substantially higher prevalence, earlier age of onset, and greater symptom burden than women of other racial backgrounds across multiple large epidemiologic studies, a disparity with recognized implications for equitable access to the fertility-sparing treatment options discussed below. This exceptionally high background prevalence of predominantly benign, often asymptomatic leiomyoma is the essential epidemiologic context underlying this chapter's diagnostic emphasis, since the clinical challenge is rarely detecting a uterine mass, which is common and usually straightforward, but rather correctly identifying the comparatively rare instance in which an apparent leiomyoma actually represents the far more consequential leiomyosarcoma.

Leiomyoma: Classification and Typical Imaging Features

Uterine leiomyoma, the most common benign uterine neoplasm and among the most common tumors overall in women of reproductive age, is classified by its location relative to the uterine wall as submucosal, projecting into the endometrial cavity and most directly relevant to abnormal uterine bleeding and fertility given its distortion of the cavity, intramural, confined within the myometrium, or subserosal, projecting outward from the uterine serosal surface and sometimes pedunculated, a classification with direct treatment planning relevance since submucosal leiomyoma is generally amenable to hysteroscopic resection while intramural and subserosal leiomyoma more often require a different surgical or interventional approach when treatment is pursued. Typical leiomyoma demonstrates homogeneous, well-defined, low T2 signal reflecting its dense smooth muscle and fibrous composition, though degenerative change, common in larger leiomyomas given their comparatively limited blood supply relative to their size, produces variable signal heterogeneity, cystic degeneration, or, in the specific context of pregnancy-associated red degeneration, elevated T1 signal from hemorrhagic infarction, each representing an expected, benign variant that should not be mistaken for a more concerning process when the overall lesion morphology and clinical context remain otherwise typical for leiomyoma.

Leiomyosarcoma: Distinguishing Features and Diagnostic Limitations

Uterine leiomyosarcoma, a rare but aggressive malignancy, presents a genuinely challenging preoperative diagnostic problem given its substantial imaging overlap with degenerated leiomyoma, and no single imaging feature reliably distinguishes the two entities with sufficient accuracy for confident preoperative exclusion, such that a combination of features, including ill-defined or irregular margins in contrast to the typically well-defined leiomyoma margin, heterogeneous, intermediate-to-high T2 signal with intratumoral hemorrhage, marked diffusion restriction with a correspondingly low apparent diffusion coefficient value, and rapid interval growth on serial imaging, together raise suspicion for leiomyosarcoma over typical or even degenerated leiomyoma. Because no single MRI feature or combination of features achieves sufficient sensitivity and specificity to entirely exclude leiomyosarcoma preoperatively, and because leiomyosarcoma is comparatively rare relative to the very high background prevalence of leiomyoma, the clinical approach for most uterine masses, even those with some atypical features, remains surgical management as though the mass is presumed benign, with a subset of higher-risk masses, particularly those demonstrating marked diffusion restriction together with rapid growth or postmenopausal presentation, warranting more cautious surgical planning, including avoiding uncontained morcellation techniques that risk disseminating an unrecognized malignancy throughout the peritoneal cavity.

Figure 16.1: Degenerated Leiomyoma with Atypical Signal Heterogeneity

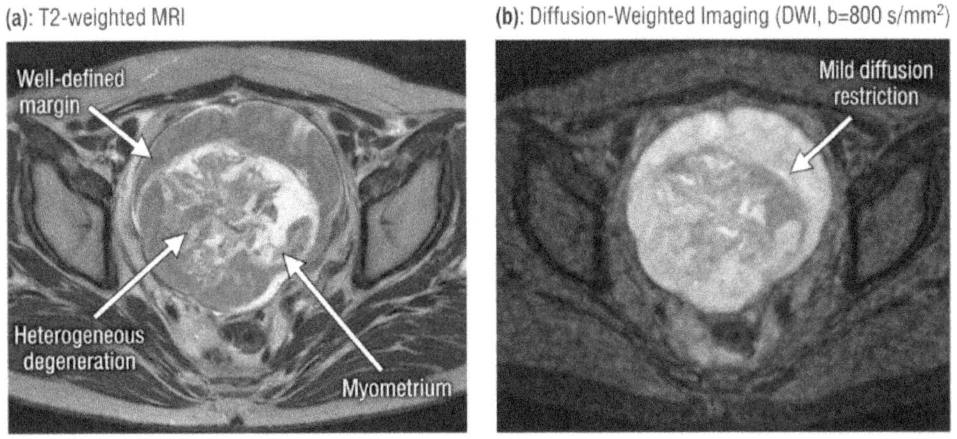

(a) T2-weighted MRI (b) Diffusion-Weighted Imaging (DWI, b=800 s/mm^2)

THE SIGNAL-TO-CATEGORY DECISION SYSTEM — Leiomyoma versus Leiomyosarcoma Triage

The Signal Pattern: A uterine mass with myometrial or endometrial cavity-distorting morphology is identified, and the reader must assess margin definition, signal heterogeneity, diffusion characteristics, and growth pattern to stratify malignant probability.

Category Signature: A well-defined, homogeneously low T2 signal mass without marked diffusion restriction is categorized as favoring typical leiomyoma; a mass with ill-defined margins, heterogeneous signal with hemorrhage, and marked diffusion restriction, particularly with a history of rapid growth or postmenopausal presentation, is categorized as higher-risk and favoring possible leiomyosarcoma.

The Decision: A typical leiomyoma proceeds to standard management per the patient's symptoms and fertility goals, including myomectomy, hysterectomy, or uterine artery embolization as clinically appropriate; a higher-risk mass prompts more cautious surgical planning, avoiding uncontained morcellation, and consideration of additional preoperative counseling about the residual, though reduced, possibility of malignancy despite the absence of a definitive preoperative diagnostic test.

Trap Logic: Degenerative change in a typical, otherwise benign leiomyoma, particularly cystic or red degeneration, can produce signal heterogeneity that superficially resembles the concerning pattern favoring leiomyosarcoma; the discriminating step is integrating the full feature combination, margin definition and diffusion characteristics specifically, together with the clinical growth trajectory, rather than reacting to signal heterogeneity in isolation, since heterogeneity alone is a common and usually benign finding in this specific organ.

Pattern Anchor: No single MRI feature excludes leiomyosarcoma; integrate margin definition, diffusion restriction, and growth trajectory together, and communicate residual uncertainty to the surgical team for a mass with atypical but not definitively malignant features.

Uterine Artery Embolization and Fertility-Sparing Treatment Options

Uterine artery embolization, an interventional radiologic procedure occluding the blood supply to leiomyoma to induce ischemic infarction and subsequent volume reduction, offers a uterus-preserving alternative to hysterectomy for symptomatic leiomyoma, and preprocedural MRI contributes essential planning information, including precise leiomyoma number, size, and location, together with assessment for any feature raising concern for leiomyosarcoma per this chapter's framework, since embolization would be an inappropriate treatment approach for a mass with concerning features warranting surgical excision and pathologic evaluation instead. Postembolization MRI, generally obtained to assess treatment response or evaluate for a suspected complication, demonstrates successful infarction as absent postcontrast enhancement within the treated leiomyoma together with progressive volume reduction on serial imaging, while a leiomyoma demonstrating persistent enhancement suggests incomplete embolization that may require additional intervention, and myomectomy, either hysteroscopic for submucosal leiomyoma or laparoscopic or open for intramural and subserosal leiomyoma, remains the preferred fertility-preserving surgical option for a patient desiring future pregnancy given uterine artery embolization's less well-established impact on subsequent fertility outcomes relative to the more extensively studied myomectomy approach.

Uterine Sarcoma Subtypes Beyond Leiomyosarcoma

Beyond leiomyosarcoma, endometrial stromal sarcoma, arising from the endometrial stroma rather than the myometrial smooth muscle, presents with a distinctive infiltrative growth pattern often extending along vascular and lymphatic channels within the myometrium, producing a characteristic worm-like or tongue-like pattern of intramyometrial extension on imaging that differs from the more discrete, expansile mass morphology of leiomyosarcoma, and carcinosarcoma, a biphasic malignancy containing both carcinomatous and sarcomatous elements and generally considered a high-grade variant of endometrial carcinoma rather than a true sarcoma despite its name, typically presents as a large, polypoid, endometrial cavity-filling mass with aggressive features including deep myometrial invasion frequently present at diagnosis. These less common uterine sarcoma subtypes share the fundamental interpretive challenge discussed throughout this chapter's Rhythm Layer, namely that no single imaging feature reliably excludes malignancy in an atypical uterine mass, reinforcing the broader principle that atypical features in any uterine mass, not solely those with the specific leiomyosarcoma-favoring pattern discussed above, warrant cautious surgical planning and multidisciplinary discussion rather than presumptive benign management.

Special Populations: Leiomyoma in Pregnancy

Leiomyoma is commonly encountered during pregnancy, either as a preexisting finding or one first identified on obstetric imaging, and while most leiomyomas remain asymptomatic throughout gestation, a subset undergo red degeneration, a form of hemorrhagic infarction related to the mass outgrowing its blood supply as it enlarges under pregnancy's hormonal stimulation, presenting with acute, localized pain and, on MRI, the elevated T1 signal from hemorrhage discussed earlier in this chapter, a benign though clinically painful process managed conservatively with analgesia rather than surgical intervention during pregnancy given the risks intervention would pose to the pregnancy itself. Leiomyoma location and size relative to the placenta and cervix carry specific obstetric relevance, since a large submucosal or lower uterine segment leiomyoma can contribute to malpresentation, labor dystocia, or, when located immediately adjacent to the placental implantation site, an elevated risk of placental abruption, considerations the radiologist's report can usefully highlight for the obstetric team's delivery planning beyond simply documenting the leiomyoma's presence and size.

Adenomyosis

Adenomyosis: Pathophysiology and Imaging Features

Adenomyosis, the presence of ectopic endometrial glands and stroma within the myometrium, produces a distinctive imaging pattern of junctional zone thickening, generally exceeding twelve millimeters when measured at its thickest point, together with small, punctate high T2 signal foci within the thickened junctional zone or adjacent myometrium representing the ectopic endometrial tissue itself or associated cystic hemorrhagic change, a combination that, once recognized, distinguishes adenomyosis from the leiomyoma differential discussed above given adenomyosis's characteristically ill-defined, infiltrative myometrial involvement rather than a discrete, well-defined mass. Diffuse adenomyosis, involving the myometrium circumferentially, and focal adenomyosis, producing a more localized, mass-like area of involvement termed an adenomyoma, represent two ends of a morphologic spectrum, with focal adenomyosis presenting a specific diagnostic challenge given its mass-like appearance that can mimic leiomyoma, though the ill-defined margins and interspersed punctate high T2 foci characteristic of adenomyosis, in contrast to the well-defined margin and homogeneous low signal of typical leiomyoma, generally allow distinction between these two entities when specifically sought.

Clinical Correlation and Treatment Implications

Adenomyosis is a common cause of dysmenorrhea and heavy menstrual bleeding, particularly in multiparous women in their late reproductive years, and its accurate preoperative diagnosis carries meaningful treatment planning relevance, since adenomyosis, unlike a discrete leiomyoma, is not amenable to focal surgical excision given its diffuse, infiltrative involvement of the myometrium, such that a patient with symptomatic adenomyosis desiring uterine preservation is generally counseled toward medical management or, for more severe cases, uterine artery embolization rather than a myomectomy-type procedure that would be appropriate for a discrete leiomyoma but ineffective for diffusely infiltrative adenomyosis. Adenomyosis and leiomyoma coexist in a substantial proportion of affected women, and when both are present, the radiologist's report should clearly distinguish and separately characterize each process, since a patient's symptoms may be attributable to either or both processes, and surgical planning, when pursued, benefits from understanding the relative contribution and location of each distinct pathology rather than a generalized description of uterine enlargement or heterogeneity alone.

Endometrioid Endometrial Carcinoma

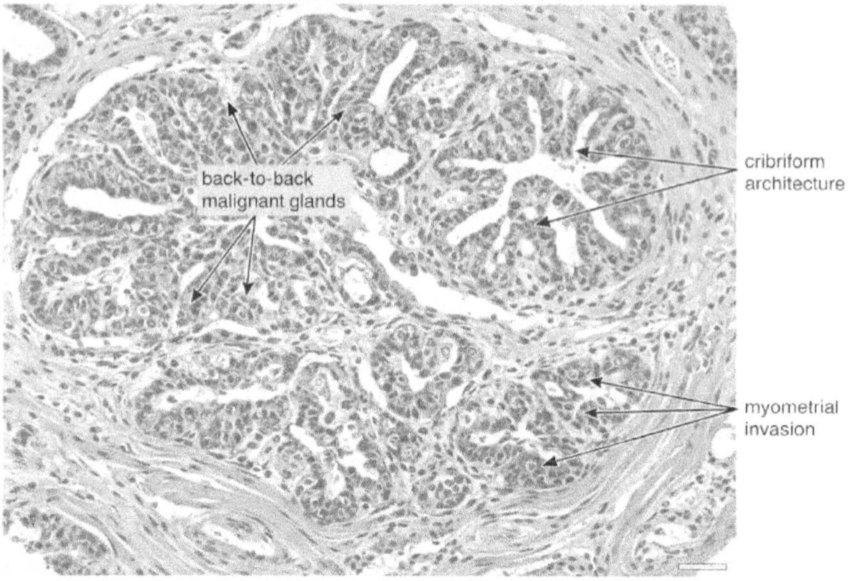

Figure 16.2 Endometrioid Endometrial Carcinoma 20x

Special Populations: Adenomyosis in Infertility Evaluation

Adenomyosis carries a recognized, if incompletely understood, association with reduced fertility and adverse pregnancy outcomes, including an elevated risk of miscarriage and preterm delivery, thought to relate to impaired uterine junctional zone contractility and an altered endometrial implantation environment, such that its identification in a woman undergoing infertility evaluation provides relevant context beyond the symptomatic dysmenorrhea and heavy bleeding presentation more typically emphasized, and should be specifically communicated to the reproductive endocrinology team given its potential relevance to the patient's overall fertility treatment planning, including consideration of medical suppression therapy before assisted reproductive technology in appropriately selected cases. The historical teaching that adenomyosis occurs predominantly in multiparous women in their fourth and fifth decades has been revised by more recent imaging-based series demonstrating a meaningful prevalence in younger, nulliparous women presenting with infertility or dysmenorrhea alone, underscoring that adenomyosis should not be dismissed from the differential in a younger patient simply because she does not fit the classic demographic profile historically associated with this diagnosis.

Endometrial Carcinoma Staging

Epidemiology and Risk Factors for Endometrial Carcinoma

Endometrial carcinoma is the most common gynecologic malignancy in many developed-world populations, with established risk factors converging substantially on the theme of unopposed estrogen exposure, including obesity, given peripheral aromatization of androgens to estrogen in adipose tissue, nulliparity, early menarche and late menopause, tamoxifen therapy, and polycystic ovary syndrome, each contributing to a prolonged or excessive estrogenic stimulation of the endometrium without the counterbalancing effect of progesterone that characterizes a normal ovulatory cycle. Postmenopausal bleeding, the dominant presenting symptom, prompts endometrial sampling in most cases given its direct diagnostic yield, with imaging, most often transvaginal ultrasound as the first-line modality followed by MRI for staging once carcinoma is confirmed, playing a complementary rather than primary diagnostic role, though the endometrial thickness threshold discussed earlier in this chapter provides useful risk stratification when ultrasound is the initial imaging study obtained for this common and important presenting complaint.

Histologic Subtypes and Molecular Classification

Endometrioid adenocarcinoma, the most common histologic subtype and generally associated with the unopposed estrogen risk factor profile discussed above, typically carries a comparatively favorable prognosis when diagnosed at an early stage, while the non-endometrioid subtypes, including serous and clear cell carcinoma, demonstrate a more aggressive clinical behavior with a greater propensity for deep myometrial invasion, lymphovascular invasion, and extrauterine spread even when the primary tumor itself appears comparatively small, such that histologic subtype, established through endometrial sampling before imaging staging is performed, provides essential context the radiologist should incorporate when characterizing invasion depth and searching for extrauterine disease, since a small serous carcinoma may still warrant the same thorough staging evaluation applied to a considerably larger endometrioid tumor given its disproportionately aggressive behavior. Contemporary molecular classification, incorporating features including microsatellite instability status and TP53 mutation status alongside traditional histologic subtyping, has refined prognostic stratification beyond histology and stage alone, though this molecular classification remains a pathologic rather than imaging-based determination, with the radiologist's role continuing to center on the anatomic staging parameters, myometrial invasion depth, cervical stromal invasion, and extrauterine extension, discussed throughout this chapter.

Lynch Syndrome and Endometrial Carcinoma Screening

Lynch syndrome, the hereditary cancer syndrome discussed in the pancreatic and renal chapters of this book, carries a substantially elevated endometrial carcinoma risk, with endometrial carcinoma representing the most common Lynch syndrome-associated malignancy in affected women and, in some cases, the sentinel cancer diagnosis that prompts the hereditary syndrome's initial identification, such that endometrial carcinoma diagnosed at a younger age than typical, or in a patient with a compatible family history, should prompt genetic counseling referral given the syndrome's implications for the patient's own additional cancer risk and for cascade testing of at-risk family members.

Myometrial Invasion Depth Assessment

Myometrial invasion depth, stratified as confined to the inner half or extending into the outer half of the myometrium, represents the central staging determination for endometrial carcinoma and the single most important MRI-derived staging parameter, since invasion depth correlates directly with lymph node metastasis risk and drives the surgical lymphadenectomy decision, with outer-half invasion carrying a substantially elevated nodal metastasis risk warranting more extensive lymph node dissection at the time of hysterectomy compared to the more limited or absent lymphadenectomy that may be appropriate for confidently inner-half-confined disease. This depth assessment relies on identifying the junctional zone-myometrial interface and tracking the tumor's deepest point of extension relative to the outer myometrial serosal margin, most reliably performed on a combination of T2-weighted and dynamic contrast-enhanced imaging, where the hypervascular, early-enhancing normal myometrium provides contrast against the comparatively hypoenhancing tumor, a technique particularly valuable when the junctional zone itself is indistinct, as is common in the postmenopausal patient population in whom endometrial carcinoma most often presents.

Cervical Stromal Invasion and Extrauterine Extension

Cervical stromal invasion, extension of tumor from the endometrial cavity into the fibrous cervical stroma, upstages disease beyond the uterine corpus-confined categories and, similar to myometrial invasion depth, is best assessed by identifying disruption of the normal low T2 signal cervical stroma by intermediate-to-high signal tumor, a distinction requiring careful attention given that cervical mucus and glandular tissue can produce signal that potentially confounds this assessment if the cervical anatomy is not carefully and systematically evaluated in its own right rather than simply extrapolated from the corpus findings. Extrauterine extension, including parametrial invasion, vaginal involvement, and adnexal spread, together with regional lymphadenopathy assessed using the same morphologic criteria applied to lymph nodes throughout this book, complete the staging assessment, and, akin to prostate cancer staging discussed in an earlier chapter, precise, structured documentation of each of these specific staging components, rather than a general impression of tumor extent, is essential information for the gynecologic oncology team's surgical and treatment planning.

THE SIGNAL-TO-CATEGORY DECISION SYSTEM — Myometrial Invasion Depth Assessment

The Signal Pattern: Endometrial carcinoma is identified, and the reader must determine the deepest point of myometrial invasion relative to the outer serosal margin to assign invasion depth category.

Category Signature: Tumor confined to the endometrium or invading no more than the inner half of the myometrial thickness is categorized as inner-half invasion; tumor extending into the outer half of the myometrial thickness, approaching or reaching the serosa, is categorized as outer-half invasion.

The Decision: Inner-half invasion supports a more limited surgical lymphadenectomy approach in an appropriately risk-stratified patient; outer-half invasion supports more extensive lymph node dissection given the substantially elevated associated nodal metastasis risk.

Trap Logic: A large, exophytic endometrial tumor can distort and thin the adjacent myometrium through mass effect alone without true invasion, an appearance that can be mistaken for deep myometrial invasion if the distinction between true invasive extension and simple mechanical thinning from an adjacent bulky mass is not deliberately considered; the discriminating step is assessing dynamic contrast-enhanced imaging, where true tumor invasion typically demonstrates lower enhancement than the adjacent, mechanically thinned but still viable normal myometrium.

Pattern Anchor: Distinguish true invasive extension from mechanical myometrial thinning by an exophytic mass using dynamic contrast enhancement; myometrial thinning alone is not equivalent to deep invasion.

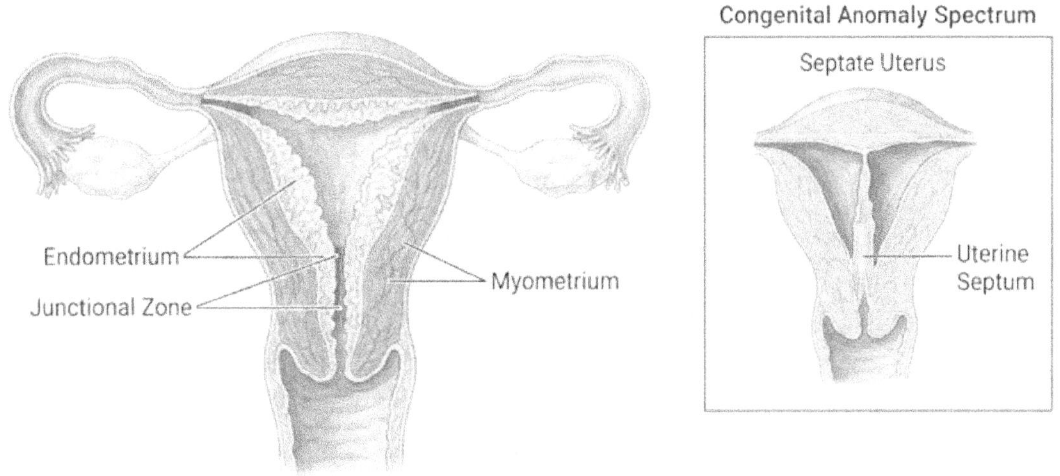

Figure 16.3: Uterine Zonal Anatomy and Congenital Anomaly Spectrum

Congenital Uterine Anomalies

Clinical Presentation and Fertility Implications of Congenital Anomalies

Congenital uterine anomalies often remain clinically silent until pregnancy-related complications, including recurrent first-trimester loss most classically associated with septate uterus given the septum's poor vascularity, or second-trimester loss and preterm delivery more classically associated with the reduced uterine cavity volume of a unicornuate or bicornuate uterus, prompt the imaging evaluation that ultimately identifies the underlying anomaly, and a minority of anomalies, particularly a non-communicating rudimentary horn in unicornuate uterus, present with cyclic pelvic pain from obstructed menstrual outflow within the isolated horn, a presentation that can mimic other causes of pelvic pain if the underlying anomaly is not specifically considered. Fertility and obstetric outcomes vary considerably by anomaly type, with septate uterus carrying the least favorable untreated reproductive prognosis among the anomalies discussed in this chapter but also the most treatable given its amenability to hysteroscopic correction, underscoring why accurate anomaly subtype classification, rather than a general diagnosis of congenital uterine anomaly, is essential for appropriate patient counseling and treatment planning in this specific population.

Anomaly	External Fundal Contour	Septum/Divider Composition	Typical Management
Septate uterus	Smooth or minimally indented	Fibrous, low T2 signal	Hysteroscopic resection

Bicornuate uterus	Deep indentation (>1 cm)	Myometrial, intermediate T2 signal	Generally conservative
Didelphys uterus	Two separate uterine bodies	Two separate cervices	Individualized; often conservative
Unicornuate uterus	Single banana-shaped horn	May have non-communicating rudimentary horn	Excision of obstructed rudimentary horn if present

Müllerian Duct Anomaly Classification

Congenital uterine anomalies arise from abnormal Müllerian duct development, fusion, or resorption during embryogenesis, and the classification system in widest current use organizes anomalies by the specific developmental defect: agenesis or hypoplasia, in which the uterus fails to develop or develops incompletely, unicornuate uterus, arising from failure of one Müllerian duct to develop with the contralateral duct forming a normal or near-normal hemiuterus, didelphys uterus, arising from complete failure of Müllerian duct fusion producing two separate uterine bodies and cervices, bicornuate uterus, arising from partial fusion failure producing two uterine horns sharing a single cervix, septate uterus, arising from normal fusion but failed resorption of the midline septum, and arcuate uterus, representing a minor, generally clinically insignificant fundal contour variant at the mild end of this anomaly spectrum. Distinguishing septate from bicornuate uterus, a clinically important distinction given their markedly different treatment implications, relies on assessing the external fundal contour, which is smooth or minimally indented in septate uterus but demonstrates a deep, greater than one-centimeter indentation in bicornuate uterus, together with the composition of the dividing septum itself, fibrous and low T2 signal in a true septate uterus versus myometrial and intermediate T2 signal in bicornuate uterus, a distinction for which MRI's superior soft tissue contrast offers a meaningful advantage over other imaging modalities.

Clinical Significance and Renal Anomaly Association

This distinction carries direct treatment relevance, since septate uterus, associated with an elevated risk of recurrent pregnancy loss related to the septum's poor vascularity and unfavorable implantation environment, is amenable to hysteroscopic septum resection, a comparatively straightforward procedure that can improve reproductive outcomes, while bicornuate uterus, reflecting a fusion defect rather than a resorption defect, is not amenable to this same hysteroscopic approach and is instead managed conservatively in most cases given the more limited surgical options and generally more favorable reproductive prognosis relative to septate uterus despite the anomaly itself. Müllerian duct anomalies carry a well-recognized association with renal anomalies, reflecting the shared embryologic origin and close developmental relationship between the Müllerian and mesonephric duct systems, most classically unilateral renal agenesis ipsilateral to a unicornuate uterus's non-communicating rudimentary horn, such that identification of a Müllerian anomaly should prompt a deliberate search for an associated renal anomaly, and conversely, an unexplained unilateral renal anomaly identified in a young woman should prompt consideration of an associated, potentially previously unrecognized uterine anomaly.

Figure 16.4: Hysteroscopic Uterine Septum Resection Technique

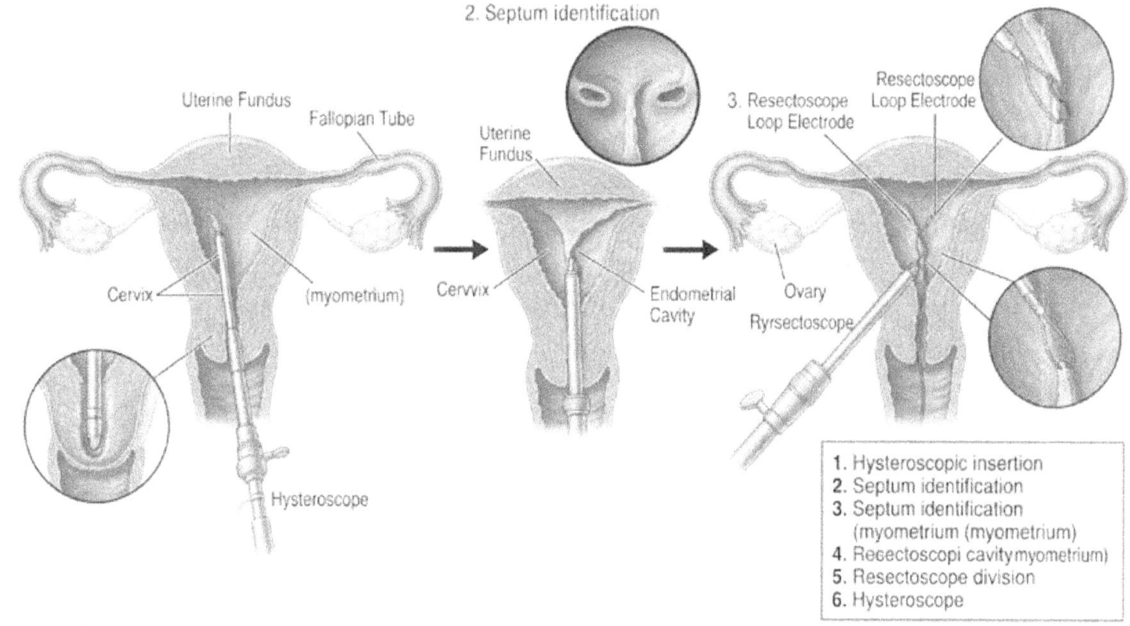

Clinical Case Presentations

Case 1. A 42-year-old woman with heavy menstrual bleeding and pelvic pressure undergoes MRI demonstrating a 6-centimeter well-defined intramural mass with homogeneous low T2 signal, without irregular margins or marked diffusion restriction. The radiologist categorizes the mass as typical leiomyoma and recommends standard management options per the patient's fertility goals, reassuring the gynecology team that the imaging features do not raise concern for leiomyosarcoma.

Case 2. A 61-year-old postmenopausal woman presents with a rapidly enlarging pelvic mass over several months, and MRI demonstrates a 9-centimeter uterine mass with ill-defined margins, heterogeneous signal with areas of hemorrhage, and marked diffusion restriction with a low apparent diffusion coefficient value. Given the rapid growth, postmenopausal presentation, and combination of concerning imaging features, the radiologist categorizes the mass as higher-risk for leiomyosarcoma and specifically recommends against uncontained morcellation during surgical management, appropriately flagging the residual malignant possibility despite the absence of a definitive preoperative diagnosis.

Case 3. A 38-year-old woman with severe dysmenorrhea undergoes MRI demonstrating diffuse thickening of the junctional zone to 16 millimeters with numerous punctate high T2 signal foci throughout the thickened zone, without a discrete, well-defined mass. The radiologist categorizes the findings as diffuse adenomyosis and counsels the gynecology team that this diffuse, infiltrative process is not amenable to focal myomectomy, directing the treatment discussion toward medical management or uterine artery embolization instead.

Case 4. A 68-year-old woman with postmenopausal bleeding undergoes MRI demonstrating an endometrial mass with tumor signal extending into the outer half of the myometrial thickness, approaching but not reaching the serosal surface, without cervical stromal invasion or lymphadenopathy. The radiologist categorizes the findings as outer-half myometrial invasion and communicates this specific staging detail to the gynecologic oncology team, supporting their planning for a more extensive lymphadenectomy given the elevated nodal metastasis risk this depth of invasion carries.

Case 5. A 24-year-old woman with recurrent first-trimester pregnancy loss undergoes MRI demonstrating a uterus with a smooth external fundal contour and a fibrous, low T2 signal septum dividing the endometrial cavity into two separate horns. Recognizing the smooth external contour and fibrous septal composition as characteristic of septate rather than bicornuate uterus, the radiologist recommends hysteroscopic septum resection evaluation given this specific anomaly's amenability to this procedure and its association with improved reproductive outcomes following correction.

Case 6. A 45-year-old woman recently diagnosed with endometrioid endometrial carcinoma at age 45, considered younger than typical for this diagnosis, has a family history notable for her mother's colorectal cancer at age 48 and an uncle's endometrial cancer at age 50. Recognizing this family history pattern together with the patient's own comparatively young age at diagnosis as suspicious for Lynch syndrome, the radiologist notes this observation in the report to prompt the gynecologic oncology team's consideration of genetic counseling referral, which subsequently confirms a pathogenic MLH1 mutation, leading to appropriate additional cancer surveillance for the patient and cascade genetic testing offered to her at-risk family members.

Case 7. A 29-year-old woman ten days postpartum presents with worsening vaginal bleeding, and MRI demonstrates heterogeneous, enhancing intracavitary tissue together with a focal tangle of abnormal, prominent flow voids within the adjacent myometrium. Recognizing the flow voids as concerning for an underlying arteriovenous malformation rather than simple retained products of conception alone, the radiologist recommends interventional radiology consultation before any curettage is performed, and subsequent angiography confirms and successfully embolizes the malformation, avoiding the potentially catastrophic hemorrhage that curettage of an unrecognized arteriovenous malformation could have caused.

THE SIGNAL-TO-CATEGORY DECISION SYSTEM — Uterine Mass and Staging Triage Arc

The Signal Pattern: This chapter's patterns span the uterine risk spectrum, from a myometrial mass whose margin and diffusion characteristics must be integrated before a benign leiomyoma label is applied, to endometrial carcinoma whose invasion depth must be precisely tracked relative to the serosal margin for staging.

Category Signature: Uterine masses are categorized as favoring leiomyoma or higher-risk for leiomyosarcoma based on margin, signal heterogeneity, diffusion restriction, and growth; endometrial carcinoma is categorized by inner-half versus outer-half myometrial invasion depth.

The Decision: Category assignment in this chapter ranges from standard leiomyoma management to cautious surgical planning avoiding morcellation, and from limited to extensive lymphadenectomy, with every category assigned only after the specific confirmatory feature combination this chapter's framework requires has been deliberately assessed.

The Trap Logic: Both patterns in this chapter share a common trap: a benign or mechanical explanation, degenerative heterogeneity or mass-effect myometrial thinning, that can superficially mimic the concerning, category-defining finding without meeting its true diagnostic criteria.

Pattern Anchor: Integrate the full feature combination, never a single signal characteristic in isolation, before assigning either category in this chapter; degenerative and mechanical mimics are common and require deliberate distinction from true pathologic findings.

Summary and Key Concepts

Uterine zonal anatomy, endometrium, junctional zone, and myometrium, varies with menstrual cycle timing and reproductive life stage and forms the foundation for nearly every diagnostic task in this chapter.

No single MRI feature excludes leiomyosarcoma; a combination of ill-defined margins, heterogeneous hemorrhagic signal, marked diffusion restriction, and rapid growth raises suspicion over typical or degenerated leiomyoma.

Adenomyosis shows junctional zone thickening exceeding 12 millimeters with punctate high T2 foci and ill-defined infiltrative margins, distinguishing it from the well-defined, homogeneous appearance of leiomyoma; it is not amenable to focal myomectomy.

Myometrial invasion depth, inner-half versus outer-half, is the central endometrial carcinoma staging determination and directly drives the lymphadenectomy decision.

True myometrial invasion should be distinguished from mechanical thinning by an exophytic mass using dynamic contrast enhancement.

Septate uterus has a smooth external fundal contour and fibrous septum, amenable to hysteroscopic resection; bicornuate uterus has a deeply indented contour and myometrial septum, not amenable to this approach.

Müllerian duct anomalies carry a well-recognized association with renal anomalies given their shared embryologic origin.

CHAPTER 17: ADNEXAL MASSES AND THE O-RADS FRAMEWORK

Learning Objectives

1. Apply the O-RADS MRI framework to stratify adnexal masses by malignant probability.
2. Recognize the imaging features of the major benign ovarian mass types, including endometrioma, dermoid, and simple cyst.
3. Recognize the imaging features of epithelial ovarian carcinoma and distinguish it from benign mimics.
4. Recognize ovarian torsion and its imaging correlates relevant to surgical urgency.
5. Characterize fallopian tube pathology and tubo-ovarian abscess.

Clinical Overview

The adnexal mass presents one of the more anxiety-provoking clinical scenarios in gynecologic imaging, given the wide gulf between the reassuringly common, entirely benign functional cyst and the comparatively rare but lethal epithelial ovarian carcinoma, and the O-RADS MRI framework discussed throughout this chapter provides the structured, standardized approach that has meaningfully improved consistency and communication around this critical triage task, mirroring the PI-RADS and VI-RADS frameworks introduced in preceding chapters for their respective organs. This chapter proceeds from the O-RADS framework and benign adnexal mass types, through epithelial ovarian carcinoma, ovarian torsion as a surgical emergency, and closes with fallopian tube pathology and tubo-ovarian abscess.

Two instances of the Signal-to-Category Decision System are applied in this chapter, the first to O-RADS category assignment itself, and the second to the ovarian torsion triage that determines surgical urgency, a time-critical decision distinct in character from the malignancy risk stratification that dominates the remainder of this chapter.

The O-RADS MRI Framework

Epidemiology and Clinical Presentation of Adnexal Masses

Adnexal masses are identified across the full span of a woman's reproductive life, with the specific differential diagnosis meaningfully shifting by age and menopausal status: in a premenopausal woman, a functional cyst is by far the most common cause of an adnexal finding and generally warrants a period of short-interval follow-up before further characterization is pursued, given the high likelihood of spontaneous resolution, while in a postmenopausal woman, functional cysts are far less common given the absence of ongoing ovulatory cycling, such that a new solid or complex adnexal mass in this population carries a correspondingly higher baseline malignant probability warranting more assertive characterization from the outset. Clinical presentation ranges from an entirely asymptomatic incidental finding on imaging performed for an unrelated indication, the most common scenario for a smaller, uncomplicated mass, to acute pelvic pain from torsion or rupture discussed later in this chapter, to the comparatively nonspecific and often insidious symptoms, bloating, early satiety, and pelvic pressure, that frequently accompany more advanced ovarian carcinoma and contribute to this malignancy's characteristically late-stage presentation relative to many other cancers discussed throughout this book.

MRI Technique and Indications for Adnexal Mass Evaluation

Ultrasound remains the first-line imaging modality for adnexal mass characterization given its excellent performance for the majority of lesions, wide availability, and lower cost, and MRI, as with several other organ systems discussed throughout this book, is generally reserved as a problem-solving tool for a mass that remains indeterminate after ultrasound, functioning specifically to further risk-stratify these indeterminate lesions using the O-RADS MRI framework discussed throughout this chapter, a role that has become increasingly standardized and guideline-supported as evidence for this specific problem-solving application has accumulated. A dedicated adnexal MRI protocol incorporates high-resolution T2-weighted imaging, fat-suppressed T1-weighted imaging both before and after contrast administration, essential for confirming both macroscopic fat, relevant to the dermoid diagnosis discussed later in this chapter, and true enhancement of any solid component, and dynamic contrast-enhanced imaging with time-intensity curve capability specifically to support the quantitative solid tissue characterization central to O-RADS category assignment.

Framework Structure and Lesion Type Determination

The O-RADS MRI framework first requires the reader to characterize the adnexal mass by its fundamental composition, purely cystic, cystic with a solid component, or purely or predominantly solid, since this initial characterization determines which of several distinct decision pathways within the framework applies, analogous in this branching logical structure to the zone-dependent dominant sequence assignment in the PI-RADS framework discussed in an earlier chapter. Within each composition-based pathway, the framework then assesses additional features, including the number and thickness of internal septations, the presence and enhancement pattern of any solid or papillary projections, and the specific tissue characteristics that may indicate a specific benign entity such as endometrioma or dermoid, discussed later in this chapter, each contributing to the final five-tier risk category assignment ranging from category 1, indicating a normal ovary or a lesion certain to be physiologic and not requiring the O-RADS system at all, through category 5, indicating a high probability of malignancy.

Solid Tissue and Time-Intensity Curve Assessment

The presence, number, and enhancement kinetics of solid tissue within a cystic or complex adnexal mass represent the single most important risk-stratifying feature within the O-RADS framework, and dynamic contrast-enhanced imaging with time-intensity curve analysis, in which the relative signal intensity of a solid component is plotted over serial postcontrast time points and compared to the enhancement curve of a reference tissue such as myometrium, provides an objective, quantifiable method for characterizing this solid tissue's likely biologic behavior, with a curve demonstrating slow, gradual enhancement generally favoring a benign process and a curve demonstrating rapid, early enhancement with subsequent washout, mirroring the malignant enhancement pattern discussed for other organs throughout this book, favoring malignancy. This time-intensity curve methodology, together with the more qualitative assessment of solid component morphology, smooth versus irregular, and diffusion characteristics, collectively inform the O-RADS category assignment for a mass with a solid component, and the framework's specific numeric size and enhancement thresholds, detailed within the O-RADS technical specification, provide the reproducible, structured criteria that reduce the interobserver variability historically associated with more subjective, gestalt-based adnexal mass characterization approaches.

O-RADS Category	Composition	Solid Component / Enhancement	Estimated Malignancy Risk	Management
O-RADS 1	Normal ovary	Not applicable	Not applicable	No further workup
O-RADS 2	Unilocular cyst, or cyst with entity-specific diagnostic signal (endometrioma, dermoid)	None	Under 0.5%	Routine follow-up or none
O-RADS 3	Multilocular cyst with thin septations, or unilocular cyst with a small smooth solid component	Smooth, slow enhancement if present	Roughly 3% to 10%	Short-interval follow-up or specialist correlation
O-RADS 4	Mass with a solid component demonstrating smooth margins and moderate enhancement	Smooth, moderate enhancement	Roughly 10% to 50%	Gynecologic oncology referral considered
O-RADS 5	Mass with an irregular solid component demonstrating rapid, washout-pattern enhancement, or peritoneal implants	Irregular, rapid washout	Greater than 50%	Urgent gynecologic oncology referral

Special Populations: Adnexal Masses in Pregnancy and Pediatric Patients

Adnexal mass evaluation during pregnancy carries distinct considerations beyond the framework discussed above, since the corpus luteum of pregnancy itself can appear as a prominent, sometimes complex or hemorrhagic-appearing cystic structure that should not be mistaken for a pathologic mass, and MRI without gadolinium contrast, given the theoretical concerns regarding gadolinium crossing the placenta and its uncertain long-term fetal effects, becomes the preferred problem-solving modality when ultrasound is indeterminate in a pregnant patient, relying more heavily on T2-weighted morphology and diffusion-weighted imaging than on the contrast-enhanced kinetics that anchor O-RADS category assignment in the nonpregnant population. A persistent, enlarging, or morphologically concerning adnexal mass identified during pregnancy warrants the same fundamental oncologic vigilance applied outside of pregnancy, with surgical management, when required, generally deferred to the second trimester when feasible to minimize both the miscarriage risk associated with first-trimester intervention and the preterm labor risk associated with later intervention. In the pediatric and adolescent population, mature cystic teratoma and functional cysts remain the dominant benign entities, mirroring the adult differential, but ovarian torsion assumes particular prominence as a diagnostic consideration given the comparatively higher torsion risk in this age group, including torsion of a structurally normal ovary without a predisposing mass, a pattern less commonly encountered in adult patients and one that should keep torsion on the differential even when no clearly predisposing lesion is identified on initial imaging.

KEY POINT: O-RADS category assignment for a mass with a solid component depends on confirmed enhancement, not simply the presence of a hyperintense or heterogeneous-appearing region on precontrast imaging; subtraction imaging or direct precontrast-to-postcontrast comparison is essential before a solid component is treated as truly enhancing tissue.

THE SIGNAL-TO-CATEGORY DECISION SYSTEM — O-RADS Category Assignment

---

The Signal Pattern: An adnexal mass is identified, and the reader must first classify its composition, purely cystic, cystic with solid component, or predominantly solid, before applying the composition-specific O-RADS decision pathway.

Category Signature: A unilocular cyst without solid components or septations, or one with signal characteristics diagnostic of a specific benign entity, is categorized as low O-RADS risk; a multilocular cyst with thin septations is categorized as intermediate; a mass with a solid component demonstrating smooth margins and slow, gradual enhancement is categorized as moderate risk; a mass with an irregular solid component demonstrating rapid, washout-pattern enhancement is categorized as high risk.

The Decision: Low-risk categories generally require no further workup or short-interval follow-up alone; intermediate categories may warrant gynecologic oncology referral or specialist ultrasound correlation depending on additional clinical factors; higher-risk categories warrant gynecologic oncology referral for surgical planning given the substantially elevated associated malignant probability.

Trap Logic: A hemorrhagic cyst or endometrioma can contain clotted blood that mimics a solid, enhancing mural nodule on a single postcontrast sequence if enhancement is not carefully confirmed with subtraction imaging or precontrast comparison, directly analogous to the hemorrhagic renal cyst pitfall discussed in an earlier chapter; the discriminating step is confirming true enhancement of any apparent solid component before assigning a higher-risk category, since a genuinely non-enhancing clot, however solid in appearance, does not carry the same risk implication as a truly enhancing solid nodule.

Pattern Anchor: Confirm true enhancement of any apparent solid component before assigning a higher O-RADS category; clotted blood within a hemorrhagic cyst is a common and important mimic of a genuine solid nodule.

Figure 17.1: O-RADS 5 Complex Adnexal Mass with Irregular Enhancing Solid Component

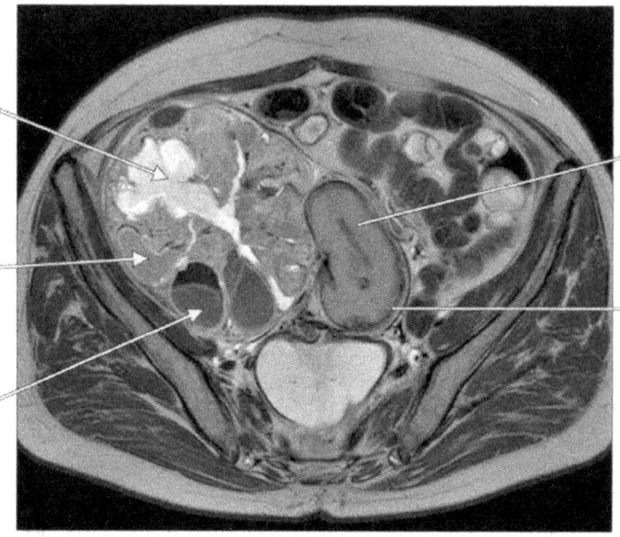

Patient Education and Counseling for Adnexal Mass Findings

Communicating an adnexal mass finding to a patient requires calibrating the language of risk carefully, since the word mass itself carries substantial emotional weight for many patients regardless of the underlying O-RADS category, and framing a low-risk finding in terms of its specific, favorable characteristics, a simple cyst with no concerning features, expected to resolve or remain stable, rather than leaving a patient to interpret the word mass in isolation, meaningfully reduces unnecessary anxiety while still conveying an accurate clinical picture. For a patient with an intermediate or higher-risk O-RADS category, clear explanation of the recommended next step, whether short-interval follow-up imaging, specialist referral, or surgical planning, together with a realistic, non-alarmist discussion of the estimated risk range associated with that category, supports informed decision-making and helps the patient understand why a particular pathway has been recommended rather than another, particularly when the recommended step involves a waiting period that can itself be a source of considerable anxiety. Patients with a personal or family history suggestive of hereditary ovarian carcinoma risk, discussed above in the context of BRCA mutation, benefit from proactive counseling regarding genetic testing referral even when the adnexal finding prompting the current evaluation is itself benign, since the imaging encounter often represents a meaningful opportunity to identify a patient who would benefit from risk assessment independent of the specific finding under evaluation, and clear documentation of this counseling recommendation in the report or accompanying clinical communication helps ensure the recommendation is not lost in the subsequent care pathway. Patients undergoing evaluation for suspected torsion require a distinctly different counseling approach given the time-critical nature of this diagnosis, with clear, direct communication of the urgency involved and the rationale for proceeding promptly to surgical exploration even when the imaging findings are not entirely classic, since patient understanding of the salvage-versus-loss stakes involved supports timely consent and reduces the anxiety associated with an unexpected emergent surgical recommendation.

Benign Adnexal Mass Types

Epidemiology of Benign Adnexal Masses

Functional cysts, endometrioma, and mature cystic teratoma together account for the substantial majority of adnexal masses encountered in clinical practice across all age groups, and this high background prevalence of predominantly benign entities, echoing the epidemiologic context established for other organ systems throughout this book, is essential to appropriately calibrating the assertiveness of the workup pathway applied to a given adnexal finding, favoring confident, criteria-based benign characterization when a specific entity's diagnostic signal pattern is clearly present rather than reflexively pursuing further workup for every adnexal finding regardless of its imaging specificity. Endometrioma specifically occurs in the context of endometriosis, a systemic condition addressed in greater anatomic detail in the following chapter's discussion of pelvic endometriosis, and its presence should prompt a search for additional endometriotic implants elsewhere in the pelvis, including the pouch of Douglas, uterosacral ligaments, and bowel serosa, rather than treating the ovarian endometrioma as an isolated finding disconnected from this broader, often multifocal disease process.

Struma Ovarii and Other Rare Benign Entities

Struma ovarii, a rare, highly specialized monodermal teratoma composed predominantly of thyroid tissue, can occasionally produce clinical hyperthyroidism from autonomous thyroid hormone secretion and demonstrates a distinctive, markedly heterogeneous, multiloculated cystic and solid appearance with variable, sometimes very low T2 signal in solid components reflecting the dense colloid content characteristic of thyroid tissue, a specific and unusual signal pattern that, together with a compatible clinical presentation of hyperthyroidism without an identifiable cervical thyroid abnormality, should prompt consideration of this specific rare entity. Fibroma and fibrothecoma, benign sex cord-stromal tumors, present as solid, markedly low T2 signal masses reflecting their dense fibrous composition, an appearance that can closely resemble a pedunculated subserosal leiomyoma discussed in the preceding chapter if the mass's precise ovarian, rather than uterine, origin is not carefully confirmed, and Meigs syndrome, the association of a benign ovarian fibroma with ascites and pleural effusion that resolve following tumor resection, is a specific and clinically satisfying pattern worth recognizing given its entirely benign nature despite the alarming combination of findings it can present.

Endometrioma

Endometrioma, an ovarian cyst containing accumulated menstrual-cycle blood products from ectopic endometrial tissue, demonstrates a highly characteristic and specific MRI appearance, homogeneous, markedly elevated T1 signal that fails to suppress on fat-suppressed sequences, distinguishing it from the fat-containing dermoid discussed below which does suppress, together with the shading sign, a subtle but characteristic decrease in T2 signal relative to simple fluid reflecting the cyst's progressively concentrated, iron-rich hemosiderin content from repeated cyclic hemorrhage, a combination sufficiently specific to allow confident diagnosis in most cases without further workup. Endometrioma carries a small but recognized malignant transformation risk, most often to clear cell or endometrioid ovarian carcinoma, and the development of an enhancing solid or mural nodular component within a previously typical, stable endometrioma should prompt concern for this specific malignant transformation pathway rather than being dismissed as an expected feature of endometrioma, making this specific finding, a new or enlarging solid component within an otherwise typical endometrioma, an important exception to the generally reassuring default management of this common benign entity.

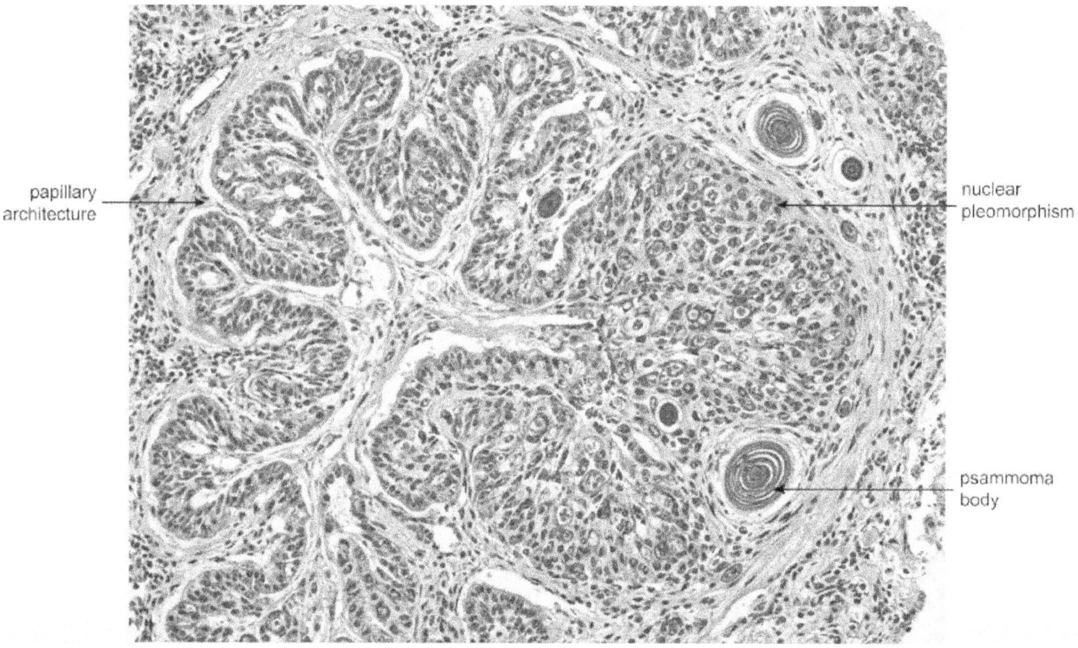

Mature Cystic Teratoma and Other Benign Findings

Mature cystic teratoma, commonly termed dermoid cyst and among the most common benign ovarian neoplasms particularly in younger women, demonstrates macroscopic fat, readily confirmed with the same fat-suppression technique discussed throughout this book, together with a characteristic mural nodule termed the Rokitansky protrusion or dermoid plug, which can contain teeth, hair, or other ectodermal, mesodermal, or endodermal derivatives reflecting the tumor's origin from totipotent germ cells, and fat-fluid or hair-fluid levels, when present, provide additional corroborating evidence for this diagnosis. Malignant transformation of a mature cystic teratoma, most often to squamous cell carcinoma arising within the dermoid plug, is rare but should be considered when a dermoid demonstrates an atypical or rapidly growing solid component distinct from the classically fatty, well-organized internal architecture, and simple functional cysts, including follicular and corpus luteum cysts, round out the benign adnexal mass differential, generally distinguished by their simple fluid signal, thin wall, and expected resolution on short-interval follow-up imaging in a woman of reproductive age, reflecting their origin from the normal, cyclic ovarian physiologic process rather than a true neoplasm.

Epithelial Ovarian Carcinoma

Epidemiology and Risk Factors of Epithelial Ovarian Carcinoma

Epithelial ovarian carcinoma remains the most lethal gynecologic malignancy despite its lower incidence relative to endometrial and cervical carcinoma, a disproportionate mortality burden that reflects the disease's characteristic late-stage presentation discussed earlier in this chapter, with the majority of cases diagnosed only after transcoelomic peritoneal spread has already occurred given the comparatively nonspecific, insidious symptom pattern and the absence of an effective population-level screening strategy analogous to cervical cytology or mammography. Advancing age represents the single strongest epidemiologic risk factor, with incidence rising sharply after menopause and peaking in the seventh decade, and nulliparity, early menarche, late menopause, and a personal or family history of breast carcinoma each contribute incrementally elevated risk through mechanisms related to cumulative ovulatory cycling and, in familial cases, shared germline mutation, most importantly BRCA1 and BRCA2 discussed below, though also including Lynch syndrome-associated mismatch repair gene mutations that confer elevated risk for both ovarian and endometrial carcinoma. Conversely, factors that reduce cumulative ovulatory cycling, including combined oral contraceptive use, multiparity, and breastfeeding, are each associated with measurably reduced lifetime ovarian carcinoma risk, an association consistent with the broader incessant ovulation hypothesis of ovarian carcinogenesis in which repeated ovulatory surface epithelial disruption and repair is thought to accumulate the genetic alterations that ultimately give rise to malignant transformation.

High-Grade Serous Carcinoma and Staging

High-grade serous carcinoma, the most common and most lethal epithelial ovarian carcinoma subtype, typically presents as a large, complex cystic and solid mass with irregular, papillary, avidly enhancing solid components, often bilateral, and frequently accompanied by ascites and peritoneal carcinomatosis at diagnosis given this subtype's characteristic pattern of early, extensive peritoneal dissemination discussed in the peritoneal disease chapter earlier in this book, a dissemination pattern that reflects this cancer's tendency toward transcoelomic spread throughout the peritoneal cavity rather than the more localized growth pattern of many other solid malignancies discussed in this book. Contemporary understanding increasingly recognizes the fallopian tube, specifically its fimbriated distal end, as the site of origin for a substantial proportion of what has traditionally been classified as primary ovarian high-grade serous carcinoma, a tubal origin theory that has reshaped risk-reducing surgical strategies in high-risk populations, discussed further below, toward salpingectomy as a component of risk reduction rather than oophorectomy alone.

BRCA Mutation and Risk-Reducing Surgery

Germline BRCA1 and BRCA2 mutation carry a substantially elevated lifetime risk of epithelial ovarian carcinoma, predominantly the high-grade serous subtype discussed above, and current guidelines generally recommend risk-reducing bilateral salpingo-oophorectomy once childbearing is complete and at an age informed by the specific mutation's associated risk trajectory, a preventive surgical strategy that has demonstrated a substantial reduction in both ovarian and, through the estrogen-reduction effect of oophorectomy, breast cancer risk in this specific high-risk population. Imaging surveillance with transvaginal ultrasound and serum CA-125, while historically employed for high-risk women who have not yet proceeded to risk-reducing surgery or who decline the procedure, has not been shown to meaningfully reduce ovarian cancer mortality given the disease's tendency to disseminate before it produces a detectable, localized ovarian abnormality, an important limitation that appropriately reframes imaging surveillance in this population as an interim measure pending definitive risk-reducing surgery rather than a fully adequate long-term substitute for it.

Non-Serous Epithelial Subtypes and FIGO Staging

Beyond high-grade serous carcinoma, several distinct epithelial ovarian carcinoma subtypes carry recognizable clinical and imaging associations worth distinguishing. Endometrioid and clear cell carcinoma each carry a recognized association with endometriosis and, specifically, with malignant transformation of a preexisting endometrioma discussed earlier in this chapter, generally present at an earlier stage than high-grade serous carcinoma, and, for clear cell carcinoma specifically, carry a relative chemoresistance that makes accurate subtype recognition clinically consequential for treatment planning. Low-grade serous carcinoma, a molecularly and clinically distinct entity from its high-grade counterpart despite the shared serous designation, follows a more indolent natural history with a lower response rate to standard platinum-based chemotherapy, while mucinous carcinoma, comparatively uncommon as a truly primary ovarian process, should prompt careful search for a gastrointestinal, most often appendiceal, primary tumor, given the substantially greater frequency of ovarian mucinous metastasis from a gastrointestinal source relative to genuinely primary ovarian mucinous carcinoma. FIGO staging, applied uniformly across epithelial ovarian carcinoma subtypes, progresses from stage I, disease confined to one or both ovaries, through stage II, pelvic extension, stage III, peritoneal spread beyond the pelvis or regional lymph node involvement, to stage IV, distant metastatic disease including malignant pleural effusion or parenchymal liver or splenic involvement, with cross-sectional imaging, MRI for the pelvic component and CT for the abdominal and thoracic component, providing essential staging information to guide the choice between primary cytoreductive surgery and neoadjuvant chemotherapy followed by interval cytoreduction in a patient whose disease burden appears unlikely to permit complete surgical resection at initial presentation.

CAUTION: A mucinous-appearing ovarian mass should prompt correlation with the appendix and remainder of the gastrointestinal tract, since ovarian mucinous metastasis from a gastrointestinal primary, particularly appendiceal, is substantially more common than truly primary ovarian mucinous carcinoma, and misattributing a metastatic mucinous mass to a primary ovarian process can result in an incomplete oncologic workup.

Figure 17.3: Adnexal and Ovarian Vascular Anatomy

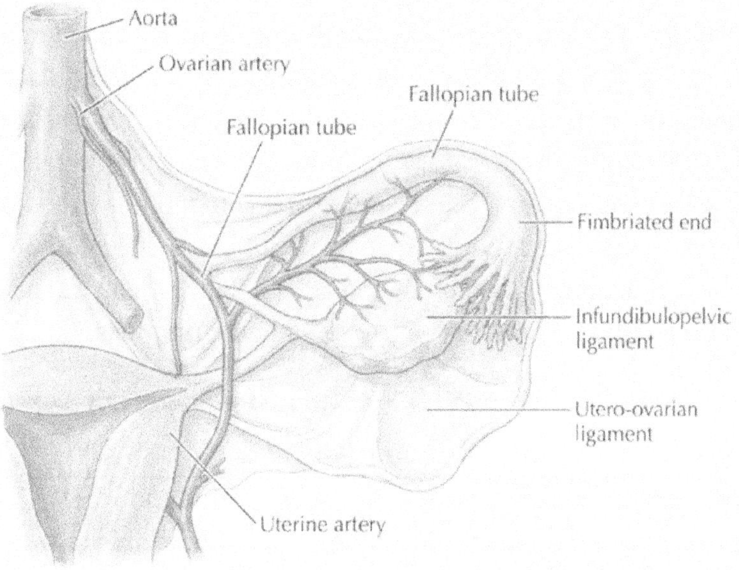

Ovarian Torsion

Epidemiology and Predisposing Factors for Ovarian Torsion

Ovarian torsion occurs across the reproductive age spectrum but demonstrates a bimodal distribution with recognized peaks in the pediatric and adolescent population, discussed above in the special populations discussion, and in women of reproductive age, with a predisposing ovarian mass, most commonly a dermoid given its characteristic size and weight distribution, identified in a substantial majority of adult cases, while torsion of a structurally normal ovary occurs disproportionately in younger patients, likely reflecting greater ovarian mobility and a more redundant utero-ovarian ligament in this population. Ovarian enlargement itself, whether from a benign mass or from ovarian hyperstimulation in the setting of assisted reproductive technology, represents the dominant predisposing mechanism, since an enlarged, heavier ovary is mechanically more prone to twisting around its vascular pedicle than a normal-sized ovary, and pregnancy itself confers modestly elevated torsion risk related to both the physiologically enlarged corpus luteum of pregnancy and the ligamentous laxity that accompanies gestation. Right-sided predominance has been repeatedly observed in torsion case series, an asymmetry generally attributed to the sigmoid colon's relative fixation on the left providing some mechanical restraint against torsion that is comparatively absent on the right, though torsion can and does occur on either side and this epidemiologic tendency does not substitute for careful bilateral evaluation in a patient with acute pelvic pain.

Ovarian Torsion: Imaging Features and Surgical Urgency

Ovarian torsion, twisting of the ovary and its supporting vascular pedicle, generally around a predisposing mass such as a dermoid or other enlarged ovarian lesion though occasionally occurring in an otherwise normal ovary particularly in a pediatric or young adult patient, represents a true surgical emergency given the time-critical risk of irreversible ischemic ovarian infarction, and its recognition on imaging, most reliably with ultrasound as the first-line modality given the same time-critical considerations discussed for testicular torsion in the preceding chapter, but with MRI contributing when ultrasound is technically limited or the presentation is atypical, centers on identifying an enlarged, edematous ovary, often displaced from its typical location, together with reduced or absent enhancement indicating compromised perfusion. The whirlpool sign, representing the twisted vascular pedicle itself visualized as a coiled, swirling structure, is a specific and helpful confirmatory finding when present, though its absence does not exclude torsion, and the overall clinical gestalt, acute pelvic pain together with the ovarian enlargement and perfusion findings discussed above, generally drives the urgent surgical exploration decision even when a fully classic, textbook imaging pattern is not present, since delayed intervention pending a more definitive imaging finding risks progression to irreversible ovarian loss.

THE SIGNAL-TO-CATEGORY DECISION SYSTEM — Ovarian Torsion Surgical Urgency Triage

The Signal Pattern: A patient presents with acute pelvic pain, and MRI or ultrasound demonstrates an enlarged, edematous ovary, and the reader must assess perfusion status to inform surgical urgency.

Category Signature: An enlarged ovary with preserved, symmetric enhancement relative to the contralateral ovary is categorized as torsion with preserved viability or an alternative, non-torsion cause of ovarian enlargement; an enlarged ovary with markedly reduced or absent enhancement is categorized as torsion with compromised viability.

The Decision: Preserved enhancement supports urgent but not maximally emergent surgical detorsion with a reasonable expectation of ovarian salvage; markedly reduced or absent enhancement still generally warrants urgent surgical exploration given the possibility of partial viability or intermittent torsion, but with more guarded counseling about the likelihood of ovarian salvage versus oophorectomy.

Trap Logic: Intermittent torsion, in which the ovary twists and spontaneously detorses, can produce a confusing, fluctuating clinical and imaging picture that does not fit the more straightforward, sustained-torsion pattern typically described, and a single examination demonstrating preserved enhancement does not exclude a torsion episode that has since spontaneously resolved or one that will recur; the discriminating step is maintaining a high index of clinical suspicion based on the symptom pattern itself, recurrent or intermittent severe pelvic pain, even when a single imaging examination is reassuring, and communicating this possibility to the clinical team rather than assuming a normal-appearing single examination definitively excludes a torsion process.

Pattern Anchor: Assess perfusion, not simply ovarian size or morphology, to inform surgical urgency and salvage likelihood; intermittent torsion can produce a reassuring single examination despite a genuine, recurring torsion process.

Figure 17.4: Laparoscopic Ovarian Detorsion Technique

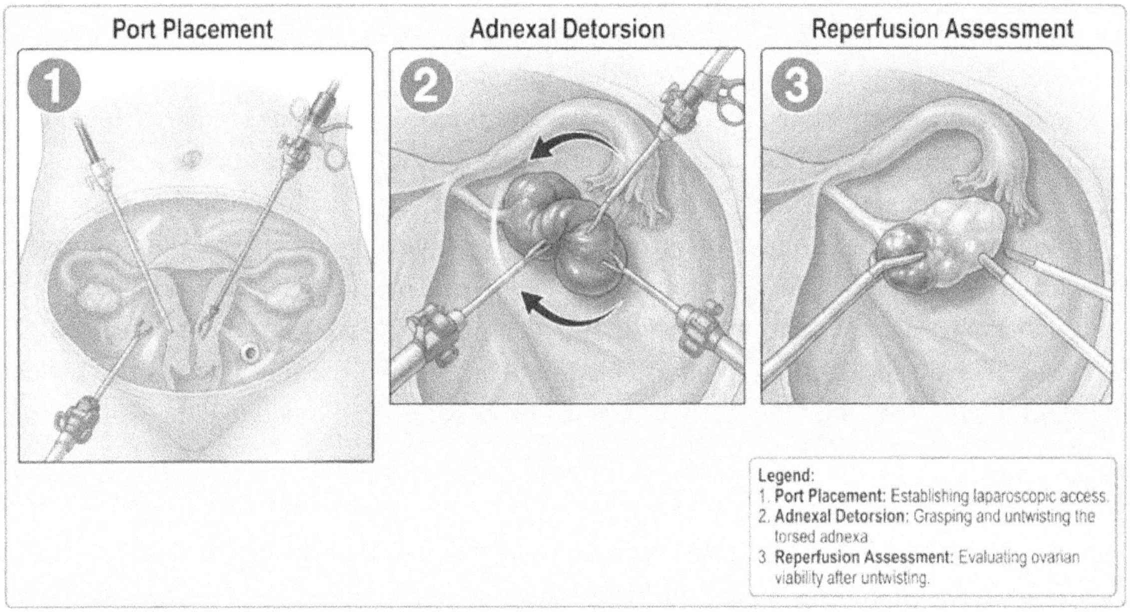

Fallopian Tube Pathology and Tubo-Ovarian Abscess

Ectopic Pregnancy and Adnexal Considerations

Ectopic pregnancy, implantation of a gestation outside the endometrial cavity most commonly within the fallopian tube itself, represents a life-threatening emergency when tubal rupture occurs and, while transvaginal ultrasound together with serial serum beta-human chorionic gonadotropin measurement remains the primary diagnostic pathway, MRI occasionally contributes a problem-solving role when ultrasound findings are equivocal in a hemodynamically stable patient, demonstrating a complex adnexal mass distinct from the ovary itself, often with a thick, hyperenhancing rind representing trophoblastic tissue, together with variable amounts of hemoperitoneum when rupture or tubal bleeding has occurred. Distinguishing a tubal ectopic mass from a corpus luteum cyst, the most common benign mimic in this clinical context, relies on confirming the mass's location distinct from and adjacent to, rather than within, the ovary itself, together with the clinical context of a positive pregnancy test without a confirmed intrauterine gestation, a combination that should prompt urgent gynecologic consultation given the substantial risk of catastrophic hemorrhage should tubal rupture occur before definitive management, whether medical with methotrexate for an unruptured, appropriately selected ectopic pregnancy or surgical for a ruptured or otherwise unsuitable case. Heterotopic pregnancy, the rare but clinically important coexistence of both an intrauterine and an ectopic gestation, occurs with disproportionately increased frequency in the setting of assisted reproductive technology relative to spontaneous conception, and its possibility should not be dismissed simply because an intrauterine gestation has already been confirmed, particularly in a patient who conceived through fertility treatment and who presents with adnexal findings or pain inconsistent with the confirmed intrauterine pregnancy alone.

Hydrosalpinx and Fallopian Tube Pathology

Hydrosalpinx, fluid distension of an obstructed fallopian tube most often related to prior pelvic inflammatory disease, endometriosis, or prior pelvic surgery, presents as a tubular, folded, or serpentine cystic structure distinct from the more rounded morphology of an ovarian cyst, with the tube's characteristic incomplete septations, representing the compressed, redundant mucosal folds of the tube's interior architecture, providing a helpful morphologic clue to its tubal rather than ovarian origin when the diagnosis is not immediately obvious from overall shape alone. Hydrosalpinx carries recognized fertility implications beyond its role as a source of chronic pelvic pain, since hydrosalpinx fluid can reflux into the endometrial cavity and adversely affect embryo implantation during assisted reproductive technology, a consideration that has led some fertility specialists to recommend salpingectomy of a hydrosalpinx before proceeding with in vitro fertilization in an affected patient, making the radiologist's clear identification and characterization of this entity clinically relevant well beyond simple pelvic pain evaluation.

Tubo-Ovarian Abscess

Tubo-ovarian abscess, a severe complication of ascending pelvic inflammatory disease in which infection produces a complex, multiloculated, rim-enhancing adnexal collection often incorporating and obliterating the normal boundary between the ovary and fallopian tube, represents a clinical and imaging pattern with substantial overlap with a complex ovarian neoplasm, making correlation with the patient's clinical presentation, fever, purulent vaginal discharge, and cervical motion tenderness on examination, together with inflammatory laboratory markers, essential to appropriately distinguishing this infectious process from malignancy in a genuinely ambiguous case. Management of tubo-ovarian abscess ranges from intravenous antibiotic therapy alone for a smaller, uncomplicated collection to image-guided or surgical drainage for a larger abscess or one failing to respond to medical therapy, and, given the imaging overlap with malignancy discussed above, a collection that fails to substantially improve on appropriate antibiotic therapy, or one presenting in a postmenopausal woman where pelvic inflammatory disease is considerably less common, should prompt reconsideration of the diagnosis and, potentially, surgical exploration to definitively exclude an underlying malignant process masquerading as infection.

Clinical Case Presentations

Case 1. A 34-year-old woman with chronic pelvic pain undergoes MRI demonstrating a 4-centimeter left ovarian cyst with homogeneous, markedly elevated T1 signal that fails to suppress on fat-suppressed sequences, together with the shading sign on T2-weighted imaging, and no enhancing solid component. The radiologist categorizes the lesion as a typical endometrioma and recommends no further workup beyond routine gynecologic follow-up, applying the specific, high-confidence signal pattern this chapter's framework describes.

Case 2. A 58-year-old postmenopausal woman undergoes MRI demonstrating a 9-centimeter complex bilateral adnexal mass with multiple irregular, avidly and rapidly enhancing solid papillary projections, together with moderate ascites and omental caking. The radiologist categorizes the mass as O-RADS 5 and recommends urgent gynecologic oncology referral, correlating the findings with the peritoneal carcinomatosis pattern discussed in an earlier chapter to support comprehensive staging evaluation for suspected high-grade serous ovarian carcinoma.

Case 3. A 19-year-old woman presents with acute-onset severe right lower quadrant pain, and MRI demonstrates a markedly enlarged, edematous right ovary containing a 5-centimeter fat-containing dermoid cyst, with absent enhancement of the ovarian parenchyma and a whirlpool sign at the adnexal pedicle. Recognizing this as ovarian torsion with compromised viability, the radiologist urgently communicates the findings, and the patient proceeds to emergent laparoscopic detorsion, with partial ovarian viability confirmed intraoperatively, allowing ovarian-sparing surgery rather than oophorectomy.

Case 4. A 27-year-old woman with fever, pelvic pain, and purulent vaginal discharge undergoes MRI demonstrating a complex, multiloculated, rim-enhancing right adnexal collection obliterating the normal ovarian-tubal boundary. Correlating the imaging findings with the compatible clinical presentation and inflammatory laboratory markers, the radiologist categorizes the findings as tubo-ovarian abscess rather than a complex neoplasm, and the patient is started on intravenous antibiotics with substantial improvement on follow-up imaging, confirming the infectious rather than neoplastic diagnosis.

Case 5. A 41-year-old woman with a confirmed BRCA1 mutation and completed childbearing undergoes risk-reducing bilateral salpingo-oophorectomy. Pathologic examination identifies a 2-millimeter focus of serous tubal intraepithelial carcinoma within the fimbriated end of the left fallopian tube, an occult malignant focus not appreciable on preoperative imaging. The radiologist's preoperative report, which had described both adnexa as unremarkable, is discussed at multidisciplinary tumor board alongside the tubal origin theory of high-grade serous carcinoma, reinforcing for the group why comprehensive fimbrial sectioning at pathology, rather than imaging alone, remains essential in this specific risk-reducing surgical context.

Case 6. A 25-year-old woman with a positive urine pregnancy test and acute right-sided pelvic pain undergoes transvaginal ultrasound showing no definite intrauterine gestation and an indeterminate right adnexal finding. Non-contrast MRI, obtained given her pregnancy status, demonstrates a thick-walled, hyperenhancing-on-T2-signal-characteristics complex mass distinct from and adjacent to a structurally normal right ovary, together with a small amount of free pelvic fluid. The radiologist characterizes the findings as consistent with tubal ectopic pregnancy rather than a corpus luteum cyst, correlating the mass's extraovarian location with the clinical presentation, and the patient is urgently referred for gynecologic evaluation and serial beta-human chorionic gonadotropin monitoring.

THE SIGNAL-TO-CATEGORY DECISION SYSTEM — Adnexal Mass Triage Arc

The Signal Pattern: This chapter's patterns span the adnexal risk spectrum, from a cystic or complex mass whose solid component enhancement must be confirmed for O-RADS category assignment, to an acutely enlarged, painful ovary whose perfusion status must be assessed for torsion surgical urgency.

Category Signature: Adnexal masses are categorized O-RADS 1 through 5 based on composition, septation, and confirmed solid component enhancement kinetics; an acutely symptomatic ovary is categorized by perfusion status as torsion with preserved or compromised viability.

The Decision: Category assignment in this chapter ranges from no further workup for a classic benign entity to urgent gynecologic oncology referral for a high-risk mass, and from urgent to maximally emergent surgical exploration for torsion, with every category assigned only after the specific confirmatory feature, true enhancement or confirmed perfusion status, has been explicitly verified.

The Trap Logic: Both patterns in this chapter share a common trap: a feature that superficially resembles the category-defining finding, clotted blood mimicking a solid nodule, or a single reassuring examination missing an intermittent or resolving torsion episode, without reflecting the true underlying process.

Pattern Anchor: Confirm true enhancement and, for torsion, true perfusion status explicitly before committing to a final category in this chapter; superficial resemblance and single-examination reassurance both carry recognized limitations addressed throughout this chapter.

Summary and Key Concepts

The O-RADS MRI framework first classifies adnexal mass composition, then applies composition-specific criteria centered on solid component presence, morphology, and enhancement kinetics to assign a five-tier malignancy risk category.

Endometrioma shows homogeneous, non-suppressing elevated T1 signal with the shading sign; a new solid component within a previously typical endometrioma raises concern for malignant transformation.

Mature cystic teratoma shows macroscopic fat with a characteristic Rokitansky protrusion; malignant transformation is rare but should be considered with an atypical, rapidly growing solid component.

High-grade serous carcinoma often presents with bilateral complex masses, ascites, and peritoneal carcinomatosis; the fallopian tube fimbria is now recognized as a common site of origin.

BRCA mutation carriers are offered risk-reducing salpingo-oophorectomy; imaging surveillance alone has not been shown to meaningfully reduce ovarian cancer mortality in this population.

Ovarian torsion surgical urgency is determined by perfusion status, not size or morphology alone; intermittent torsion can produce a falsely reassuring single examination.

Tubo-ovarian abscess can closely mimic a complex ovarian neoplasm; clinical correlation and response to antibiotic therapy help distinguish infection from malignancy, particularly in a postmenopausal woman where pelvic inflammatory disease is uncommon.

CHAPTER 18: FEMALE PELVIC FLOOR AND ENDOMETRIOSIS IMAGING

Learning Objectives

1. Describe the three-compartment model of the female pelvic floor and its application to MR defecography interpretation.
2. Grade pelvic organ prolapse using standardized reference-line criteria and correlate imaging findings with surgical planning.
3. Recognize the imaging features of deep infiltrating endometriosis across the anterior, middle, and posterior pelvic compartments.
4. Apply a systematic, compartment-based search pattern for endometriosis to avoid missing multifocal disease.
5. Recognize levator ani injury and its association with pelvic organ prolapse and pelvic floor dysfunction.

Clinical Overview

Female pelvic floor and endometriosis imaging represent two of the more technically demanding domains in body MRI, both requiring meticulous attention to imaging technique, patient preparation, and a systematic search pattern to reliably detect the subtle findings that meaningfully guide surgical decision-making. Pelvic organ prolapse and its functional consequences, addressed in the first portion of this chapter through MR defecography, and deep infiltrating endometriosis, addressed in the chapter's second portion, differ substantially in underlying pathophysiology but share a common imaging philosophy: a dedicated, protocol-specific approach applied with the same rigor as the organ-specific frameworks discussed throughout this book, since a general, non-dedicated pelvic MRI performed for an unrelated indication will reliably miss the majority of clinically significant findings in both domains.

Two instances of the Signal-to-Category Decision System are applied in this chapter, the first to pelvic organ prolapse compartment grading during MR defecography, and the second to deep infiltrating endometriosis compartment mapping, reflecting this chapter's shared emphasis on systematic, compartment-based evaluation across two otherwise distinct pelvic floor conditions.

Pelvic Floor Anatomy and MR Defecography Technique

Three-Compartment Pelvic Floor Anatomy

The pelvic floor is conventionally divided into three functional compartments for the purpose of prolapse evaluation, the anterior compartment comprising the bladder and urethra, the middle compartment comprising the uterus, cervix, and vaginal apex, or the vaginal cuff in a patient who has undergone prior hysterectomy, and the posterior compartment comprising the rectum, and this compartmental framework, directly analogous in organizing principle to the compartment-based approach applied to endometriosis later in this chapter, allows the reader to systematically assess for descent or herniation within each region independently rather than relying on a single, undifferentiated global impression of pelvic floor competence. The levator ani muscle complex, principally the puborectalis and pubococcygeus components, together with the endopelvic fascial support structures, provides the structural support upon which normal positioning of all three compartments depends, and injury or attenuation of these supporting structures, whether from vaginal delivery, chronic straining, or age-related connective tissue changes, underlies the great majority of clinically significant pelvic organ prolapse encountered in practice.

MR Defecography Technique and Patient Preparation

MR defecography requires deliberate protocol modifications beyond a standard pelvic MRI, most fundamentally the acquisition of dynamic, real-time sequences during rest, squeeze, and maximal Valsalva or straining maneuvers, and, in many though not all protocols, during actual rectal evacuation of an instilled ultrasound gel or specialized rectal contrast, since prolapse and pelvic floor dysfunction are inherently dynamic processes that a static, single-timepoint acquisition will systematically underestimate or entirely miss.

Figure 18.1 – Diagnostic Imaging: MR Defecography During Maximal Valsalva – Multicompartment Pelvic Organ Prolapse

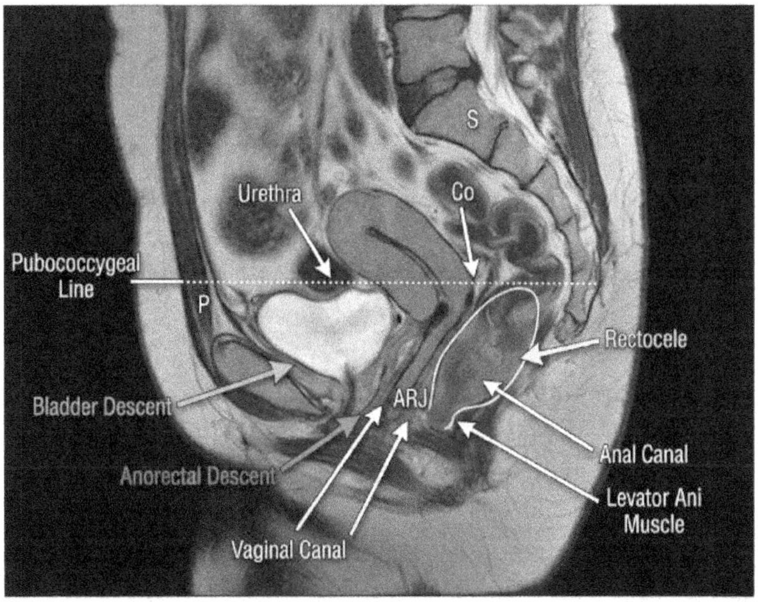

Patient positioning, whether supine within a conventional closed-bore magnet or upright in an open-configuration magnet that more closely approximates physiologic defecation posture, represents an ongoing technical consideration, with supine imaging remaining the more widely available approach despite the theoretical advantage of upright positioning in maximizing gravitational contribution to prolapse severity, and clear, structured patient coaching before and during the examination, given the inherently unnatural and sometimes challenging nature of performing a genuine, maximal Valsalva or evacuation maneuver within the scanner environment, is essential to obtaining a technically adequate, clinically representative study.

Reference Lines and Compartment Descent Measurement

Pelvic organ descent during maximal straining is quantified relative to the pubococcygeal line, drawn from the inferior margin of the pubic symphysis to the last coccygeal joint, providing a stable bony reference framework unaffected by the soft tissue changes under evaluation, with the degree of descent of the bladder base, cervix or vaginal cuff, and anorectal junction below this reference line during maximal strain, relative to their position at rest, forming the quantitative basis for prolapse grading discussed in the following section. The H-line, measuring the anteroposterior width of the levator hiatus from the pubic symphysis to the posterior anorectal junction, and the M-line, measuring the vertical descent of the levator plate from the pubococcygeal line, provide complementary measurements specifically characterizing levator hiatus widening and levator plate descent, both directly reflecting the structural pelvic floor support integrity discussed above, and together with the individual compartment measurements, these reference lines constitute the complete, reproducible quantitative framework that distinguishes MR defecography from a more subjective, purely qualitative assessment of pelvic floor descent.

Compartment	Structure Assessed	Mild Descent	Moderate Descent	Severe Descent
Anterior	Bladder base relative to pubococcygeal line	Less than 1 cm below	1 to 3 cm below	Greater than 3 cm below
Middle	Cervix or vaginal cuff relative to pubococcygeal line	Less than 1 cm below	1 to 3 cm below	Greater than 3 cm below
Posterior	Anorectal junction relative to pubococcygeal line	Less than 1 cm below	1 to 3 cm below	Greater than 3 cm below

Special Populations: Pelvic Floor Imaging in the Postpartum and Perimenopausal Patient

MR defecography performed in the early postpartum period requires cautious interpretation given that a degree of pelvic floor laxity and mild compartment descent can represent a normal, transient physiologic state during tissue recovery rather than an established, fixed pelvic floor injury, and deferring dedicated pelvic floor imaging until at least several months postpartum, allowing this initial physiologic recovery process to complete, generally provides a more clinically representative assessment of a patient's true, lasting pelvic floor status than an examination obtained in the immediate postpartum window. The perimenopausal and postmenopausal transition, by contrast, is associated with progressive, estrogen-deficiency-related connective tissue quality decline that can unmask or accelerate previously subclinical or compensated pelvic floor support deficits, meaning that a patient with a remote, decades-old obstetric injury may first become symptomatic only during this later hormonal transition, and eliciting a comprehensive obstetric history, including delivery mode and any known perineal or sphincter injury, remains clinically relevant when interpreting a pelvic floor MRI performed many years after the inciting obstetric event, since the imaging findings and the timing of symptom onset together provide a more complete clinical picture than either consideration in isolation.

Pelvic Organ Prolapse

PATIENT EDUCATION: A pessary is a removable, non-surgical device fitted to support prolapsed pelvic organs and can be an effective, reversible option for a patient who wishes to avoid or delay surgery, requires only periodic follow-up for fitting adjustment and vaginal tissue monitoring, and does not preclude a future surgical repair should symptoms progress or the device become unsuitable over time.

Epidemiology and Risk Factors for Pelvic Organ Prolapse

Pelvic organ prolapse affects a substantial proportion of parous women over the course of their lifetime, with vaginal delivery, particularly a delivery complicated by a prolonged second stage, instrumented delivery, or a large-for-gestational-age infant, representing the single most significant modifiable risk factor through direct mechanical injury to the levator ani and endopelvic fascial support structures discussed above, an injury pattern addressed in greater biomechanical detail later in this chapter. Advancing age, chronic elevation in intra-abdominal pressure from chronic cough, constipation, or occupational heavy lifting, obesity, and connective tissue disorders affecting collagen quality each contribute incremental risk through mechanisms related either to progressive support structure attenuation over time or to sustained excessive mechanical loading of an already compromised support system, and family history confers additional risk through a heritable connective tissue quality component that parallels the genetic contribution recognized in other pelvic floor and connective tissue-related conditions discussed elsewhere in gynecologic practice.

Cystocele, Rectocele, and Enterocele Differentiation

Cystocele, descent or herniation of the bladder base into the anterior vaginal wall, and rectocele, herniation of the anterior rectal wall into the posterior vaginal wall, together represent the most common individual compartment findings, with rectocele specifically often accompanied by incomplete rectal evacuation on defecatory-phase imaging, a functional consequence directly relevant to the frequent presenting symptom of a sensation of incomplete emptying requiring digital splinting for defecation. Enterocele, herniation of small bowel or, less commonly, sigmoid colon into the rectovaginal space, requires careful distinction from a simple rectocele given the differing surgical repair approach each requires, with the presence of bowel loops, rather than rectal wall alone, within the herniated tissue on sagittal dynamic imaging providing the key discriminating feature, and a peritoneocele, herniation of pelvic peritoneum alone without bowel content, represents a comparatively subtle variant along this same anatomic spectrum that can be similarly overlooked without deliberate, systematic search during the straining phase of the examination.

Management Implications of Prolapse Severity and Compartment Involvement

Management of pelvic organ prolapse spans a spectrum from conservative pelvic floor physical therapy and pessary fitting for milder, single-compartment prolapse, to surgical repair, whether native tissue repair or mesh-augmented reconstruction, for more severe or multicompartment prolapse, with the specific compartments involved and their individual severity, rather than a single global prolapse impression, directly informing the surgical approach selected and the specific anatomic structures targeted for repair. Multicompartment prolapse, in which two or three compartments demonstrate at least moderate descent, is a common finding given the shared underlying support structure across compartments, and comprehensive preoperative characterization of every involved compartment is essential to surgical planning, since addressing a single compartment in isolation while leaving a second, comparably severe compartment defect unaddressed frequently results in prolapse recurrence or unmasking of a previously compensated defect following surgery, a well-recognized clinical phenomenon that underscores the value of the systematic, three-compartment MR defecography assessment discussed throughout this section.

Patient Education and Counseling for Pelvic Organ Prolapse

Counseling a patient regarding a newly identified pelvic organ prolapse finding benefits from framing the discussion around functional impact and treatment options rather than severity grading in isolation, since a moderate-grade prolapse that is minimally symptomatic may reasonably be managed conservatively with monitoring alone, while a milder-grade prolapse that is substantially impacting a patient's quality of life through bothersome bulge sensation or sexual function concerns may warrant more assertive intervention, making the correlation between imaging severity and the patient's actual symptom burden, rather than the grading alone, central to a well-informed shared decision-making conversation. Pelvic floor physical therapy, emphasizing supervised, progressive pelvic floor muscle strengthening under the guidance of a specialized therapist, represents a genuinely effective first-line intervention for mild to moderate prolapse and for prevention of progression in an at-risk patient, and clear communication that this conservative option exists and carries a reasonable likelihood of symptomatic benefit, before proceeding directly to a pessary or surgical discussion, supports patient autonomy and avoids the impression that surgery represents the only meaningful treatment pathway. For a patient for whom surgical mesh-augmented repair is under consideration, balanced counseling addressing both the durability advantages of mesh augmentation for more severe or recurrent prolapse and the recognized, though comparatively uncommon, mesh-related complication profile, including erosion and chronic pain, supports informed consent that reflects the genuine, evolving evidence base regarding this specific surgical technique choice.

THE SIGNAL-TO-CATEGORY DECISION SYSTEM — Pelvic Organ Prolapse Compartment Grading

The Signal Pattern: A patient with pelvic floor symptoms undergoes MR defecography, and the reader must measure descent of the anterior, middle, and posterior compartments relative to the pubococcygeal line during maximal straining.

Category Signature: Descent less than 1 centimeter below the pubococcygeal line is categorized as mild; descent 1 to 3 centimeters below is categorized as moderate; descent greater than 3 centimeters below is categorized as severe, applied independently to each of the three compartments.

The Decision: Mild, single-compartment descent generally supports conservative management with pelvic floor physical therapy or pessary fitting; moderate to severe or multicompartment descent supports surgical referral, with the specific compartments and severities identified directly informing the surgical repair approach selected.

Trap Logic: An inadequate Valsalva or straining effort during image acquisition can systematically understate true prolapse severity, producing a falsely reassuring examination that does not reflect the patient's actual symptomatic descent; the discriminating step is confirming, through direct observation of pelvic floor descent and diaphragmatic excursion during the dynamic sequence itself, that a genuine maximal effort was achieved before accepting a mild-appearing examination as representative.

Pattern Anchor: Confirm genuine maximal straining effort before accepting a mild-appearing examination; measure and report all three compartments independently, since multicompartment involvement directly changes the surgical approach.

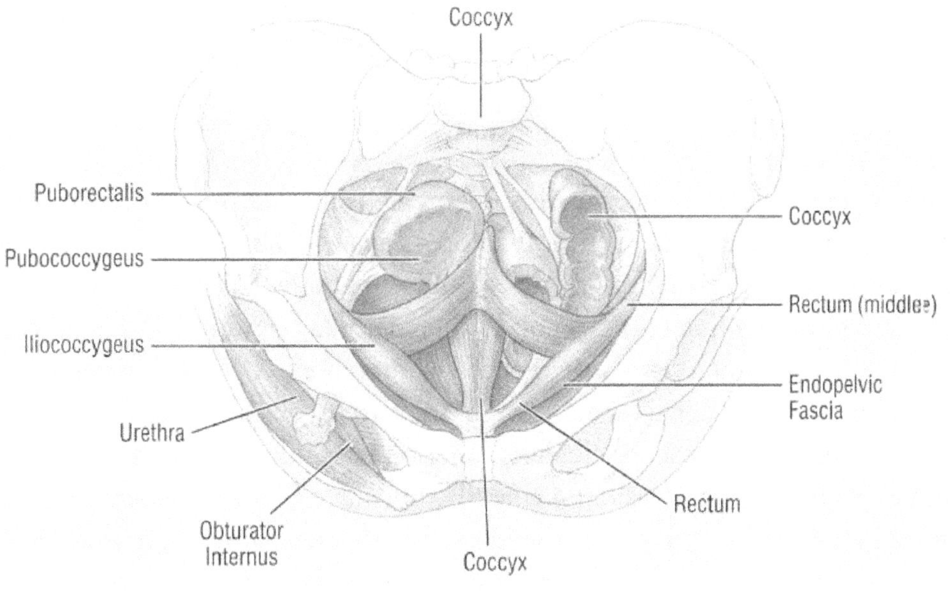

Figure 18.2 — Anatomical Illustration: Levator Ani and Pelvic Floor Support Structures

CLINICAL PEARL: A rectocele with a substantial fecal trap, retained rectal contrast within the rectocele following attempted evacuation, correlates strongly with the patient's symptomatic sensation of incomplete emptying and supports a surgical, rather than purely conservative, management recommendation even for an otherwise moderate-sized rectocele.

Levator Ani Injury and Pelvic Floor Dysfunction

EVIDENCE: Prospective cohort studies applying standardized MR and translabial ultrasound criteria have found levator ani avulsion in a substantial minority of women following forceps-assisted delivery, a rate several-fold higher than following spontaneous vaginal delivery, findings that have informed increasing interest in intrapartum decision-making around instrumented delivery in patients with additional identifiable pelvic floor risk factors.

Epidemiology of Levator Ani Injury

Levator ani injury, spanning the spectrum from diffuse attenuation to frank avulsion discussed below, occurs with disproportionately greater frequency following operative vaginal delivery, whether forceps- or vacuum-assisted, relative to spontaneous vaginal delivery, with forceps-assisted delivery specifically carrying the highest reported avulsion rates among delivery modes, a risk gradient that has informed increasing clinical interest in identifying modifiable intrapartum risk factors and in counseling patients with recognized risk factors regarding delivery mode considerations, while acknowledging that levator injury also occurs, albeit less frequently, following uncomplicated spontaneous vaginal delivery and that cesarean delivery, while associated with a lower levator injury rate, is not itself free of pelvic floor risk given its own distinct complication profile. A first vaginal delivery carries disproportionately elevated levator injury risk relative to subsequent deliveries, reflecting the comparatively greater tissue distensibility acquired after an initial delivery, and this parity-dependent risk pattern is a further consideration in counseling nulliparous patients, particularly those with additional risk factors such as a anticipated large-for-gestational-age infant, regarding realistic expectations for pelvic floor outcomes across their reproductive course.

Levator Ani Avulsion and Its Imaging Recognition

Levator ani avulsion, traumatic detachment of the puborectalis muscle from its pubic bone origin, occurs in a meaningful minority of vaginal deliveries, disproportionately those complicated by forceps-assisted delivery, and represents a distinct and more severe injury pattern than the diffuse levator thinning or stretching more commonly encountered, recognized on axial imaging through the pubovisceral muscle's abnormal, discontinuous appearance and asymmetric insertion relative to the pubic bone when compared to the contralateral, uninjured side. This specific injury pattern carries a substantially elevated association with subsequent pelvic organ prolapse, particularly anterior and middle compartment prolapse, relative to a patient with an intact, though possibly generally attenuated, levator complex, making avulsion recognition clinically relevant both for individual patient counseling regarding prolapse risk and, increasingly, for research characterizing which specific injury patterns most strongly predict long-term pelvic floor dysfunction.

Levator Hiatus Widening and Functional Consequences

Levator hiatus widening, quantified using the H-line measurement discussed earlier in this chapter, reflects the combined effect of levator muscle bulk loss, whether from avulsion or diffuse attenuation, and connective tissue support structure laxity, and a widened hiatus is mechanically permissive of greater pelvic organ descent under the same degree of intra-abdominal pressure elevation relative to a normal-caliber hiatus, functioning as a structural risk amplifier for the prolapse severity discussed throughout this chapter rather than existing as an isolated finding without functional consequence. Pelvic floor dysfunction extends beyond prolapse alone to include fecal incontinence and obstructed defecation syndrome, both of which share substantial imaging and risk factor overlap with the levator injury and prolapse findings discussed in this chapter, and a comprehensive MR defecography report addressing not only compartment-specific descent but also levator integrity and hiatal dimensions provides the referring clinician with the complete structural picture needed to counsel a patient across this full spectrum of related pelvic floor symptoms rather than addressing prolapse in isolation from these frequently coexisting functional complaints.

Fecal Incontinence and Obstructed Defecation Syndrome

Fecal incontinence, involuntary loss of stool or flatus, shares substantial risk factor overlap with the levator ani injury and prolapse findings discussed throughout this chapter, with obstetric anal sphincter injury, direct disruption of the internal or external anal sphincter complex during vaginal delivery, representing a distinct though related injury pattern from the levator avulsion discussed above, and endoanal MRI or dedicated high-resolution pelvic MRI sequences can identify sphincter defects contributing to incontinence symptoms with a precision that complements the compartment-based prolapse assessment that is this chapter's primary MR defecography focus. Obstructed defecation syndrome, the functional inability to adequately evacuate the rectum despite normal or near-normal stool consistency, frequently coexists with the rectocele and enterocele findings discussed earlier in this chapter, though it can also occur in their absence through a primary functional mechanism termed paradoxical puborectalis contraction, in which the puborectalis fails to relax, or actively contracts, during attempted defecation rather than relaxing as normally occurs, a functional abnormality directly observable on the dynamic phase of MR defecography as persistent or worsening anorectal angle narrowing during the straining and evacuation maneuvers, providing a specific, actionable finding distinct from the structural prolapse findings that dominate the remainder of this chapter's discussion.

Deep Infiltrating Endometriosis

Epidemiology and Clinical Presentation of Endometriosis

Endometriosis, the presence of endometrial-type tissue outside the uterine cavity, affects a substantial proportion of women of reproductive age and represents one of the more common causes of chronic pelvic pain and infertility evaluated in gynecologic practice, with a notoriously long average interval between symptom onset and definitive diagnosis reflecting both the nonspecific nature of many presenting symptoms, dysmenorrhea, dyspareunia, and chronic pelvic pain each individually common in the absence of endometriosis, and, historically, the comparative technical difficulty of reliably imaging deep infiltrating disease relative to the more readily identified ovarian endometrioma discussed in the preceding chapter. Deep infiltrating endometriosis specifically, defined as endometriotic infiltration extending more than 5 millimeters beneath the peritoneal surface, represents the disease subtype most directly relevant to MRI given its comparatively subtle, often peritoneal-surface or subperitoneal location that can elude both direct visual inspection at surgery without deliberate palpation and standard, non-dedicated pelvic imaging performed without the specific technique discussed in the following section.

Dedicated Endometriosis MRI Protocol

A dedicated endometriosis MRI protocol incorporates high-resolution T2-weighted imaging in multiple planes, essential for the fine anatomic detail required to identify subtle deep infiltrating lesions, together with fat-suppressed T1-weighted imaging both before and after contrast to confirm the presence of hemorrhagic content characteristic of endometriotic implants, and, in many though not all protocols, bowel preparation and administration of an antiperistaltic agent to reduce bowel motion artifact that would otherwise degrade the fine spatial resolution required for reliable deep infiltrating disease detection. Timing of the examination relative to the menstrual cycle, while historically debated, is generally recommended to avoid the immediate perimenstrual period when physiologic hemorrhagic change can confound interpretation, and clear communication of prior surgical history, including any previous endometriosis resection, is essential context for the interpreting radiologist given the altered postsurgical anatomy and scar tissue that can otherwise mimic or obscure recurrent or persistent disease.

Posterior Compartment Deep Infiltrating Endometriosis

The posterior compartment, encompassing the uterosacral ligaments, rectovaginal septum, posterior vaginal fornix, and anterior rectal wall, represents the single most common site of deep infiltrating endometriosis, with uterosacral ligament involvement classically appearing as focal or diffuse thickening and nodularity, often with low T2 signal reflecting the dense fibrotic component characteristic of chronic endometriotic infiltration, and rectovaginal septum or bowel wall involvement, when present, requiring careful characterization of the depth of infiltration, mucosal versus muscularis propria versus full-thickness, given the direct implications for surgical approach, whether shaving, discoid resection, or segmental bowel resection, discussed further below. Obliteration of the pouch of Douglas, in which adhesions fuse the posterior uterine serosa to the anterior rectum, eliminating the normally present free fluid or fat plane in this location, represents both a common finding in advanced deep infiltrating endometriosis and an important surgical planning consideration given the substantially increased technical complexity and bowel injury risk this obliteration confers during subsequent laparoscopic surgery.

Anterior and Lateral Compartment Deep Infiltrating Endometriosis

The anterior compartment, principally the bladder, and lateral compartment, principally the ureters and pelvic sidewall, are involved less frequently than the posterior compartment discussed above but carry distinct clinical significance when present, with bladder endometriosis typically involving the posterior bladder wall or dome and appearing as a focal, often low T2 signal nodule with variable hemorrhagic foci, occasionally producing cyclic hematuria when the lesion extends to the bladder mucosa. Ureteral endometriosis, whether extrinsic, from adjacent fibrotic disease compressing the ureter without direct wall invasion, or the less common intrinsic form, with actual endometriotic infiltration of the ureteral wall itself, carries particular clinical importance given the risk of silent, progressive hydronephrosis and eventual renal function loss if unrecognized, making deliberate assessment of the ureters for both direct endometriotic involvement and secondary hydronephrosis, mirroring the systematic ureteral assessment discussed in the urinary tract imaging chapter earlier in this book, an essential component of any comprehensive deep infiltrating endometriosis MRI evaluation regardless of whether ureteral symptoms are specifically reported.

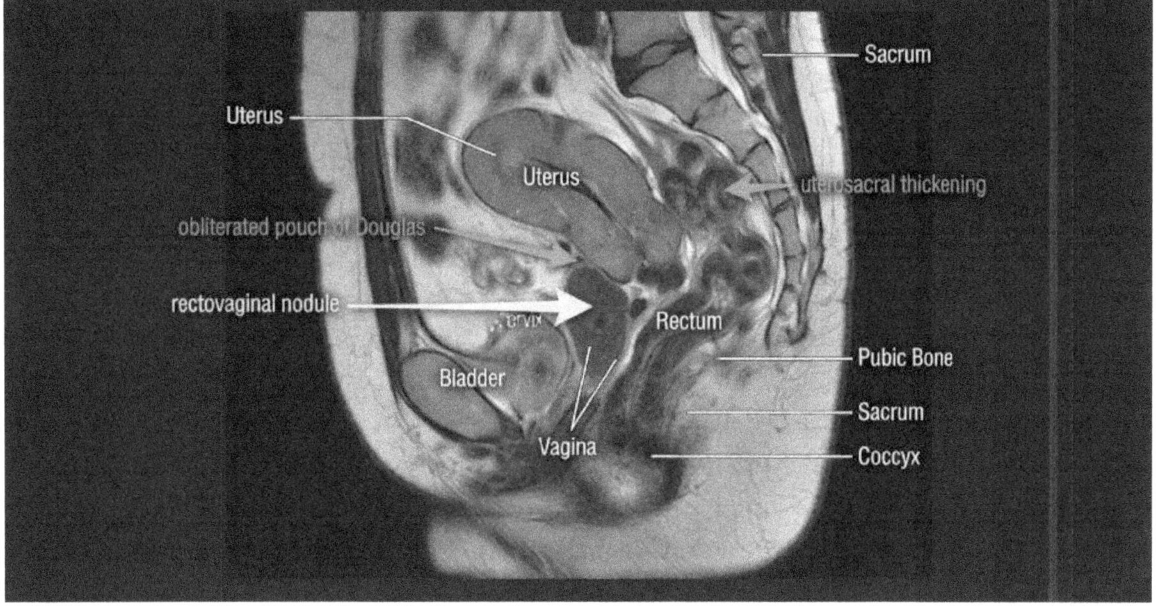

Figure 18.3: Deep Infiltrating Endometriosis of the Rectovaginal Septum

Endometriosis Staging and Surgical Mapping

Differential Diagnosis of Chronic Pelvic Pain

Chronic pelvic pain, the presenting symptom that most commonly triggers dedicated endometriosis MRI, carries a broad differential extending well beyond endometriosis alone, and a comprehensive evaluation should systematically consider adenomyosis, discussed further below given its frequent coexistence with endometriosis, uterine leiomyoma addressed in the preceding uterine imaging chapter, pelvic congestion syndrome from ovarian and pelvic venous insufficiency, interstitial cystitis or bladder pain syndrome, and, when a gynecologic and pelvic imaging evaluation is unrevealing, musculoskeletal and gastrointestinal contributors including pelvic floor myofascial pain and irritable bowel syndrome, each capable of producing a clinical picture that overlaps substantially with endometriosis-related pain. This broad differential underscores why a negative or unrevealing dedicated endometriosis MRI, performed with meticulous technique and interpreted by an experienced reader, meaningfully informs the subsequent diagnostic pathway toward these alternative etiologies rather than representing simply a failed or inconclusive study, and clear communication of a genuinely negative examination, distinct from a technically inadequate one, supports appropriate downstream evaluation rather than repeated, low-yield endometriosis-focused reimaging.

Medical Management and Hormonal Suppression

Medical management of endometriosis, whether as primary therapy for a patient not pursuing surgery or as an adjunct before or after surgical intervention, centers on hormonal suppression of the cyclic estrogen stimulation that drives endometriotic tissue activity, spanning combined oral contraceptives, progestin-only therapy, and gonadotropin-releasing hormone agonists or antagonists for more refractory disease, each functioning through a related though mechanistically distinct suppression of the hypothalamic-pituitary-ovarian axis or direct progestational effect on endometriotic tissue. Medical management is generally most effective for symptom control in superficial or lower-volume disease and is comparatively less effective at addressing the mechanical, space-occupying effects of substantial deep infiltrating nodules or the anatomic distortion from dense adhesive disease discussed throughout this chapter, a distinction that reinforces why the imaging-based categorization between superficial and deep infiltrating disease this chapter's framework provides carries direct treatment-pathway implications rather than functioning purely as a descriptive or academic classification exercise.

Structured Reporting for Surgical Planning

Structured, compartment-based MRI reporting for deep infiltrating endometriosis, systematically addressing the posterior, anterior, and lateral compartments discussed above together with ovarian involvement and pouch of Douglas status, has become increasingly standardized given the direct correlation between comprehensive preoperative mapping and successful, complete surgical resection, since multidisciplinary surgical planning for extensive deep infiltrating endometriosis, frequently involving gynecologic surgery, colorectal surgery, and urology in combination for disease spanning multiple compartments, depends fundamentally on an accurate, complete preoperative roadmap rather than reliance on intraoperative discovery alone. The distinction between superficial peritoneal endometriosis, generally addressed through simpler excision or ablation, and deep infiltrating disease requiring more extensive, compartment-specific surgical technique, discussed throughout this section, represents the single most clinically consequential categorization the interpreting radiologist provides, directly determining both the surgical complexity anticipated and the specific surgical subspecialties that should be involved in preoperative planning.

Adenomyosis and Endometriosis Coexistence

Adenomyosis, addressed in greater technical detail in the uterine imaging chapter earlier in this section, coexists with deep infiltrating endometriosis with substantial frequency, sharing overlapping proposed pathophysiologic mechanisms and risk factors, and the interpreting radiologist evaluating a patient for suspected deep infiltrating endometriosis should systematically assess the myometrium for adenomyosis's characteristic junctional zone thickening and T2 hyperintense myometrial foci alongside the compartment-based endometriosis evaluation discussed throughout this chapter, since adenomyosis, when present and unaddressed, can contribute independently to the patient's presenting pain and bleeding symptoms and may itself warrant surgical or medical management consideration distinct from the deep infiltrating disease evaluation that prompted the examination.

Special Populations: Endometriosis and Infertility

Endometriosis carries a well-recognized association with infertility, through mechanisms spanning distorted pelvic anatomy and tubal function from adhesive disease, direct ovarian reserve compromise from endometrioma or its surgical excision, discussed in the preceding chapter's endometrioma malignant transformation risk discussion, and a proposed inflammatory, implantation-impairing pelvic environment independent of anatomic distortion alone, and a patient presenting for fertility evaluation with imaging findings of deep infiltrating endometriosis benefits from coordinated counseling addressing both the endometriosis-specific surgical or medical management options discussed throughout this chapter and their potential interaction with planned or ongoing assisted reproductive technology, given that surgical intervention for endometriosis in a patient with diminished ovarian reserve requires particularly careful risk-benefit discussion regarding further reserve compromise from the surgery itself.

THE SIGNAL-TO-CATEGORY DECISION SYSTEM — Deep Infiltrating Endometriosis Compartment Mapping

---

The Signal Pattern: A patient with chronic pelvic pain undergoes dedicated endometriosis MRI, and the reader must systematically search the posterior, anterior, and lateral compartments for deep infiltrating disease.

Category Signature: A focal low T2 signal nodule confined to the peritoneal surface without deep infiltration is categorized as superficial disease; infiltration extending beyond 5 millimeters beneath the peritoneal surface into the uterosacral ligament, rectovaginal septum, bladder, bowel wall, or ureter is categorized as deep infiltrating disease, specifying the involved structure and depth.

The Decision: Superficial disease generally supports medical management or straightforward laparoscopic excision; deep infiltrating disease, particularly with bowel, bladder, or ureteral involvement, supports multidisciplinary surgical planning with the relevant surgical subspecialties identified based on the specific compartments involved.

Trap Logic: Dense pelvic adhesions can obliterate the normal fat plane and fluid interfaces the reader relies upon to identify individual structures, producing a fused, distorted anatomic picture that can cause a deep infiltrating nodule to be overlooked within the surrounding fibrotic tissue rather than recognized as a distinct, targetable lesion; the discriminating step is deliberately searching each compartment individually rather than relying on a single global gestalt impression of a distorted, adhesion-laden pelvis.

Pattern Anchor: Search each compartment individually and explicitly state involved structures and infiltration depth; a fused, adhesion-distorted pelvis is precisely the setting most likely to conceal a deep infiltrating nodule if a systematic, compartment-by-compartment search is not applied.

CAUTION: Ureteral endometriosis can produce silent, progressive hydronephrosis without corresponding flank pain or other localizing ureteral symptoms; deliberate assessment of both ureters for caliber and hydronephrosis is warranted in every deep infiltrating endometriosis evaluation regardless of the specific symptoms prompting the examination.

Complications and Prognosis Following Deep Infiltrating Endometriosis Surgery

Surgical excision of deep infiltrating endometriosis, particularly disease involving segmental bowel resection or extensive ureterolysis, carries a recognized complication profile including anastomotic leak, rectovaginal fistula formation, and ureteral injury, each reflecting the technical complexity of dissecting through the dense, fibrotic, adhesion-laden tissue planes characteristic of advanced disease, and preoperative imaging that clearly delineates the depth and extent of bowel and ureteral involvement, discussed throughout this chapter, directly supports the surgical team's ability to anticipate and specifically plan for these technically demanding dissection planes rather than encountering them unexpectedly during the procedure. Symptomatic recurrence following surgical excision occurs in a meaningful minority of patients over long-term follow-up, and postoperative imaging in a patient with recurrent symptoms benefits from direct comparison with the preoperative study and, when available, operative notes, since distinguishing genuine disease recurrence from expected postsurgical fibrotic change at a prior resection site requires this longitudinal comparison rather than interpretation of the postoperative study in isolation. Prognosis following comprehensive, complete surgical excision is generally favorable for pain symptom improvement, though fertility outcomes following surgery remain more variable and depend substantially on the extent of disease, the degree of adhesive distortion present preoperatively, and the patient's baseline ovarian reserve, considerations that reinforce the value of the coordinated, multidisciplinary counseling approach discussed earlier in this chapter's special populations discussion of endometriosis and infertility.

Clinical Case Presentations

Case 1. A 52-year-old woman with a sensation of vaginal bulge and incomplete rectal emptying undergoes MR defecography demonstrating descent of the bladder base 2 centimeters and the anorectal junction 4 centimeters below the pubococcygeal line during maximal straining, together with a large rectocele containing retained rectal contrast following attempted evacuation. The radiologist categorizes the findings as moderate anterior and severe posterior compartment prolapse with a significant fecal trap, and the patient proceeds to combined anterior and posterior compartment surgical repair.

Case 2. A 29-year-old woman with severe dysmenorrhea and dyspareunia undergoes dedicated endometriosis MRI demonstrating a low T2 signal nodule infiltrating the rectovaginal septum and anterior rectal wall muscularis propria, together with bilateral uterosacral ligament thickening and an obliterated pouch of Douglas. The radiologist categorizes the findings as deep infiltrating endometriosis with bowel involvement and recommends multidisciplinary surgical planning incorporating colorectal surgery, and the patient undergoes combined laparoscopic excision with discoid rectal resection.

Case 3. A 38-year-old woman with a history of forceps-assisted vaginal delivery and new-onset vaginal bulge undergoes MR defecography demonstrating asymmetric discontinuity of the right puborectalis muscle at its pubic bone insertion, together with moderate middle compartment prolapse. The radiologist categorizes the findings as right levator ani avulsion with associated prolapse, correlating the structural injury with the patient's symptomatic descent to support the pelvic floor reconstruction discussion at her subsequent urogynecology consultation.

Case 4. A 34-year-old woman undergoing infertility evaluation is found to have a left ovarian endometrioma on prior ultrasound, and dedicated endometriosis MRI additionally demonstrates a focal low T2 signal nodule involving the left ureter with mild proximal hydronephrosis, not suspected clinically given the absence of flank pain. The radiologist categorizes the findings as deep infiltrating endometriosis with ureteral involvement, prompting urgent urology referral to address the silent hydronephrosis alongside her fertility-focused endometriosis management.

Case 5. A 45-year-old woman with chronic pelvic pain and heavy menstrual bleeding undergoes dedicated endometriosis MRI demonstrating diffuse junctional zone thickening to 14 millimeters with scattered T2 hyperintense myometrial foci, together with a separate small deep infiltrating nodule at the right uterosacral ligament. The radiologist categorizes the findings as coexisting adenomyosis and deep infiltrating endometriosis, recommending that both conditions be addressed in the treatment planning discussion given each condition's independent contribution to her presenting symptoms.

Case 6. A 61-year-old woman with a sensation of obstructed defecation requiring digital splinting undergoes MR defecography demonstrating persistent narrowing of the anorectal angle during attempted evacuation, without the rectocele or enterocele that would typically explain her symptoms, together with only mild posterior compartment descent. The radiologist recognizes the pattern as paradoxical puborectalis contraction rather than a structural evacuation obstruction, and the patient is referred for biofeedback-based pelvic floor physical therapy rather than surgical repair, targeting the functional rather than structural basis of her symptoms.

THE SIGNAL-TO-CATEGORY DECISION SYSTEM — Pelvic Floor and Endometriosis Compartment Arc

---

The Signal Pattern: This chapter's patterns share a compartment-based search structure, from three-compartment descent measurement during MR defecography to posterior, anterior, and lateral compartment mapping for deep infiltrating endometriosis.

Category Signature: Prolapse is categorized mild, moderate, or severe independently by compartment relative to the pubococcygeal line; endometriosis is categorized superficial or deep infiltrating by depth and specific structure involved within each compartment.

The Decision: Category assignment in this chapter ranges from conservative pelvic floor therapy for mild, single-compartment prolapse to multicompartment surgical repair, and from medical management for superficial endometriosis to multidisciplinary surgical planning for deep infiltrating disease with bowel, bladder, or ureteral involvement.

The Trap Logic: Both patterns in this chapter share a common trap: an inadequate technical effort or a distorted anatomic field, an insufficient Valsalva or an adhesion-fused pelvis, that conceals the true severity or extent of disease from a reader who does not deliberately confirm technique adequacy or search each compartment individually.

Pattern Anchor: Confirm technical adequacy and search every compartment individually and explicitly in both patterns this chapter describes; a single global impression, without compartment-specific verification, risks missing the finding that most changes management.

Summary and Key Concepts

MR defecography quantifies pelvic organ descent relative to the pubococcygeal line across three compartments, bladder, vaginal cuff or cervix, and anorectum, during rest, squeeze, and maximal straining.

Cystocele, rectocele, and enterocele require careful differentiation given differing surgical repair approaches; enterocele is distinguished by herniated bowel content rather than rectal wall alone.

Levator ani avulsion, most often related to forceps-assisted vaginal delivery, carries a substantially elevated association with subsequent pelvic organ prolapse relative to diffuse levator attenuation alone.

Deep infiltrating endometriosis is defined by infiltration beyond 5 millimeters below the peritoneal surface and most commonly involves the posterior compartment, particularly the uterosacral ligaments and rectovaginal septum.

Ureteral endometriosis can cause silent, progressive hydronephrosis without localizing symptoms, making deliberate ureteral assessment essential in every deep infiltrating endometriosis evaluation.

Structured, compartment-based reporting for deep infiltrating endometriosis directly supports multidisciplinary surgical planning and correlates with more complete surgical resection.

Adenomyosis coexists with deep infiltrating endometriosis with substantial frequency and should be systematically assessed alongside compartment-based endometriosis evaluation.

CHAPTER 19: BOWEL MRI AND MR ENTEROGRAPHY IN INFLAMMATORY BOWEL DISEASE

Learning Objectives

1. Describe the technical requirements of MR enterography and MR pelvis protocols for inflammatory bowel disease evaluation.
2. Distinguish active inflammatory from fibrotic bowel wall change in Crohn disease using mural enhancement pattern and diffusion-weighted imaging.
3. Classify perianal fistulizing disease relative to the anal sphincter complex and recognize associated abscess.
4. Differentiate the characteristic distribution and imaging patterns of Crohn disease from ulcerative colitis.
5. Recognize bowel obstruction, stricture, and their surgical implications on MR enterography.

Clinical Overview

Inflammatory bowel disease imaging has been transformed over the past two decades by MR enterography, which now provides comprehensive small bowel and, with a dedicated pelvic protocol, perianal disease assessment without the ionizing radiation burden that repeated CT enterography would otherwise impose on a young patient population requiring lifelong surveillance for a chronic, relapsing-remitting condition. This chapter proceeds from MR enterography technique and Crohn disease activity assessment, through fistulizing and penetrating disease, ulcerative colitis and IBD subtype differentiation, and closes with bowel obstruction and stricture evaluation.

Two instances of the Signal-to-Category Decision System are applied in this chapter, the first to Crohn disease bowel wall activity assessment, distinguishing active inflammatory from fibrotic chronic change, and the second to perianal fistula classification relative to the sphincter complex, reflecting this chapter's two most surgically consequential categorization tasks.

MR Enterography Technique and Indications

Oral Contrast and Bowel Distension

Adequate small bowel distension represents the single most important technical prerequisite for a diagnostically useful MR enterography examination, since a collapsed, undistended bowel loop can both obscure genuine wall thickening and mimic pathologic thickening through simple luminal apposition, and this distension is achieved through ingestion of a large volume of a biphasic oral contrast agent, most commonly a low-density, non-absorbable solution such as polyethylene glycol or mannitol-based preparation, administered over 45 to 60 minutes before imaging to allow adequate transit and distension throughout the small bowel by the time of acquisition. An antiperistaltic agent, most commonly glucagon, administered immediately before the dynamic imaging sequences, reduces bowel motion artifact that would otherwise degrade image quality and obscure the fine mural detail required for reliable activity assessment, and this combination of adequate oral distension and pharmacologic peristalsis suppression together constitute the foundational technical requirements distinguishing a genuine MR enterography examination from a standard abdominal MRI performed without these dedicated preparations.

Sequence Protocol and the Role of Diffusion-Weighted Imaging

A comprehensive MR enterography protocol incorporates multiplanar T2-weighted imaging, both with and without fat suppression, to assess bowel wall thickening and mesenteric changes, together with dynamic contrast-enhanced T1-weighted imaging to characterize mural enhancement pattern, the single most important feature for distinguishing active inflammatory from fibrotic chronic disease discussed in the following section, and diffusion-weighted imaging, which has assumed an increasingly central role in this protocol given its ability to detect active inflammation-related restricted diffusion without requiring intravenous contrast administration, a meaningful advantage for the pediatric and young adult population disproportionately affected by inflammatory bowel disease who will require repeated surveillance imaging over a lifetime. Cine, or true dynamic, imaging sequences, acquired over several seconds per slice location, additionally allow direct visualization of bowel peristalsis and can help distinguish a genuinely fixed, non-peristalsing segment, suggesting a fibrotic stricture or adhesion, from a transiently non-distended segment that peristalses normally on subsequent frames and does not represent fixed pathology.

Indications and the Role of MR Enterography in Disease Monitoring

MR enterography serves both the initial diagnostic evaluation of suspected small bowel Crohn disease, particularly relevant given ileocolonoscopy's inherent inability to directly visualize the mid small bowel beyond the reach of the endoscope, and, with increasing frequency, longitudinal disease activity monitoring in a patient with established Crohn disease, an application supported by growing recognition that mucosal healing and objective imaging-based remission, rather than symptom control alone, represent the more clinically meaningful treatment target associated with improved long-term outcomes including reduced surgical intervention rates. This monitoring application places particular emphasis on the reproducibility and objectivity of the activity assessment framework discussed in the following section, since serial comparison across multiple examinations over a patient's treatment course requires a consistent, standardized approach to mural characterization rather than a purely subjective, examination-to-examination gestalt impression that would introduce unacceptable interobserver and intraobserver variability into a monitoring pathway intended to guide real treatment escalation or de-escalation decisions.

Special Populations: Pediatric and Pregnant Patients With Inflammatory Bowel Disease

Pediatric-onset inflammatory bowel disease, disproportionately affecting the small bowel and demonstrating a more extensive, aggressive disease phenotype at presentation relative to adult-onset disease, benefits particularly from MR enterography's absence of ionizing radiation given the substantial cumulative radiation exposure that repeated CT-based surveillance would otherwise impose over a young patient's expected decades of subsequent monitoring, and technical adaptations, including age-appropriate oral contrast volume dosing and, for a younger or more anxious child, procedural sedation consideration, support successful examination completion in this population without compromising the same technical rigor, adequate distension and antiperistaltic administration, discussed earlier in this chapter for the adult protocol. Pregnancy presents a distinct set of technical and interpretive considerations, with gadolinium contrast generally avoided given the theoretical placental transfer concerns discussed in the preceding chapter's endometriosis imaging context, favoring a non-contrast protocol relying more heavily on T2-weighted and diffusion-weighted sequences for activity assessment, an approach that retains meaningful diagnostic value for distinguishing active from quiescent disease even without the mural enhancement characterization that anchors the standard, non-pregnant activity assessment framework discussed throughout this chapter, and close collaboration between the radiologist, gastroenterologist, and obstetric team supports appropriately timed, technically optimized imaging when a pregnant patient with inflammatory bowel disease requires evaluation for a suspected flare.

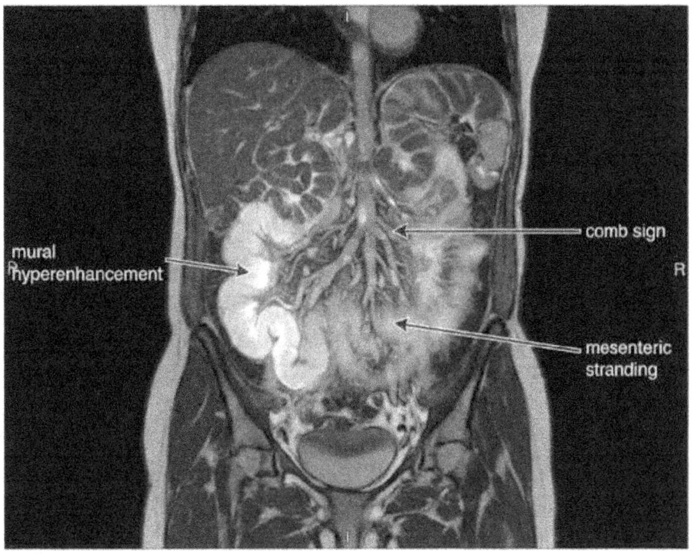

Figure 19.1
Coronal postcontrast MR Enterography showing active terminal ileal Crohn disease with mural hyperenhancement, comb sign, and mesenteric stranding.

Crohn Disease: Imaging Features and Activity Assessment

Epidemiology and Distribution of Crohn Disease

Crohn disease characteristically demonstrates a discontinuous, skip-lesion distribution pattern, with segments of diseased bowel interspersed among segments of entirely normal-appearing bowel, most classically and most commonly involving the terminal ileum, though disease can affect any portion of the gastrointestinal tract from mouth to anus, a transmural, full bowel wall thickness involvement distinct from the mucosa-predominant involvement characteristic of ulcerative colitis discussed later in this chapter. Peak incidence occurs in adolescence and early adulthood, though a meaningful proportion of cases present later in life, and a family history of inflammatory bowel disease, cigarette smoking, which paradoxically increases Crohn disease risk while appearing protective against ulcerative colitis, and specific identified genetic susceptibility loci each contribute to an individual patient's overall risk, though the precise underlying etiology remains understood as a complex interaction between genetic susceptibility, gut microbiome composition, and immune dysregulation rather than attributable to any single causative factor.

Active Inflammatory Mural Signal Characteristics

Active Crohn disease demonstrates a characteristic constellation of mural findings, mural hyperenhancement on postcontrast imaging, most pronounced in the mucosal and submucosal layers producing a stratified, layered enhancement pattern in earlier or milder disease, restricted diffusion on diffusion-weighted imaging reflecting the dense inflammatory cellularity within the thickened wall, and mesenteric hypervascularity, the comb sign, representing engorged, prominent vasa recta extending perpendicular from the mesenteric border toward the involved bowel segment, together with surrounding mesenteric fat stranding and often reactive regional lymphadenopathy. Wall thickening itself, while a sensitive marker of disease presence, is a comparatively nonspecific finding that alone cannot reliably distinguish active from fibrotic chronic disease discussed in the following section, making the enhancement pattern and diffusion characteristics, rather than thickness measurement alone, the primary features driving accurate activity categorization within this chapter's framework.

Fibrotic Chronic Change and the Active-Fibrotic Distinction

Fibrotic chronic bowel wall change, representing the reparative, scarring end-stage of longstanding or repeatedly active disease, demonstrates a distinctly different imaging signature from the active inflammatory pattern discussed above, with the wall appearing thickened but demonstrating homogeneous, delayed, comparatively mild enhancement rather than the pronounced early hyperenhancement of active disease, low T2 signal reflecting the dense, relatively acellular fibrous tissue composition, and notably absent or minimal diffusion restriction given the reduced cellular density relative to active inflammation. This active-fibrotic distinction carries direct, substantial treatment implications, since active inflammatory disease is expected to respond to escalated medical therapy, whether biologic or immunomodulator, while a predominantly fibrotic stricture, discussed further in the bowel obstruction section later in this chapter, will not meaningfully improve with medical therapy alone and instead requires either endoscopic balloon dilation or surgical resection, making accurate mural characterization, rather than symptom severity or wall thickness alone, the pivotal determinant of appropriate next-step management for a patient with a Crohn disease-related stricture.

Medical Management and Treat-to-Target Strategy

Contemporary Crohn disease management has increasingly adopted a treat-to-target strategy, in which the therapeutic endpoint is defined as objective evidence of mucosal and, increasingly, transmural healing on imaging or endoscopy rather than symptom control alone, a shift in treatment philosophy that has elevated the role of the mural activity characterization discussed throughout this section from a purely diagnostic exercise to an ongoing treatment-monitoring tool directly informing escalation, maintenance, or de-escalation decisions across a patient's treatment course. Biologic therapy, principally anti-tumor necrosis factor agents, anti-integrin agents, and interleukin-targeted agents, together with, for appropriately selected patients, small-molecule agents including Janus kinase inhibitors, form the backbone of medical therapy for active inflammatory disease, with the specific agent selected informed by disease location, severity, prior treatment history, and individual patient risk factors, and serial MR enterography, applying the same active-versus-fibrotic framework discussed throughout this chapter, provides an objective, radiation-free method for confirming genuine treatment response beyond symptom improvement alone, since clinical symptom improvement can occasionally precede or, in some cases, diverge from genuine mucosal and transmural healing, making the imaging-confirmed treat-to-target endpoint a meaningfully more rigorous marker of durable disease control.

THE SIGNAL-TO-CATEGORY DECISION SYSTEM — Crohn Disease Mural Activity Assessment

---

The Signal Pattern: A thickened bowel wall segment is identified on MR enterography, and the reader must characterize its mural enhancement pattern, T2 signal, and diffusion characteristics to determine disease activity.

Category Signature: Mural hyperenhancement with a stratified pattern, restricted diffusion, and surrounding mesenteric hypervascularity is categorized as active inflammatory disease; homogeneous, mild, delayed enhancement with low T2 signal and absent diffusion restriction is categorized as fibrotic chronic disease; a mixed pattern with features of both is categorized as mixed inflammatory-fibrotic disease.

The Decision: Active inflammatory disease supports escalation of medical therapy, whether biologic or immunomodulator, with an expectation of treatment response; predominantly fibrotic disease, particularly a fibrotic stricture, warrants endoscopic or surgical intervention given the expected lack of response to medical therapy alone; mixed disease supports a trial of medical therapy with close interval imaging follow-up to reassess the balance of activity.

Trap Logic: Wall thickness alone does not distinguish active from fibrotic disease, and a chronically thickened, predominantly fibrotic segment can appear qualitatively similar to an actively inflamed segment if the reader relies on thickness measurement rather than enhancement pattern and diffusion characteristics; the discriminating step is explicitly characterizing the enhancement kinetics and diffusion signal of the wall rather than anchoring the activity assessment on thickness alone.

Pattern Anchor: Characterize mural enhancement pattern and diffusion signal, not wall thickness alone, to distinguish active from fibrotic disease; this distinction directly determines whether medical escalation or mechanical intervention is the appropriate next step.

Figure 19.2 — Anatomical Illustration: Bowel Wall Layers in Active Versus Fibrotic Crohn Disease

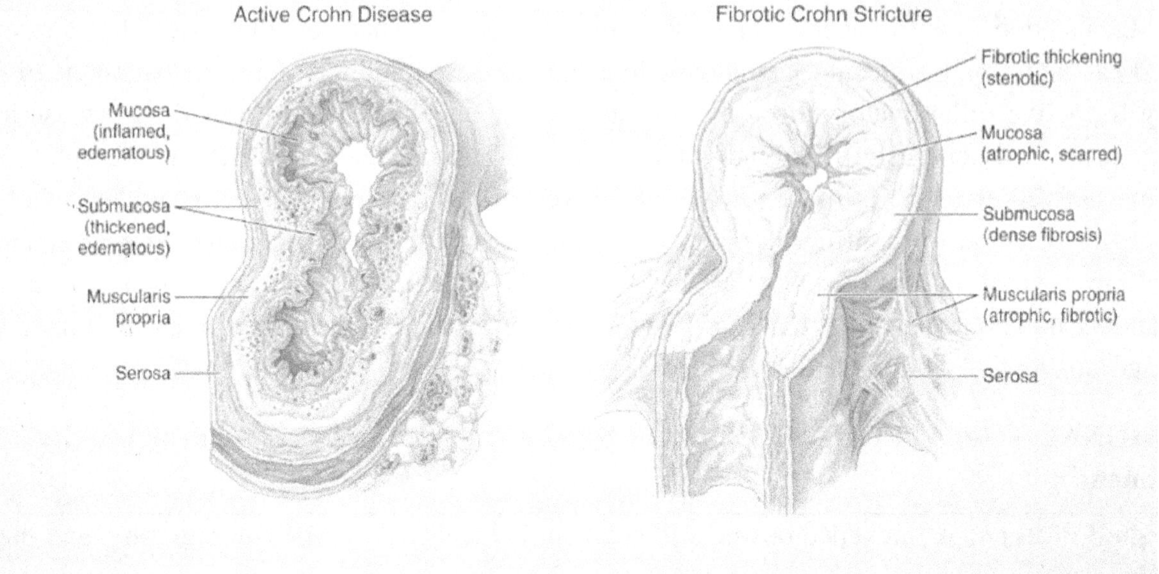

CLINICAL PEARL: A stratified, layered mural enhancement pattern, with pronounced inner-layer hyperenhancement relative to a comparatively less enhancing outer muscularis layer, favors active inflammatory disease, while homogeneous, transmural enhancement of similar intensity throughout the wall favors fibrotic chronic change; this layered-versus-homogeneous distinction complements the diffusion-weighted assessment discussed in this chapter's framework.

Fistulizing and Penetrating Crohn Disease

Complications and Prognosis of Fistulizing and Perianal Disease

Perianal fistulizing disease, discussed throughout this section, carries a recognized association with reduced quality of life and, for the more complex transsphincteric and suprasphincteric patterns, a meaningful risk of fecal incontinence following surgical intervention if sphincter-preserving technique is not carefully applied, making the accurate, complete tract classification this chapter's framework emphasizes directly relevant not only to initial surgical planning but to long-term functional outcome counseling as well. Long-term prognosis for fistulizing disease has improved substantially with the combined medical and surgical approach now standard in most treatment centers, staged seton drainage and medical therapy optimization followed by definitive sphincter-preserving repair once inflammation has been adequately controlled, relative to the historical approach of earlier, more aggressive primary surgical repair attempted before adequate medical control had been achieved, an older sequencing associated with substantially higher rates of both fistula recurrence and surgical complication. A minority of patients with severe, refractory, multiply recurrent perianal fistulizing disease ultimately require fecal diversion, temporary or permanent colostomy, to achieve adequate symptom control and allow perianal tissue healing, a comparatively drastic intervention generally reserved for the most severe, treatment-refractory presentations after the staged medical and sphincter-preserving surgical approaches discussed above have been exhausted.

PATIENT EDUCATION: MR enterography and dedicated pelvic MRI, unlike CT enterography, use no ionizing radiation, an important consideration to communicate to a patient, particularly a younger patient, who will likely require multiple surveillance examinations over the course of a lifelong, relapsing-remitting condition, and adequate preparation, completing the full oral contrast volume within the instructed time window, meaningfully improves image quality and reduces the likelihood of a technically limited examination requiring repeat imaging.

Enteroenteric and Enterocutaneous Fistula

Fistula formation, an abnormal communication tract between the bowel and an adjacent structure, represents a manifestation of the transmural, full-thickness inflammation characteristic of Crohn disease, discussed earlier in this chapter, distinguishing this condition from the mucosa-predominant ulcerative colitis discussed later, and enteroenteric fistula, communication between two bowel loops, appears on MR enterography as an abnormal, often star-shaped or linear tract of T2 hyperintense fluid or enhancing tissue directly connecting the two involved loops, occasionally producing a bypass effect in which luminal contrast preferentially flows through the fistulous tract rather than the native bowel lumen. Enterocutaneous fistula, communication between bowel and the skin surface, most often occurring at a prior surgical incision site, and enterovesical fistula, communication with the bladder, each carry distinct clinical presentations, cutaneous drainage for the former and recurrent urinary tract infection or pneumaturia, air within the urine, for the latter, and MR enterography's multiplanar capability provides essential preoperative roadmapping of these fistulous tracts and their relationship to adjacent structures for the surgical team planning definitive resection.

Abscess and Penetrating Complications

Intra-abdominal abscess, a walled-off collection of pus typically arising from bowel wall perforation or fistula tract-associated infection, appears as a rim-enhancing fluid collection, often with internal restricted diffusion reflecting the purulent content, and its identification carries urgent management implications distinct from the more indolent inflammatory and fibrotic findings discussed elsewhere in this chapter, since an abscess generally requires percutaneous or surgical drainage, often as a staged approach preceding rather than accompanying any planned bowel resection, given the substantially elevated anastomotic complication risk associated with attempting primary resection and anastomosis in the setting of active, undrained infection. Free perforation, while comparatively uncommon in Crohn disease relative to the more frequently encountered contained, fistulizing, or abscess-forming penetrating complications discussed above, represents a surgical emergency when it occurs, and any free intraperitoneal air or gross peritoneal contamination identified on imaging in a patient with known or suspected Crohn disease warrants immediate surgical consultation rather than the more measured, staged approach appropriate for contained penetrating disease.

Perianal Fistula Classification

Perianal fistulizing disease, a distinct and clinically significant Crohn disease phenotype affecting a substantial proportion of patients over their disease course, requires a dedicated pelvic MRI protocol with high-resolution, small field-of-view T2-weighted imaging in multiple planes specifically targeting the anal sphincter complex, and fistula classification relative to this sphincter complex, following the widely adopted framework distinguishing intersphincteric, transsphincteric, suprasphincteric, and extrasphincteric tract courses based on the tract's relationship to the internal and external anal sphincter, directly determines the surgical approach, ranging from simple fistulotomy for a straightforward intersphincteric tract to staged seton placement and, potentially, advancement flap or other sphincter-preserving technique for a more complex transsphincteric tract involving a substantial proportion of the sphincter musculature.

THE SIGNAL-TO-CATEGORY DECISION SYSTEM — Perianal Fistula Sphincter Classification

---

The Signal Pattern: Dedicated pelvic MRI is performed for suspected perianal fistulizing disease, and the reader must trace the fistula tract's complete course, including any secondary extensions, relative to the internal and external anal sphincter.

Category Signature: A tract confined between the internal and external sphincter is categorized intersphincteric; a tract crossing through both sphincters into the ischioanal fossa is categorized transsphincteric; a tract passing above the puborectalis is categorized suprasphincteric; a tract bypassing the sphincter complex entirely is categorized extrasphincteric, with any associated abscess or secondary extension separately noted.

The Decision: A simple intersphincteric tract without abscess may support straightforward fistulotomy; a transsphincteric or more complex tract, particularly with a secondary extension or abscess, supports staged management with seton placement and medical therapy optimization before definitive sphincter-preserving repair, given the elevated incontinence risk associated with primary fistulotomy of a tract involving substantial sphincter musculature.

Trap Logic: A horseshoe-configuration secondary extension, tracking circumferentially around the anal canal from a primary tract, can be easily overlooked if the reader traces only the most obvious primary tract identified on a single image without systematically following the tract through its complete multiplanar course; the discriminating step is deliberately tracing every fistula tract to its full termination across all acquired planes before finalizing the classification.

Pattern Anchor: Trace the complete fistula tract, including any secondary extensions or horseshoe configuration, across all planes before finalizing sphincter classification; an incompletely traced tract risks an incomplete surgical repair and disease recurrence.

Figure 19.3: Transsphincteric Perianal Fistula on Pelvic MRI

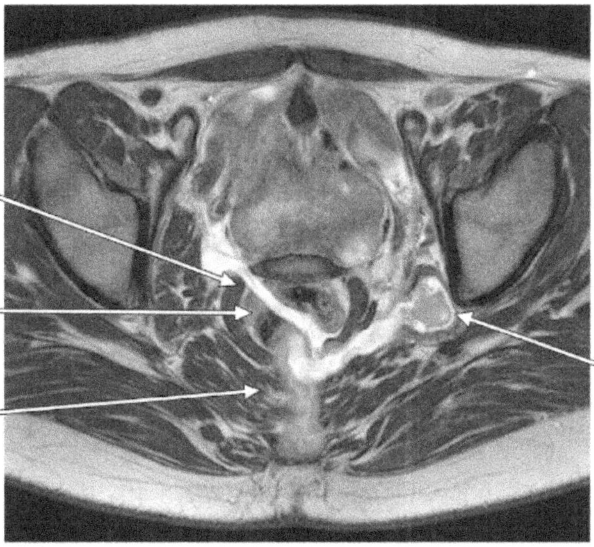

Ulcerative Colitis and Differentiating IBD Subtypes

CAUTION: Colonic wall thinning with marked dilation, rather than the wall thickening characteristic of typical active colitis, is the key imaging feature of toxic megacolon and reflects an advanced, perforation-prone disease state warranting immediate communication to the clinical team rather than routine, non-urgent reporting.

Feature	Crohn Disease	Ulcerative Colitis
Distribution	Discontinuous, skip lesions, mouth to anus	Continuous, rectum-originating, colon only
Wall involvement	Transmural	Mucosa-predominant
Fistula and abscess	Common	Rare, generally absent
Perianal disease	Common	Absent
Small bowel involvement	Common, especially terminal ileum	Absent
Characteristic complication	Stricture, fistula, abscess	Toxic megacolon, fulminant colitis

Epidemiology and Risk Factors for Ulcerative Colitis

Ulcerative colitis shares substantial epidemiologic overlap with Crohn disease, including peak incidence in adolescence and early adulthood, a genetic susceptibility component with recognized family clustering, and a proposed underlying mechanism of gut microbiome-immune dysregulation interaction, but diverges in its relationship with cigarette smoking, which, in a pattern that has long attracted mechanistic interest without full explanation, appears modestly protective against ulcerative colitis development and, in some studies, associated with a milder disease course, in direct contrast to smoking's risk-elevating and disease-worsening association with Crohn disease discussed earlier in this chapter. Appendectomy performed for confirmed appendicitis earlier in life has similarly been associated with reduced subsequent ulcerative colitis risk in multiple epidemiologic studies, a further point of mechanistic interest paralleling the smoking association, while a family history of inflammatory bowel disease of either subtype confers elevated risk for both Crohn disease and ulcerative colitis in a first-degree relative, reflecting shared, overlapping genetic susceptibility loci between the two conditions despite their distinct clinical and imaging phenotypes.

Ulcerative Colitis Distribution and Imaging Features

Ulcerative colitis, in contrast to the transmural, skip-lesion pattern characteristic of Crohn disease discussed throughout the preceding sections, demonstrates continuous, mucosa-predominant inflammation beginning at the rectum and extending proximally for a variable distance without the intervening segments of normal bowel characteristic of Crohn disease, and this continuous, rectum-originating distribution pattern, together with the disease's confinement to the colon without small bowel or perianal fistulizing involvement, discussed further below, together constitute the primary features distinguishing ulcerative colitis from Crohn disease on cross-sectional imaging and endoscopic evaluation alike. MRI findings in active ulcerative colitis include mural thickening, generally less pronounced than the often more substantial thickening of active Crohn disease, mucosal hyperenhancement, and, in more severe or fulminant disease, loss of the normal haustral pattern producing the featureless, tubular colonic appearance classically associated with longstanding disease, together with, in the most severe presentations, findings suggesting toxic megacolon, a surgical emergency characterized by marked colonic dilation with wall thinning rather than thickening, reflecting the loss of normal muscular wall integrity in this fulminant presentation.

IBD-Unclassified and the Overlap Presentation

A meaningful minority of inflammatory bowel disease presentations do not cleanly fit the classic Crohn disease or ulcerative colitis pattern discussed above, demonstrating overlapping or indeterminate features, a scenario termed IBD-unclassified, and the imaging findings in this indeterminate presentation, whether isolated colonic involvement with atypical distribution or subtle features suggesting transmural involvement without frank fistulizing disease, contribute alongside endoscopic, histologic, and serologic evaluation to the multidisciplinary diagnostic process, with definitive subtype classification sometimes only achieved over a longer period of clinical observation as the disease's characteristic behavior and distribution pattern become more apparent over time. This diagnostic uncertainty carries genuine clinical significance beyond simple nomenclature, since specific therapeutic and surgical decisions, most notably the appropriateness of restorative proctocolectomy with ileal pouch-anal anastomosis, a definitive surgical option generally reserved for ulcerative colitis given the substantially elevated pouch complication rate when Crohn disease is later identified in a patient who has undergone this procedure, depend meaningfully on accurate subtype classification, reinforcing the clinical value of the careful, systematic imaging distribution assessment this chapter's discussion emphasizes.

Extraintestinal Manifestations of Inflammatory Bowel Disease

Inflammatory bowel disease, whether Crohn disease or ulcerative colitis, carries recognized extraintestinal manifestations that can occasionally prompt the imaging evaluation that ultimately leads to IBD diagnosis, or that require specific attention in a patient with established disease, including primary sclerosing cholangitis, a fibrosing biliary tract condition disproportionately associated with ulcerative colitis and addressed in greater technical detail in the hepatobiliary imaging chapters earlier in this book, sacroiliitis and axial spondyloarthropathy, and a range of ocular, dermatologic, and hepatobiliary associations including episcleritis, erythema nodosum, pyoderma gangrenosum, and, less commonly, autoimmune hepatitis overlap. Recognition of these extraintestinal associations carries practical value for the interpreting radiologist beyond simple academic interest, since an incidental finding of sacroiliitis on a pelvic MRI performed for an unrelated indication, or biliary duct irregularity suggesting primary sclerosing cholangitis on an abdominal MRI, in a patient with known or suspected inflammatory bowel disease warrants explicit mention and correlation given the direct diagnostic and management relevance these associated conditions carry, and, conversely, an incidental finding of one of these extraintestinal manifestations in a patient without an established inflammatory bowel disease diagnosis should prompt consideration of otherwise unrecognized IBD as a potential unifying explanation.

Toxic Megacolon and Fulminant Colitis

Toxic megacolon, a severe, life-threatening complication of fulminant colitis, most classically associated with ulcerative colitis though occasionally occurring in Crohn colitis or infectious colitis, represents a distinct imaging and clinical emergency requiring recognition separate from the more indolent activity assessment framework this chapter otherwise emphasizes, with imaging demonstrating marked colonic dilation, generally exceeding 6 centimeters in transverse diameter for the transverse colon specifically, together with mural thinning rather than the thickening characteristic of the active disease patterns discussed throughout this chapter, reflecting a loss of normal smooth muscle wall integrity and tone from the severe, fulminant inflammatory process, and loss of the normal haustral pattern producing a smooth, featureless colonic contour. This mural thinning, rather than thickening, represents a critical distinguishing feature the reader must specifically recognize, since it reflects an ominous, more advanced disease state carrying substantial perforation risk, distinct from and considerably more urgent than the thickened, actively inflamed but structurally intact bowel wall of typical active colitis discussed earlier in this chapter, and any identification of this pattern warrants immediate communication to the clinical team given the surgical emergency it represents, generally necessitating urgent colectomy when conservative medical management fails to achieve rapid improvement.

Bowel Obstruction and Strictures

Stricture Identification and Upstream Dilation

Bowel stricture, a fixed luminal narrowing, is identified on MR enterography through the combination of a persistently narrowed segment across the dynamic imaging sequences, discussed earlier in this chapter's technique section, together with upstream bowel dilation proportional to the degree and chronicity of the obstruction, and distinguishing a genuine fixed stricture from a transiently narrowed but normally peristalsing segment relies on this combination of persistent narrowing across multiple dynamic frames together with the presence of proportionate upstream dilation, since a segment that appears narrowed on a single static image but demonstrates normal distension and peristalsis on the cine sequences does not represent a fixed, clinically significant stricture. The mural characterization framework discussed earlier in this chapter, distinguishing active inflammatory from fibrotic chronic change, applies directly to stricture evaluation, since the management pathway diverges substantially between a predominantly inflammatory stricture, which may improve with escalated medical therapy, and a predominantly fibrotic stricture, which will require mechanical intervention, whether endoscopic balloon dilation for a shorter, more accessible stricture or surgical resection for a longer or less accessible one.

Prestenotic Dilation and Surgical Decision-Making

The degree of prestenotic, or upstream, bowel dilation carries direct prognostic and management significance, with a markedly dilated prestenotic segment, generally accepted as exceeding roughly 3 centimeters in diameter, suggesting a more longstanding, hemodynamically significant obstruction less likely to respond adequately to medical therapy alone regardless of the underlying inflammatory-versus-fibrotic composition of the stricture itself, and this prestenotic dilation measurement, together with stricture length and the mural activity characterization discussed above, collectively inform the surgical decision between a shorter segmental resection for a focal, isolated stricture and a more extensive resection or strictureplasty, a bowel-sparing surgical technique that widens rather than resects a stricture, for multifocal or longer-segment stricturing disease. Bowel obstruction from Crohn disease-related stricture must additionally be distinguished from adhesive obstruction related to prior abdominal surgery, a distinction relying on the presence or absence of the mural thickening and enhancement characteristics of active or fibrotic Crohn disease discussed throughout this chapter at the transition point itself, since a purely adhesive band, without associated bowel wall thickening, represents a mechanically distinct and generally more straightforward surgical problem than a true Crohn disease stricture.

Postoperative Recurrence Assessment

Surgical resection, while effective for the fibrotic stricture and penetrating complications discussed throughout this chapter, is not curative for Crohn disease, and disease recurrence at or adjacent to the surgical anastomosis occurs with substantial frequency over long-term follow-up, making postoperative surveillance imaging, generally performed at a defined interval following surgery together with endoscopic evaluation, an important component of ongoing disease management rather than a discretionary add-on reserved only for a patient with recurrent symptoms. MR enterography interpretation in the postoperative setting requires familiarity with expected postsurgical anatomy, the surgical anastomosis itself, whether end-to-end, side-to-side, or another configuration, and any associated surgical clips or other hardware, to avoid misattributing normal postsurgical change to recurrent disease, and the same active-versus-fibrotic mural characterization framework discussed throughout this chapter applies directly to the neoterminal ileum immediately proximal to the anastomosis, the site of disease recurrence in the substantial majority of cases, with early recurrent mural hyperenhancement and diffusion restriction at this specific location warranting close clinical correlation and consideration of medical therapy optimization before more extensive recurrent disease and a repeat cycle toward stricture or penetrating complication has the opportunity to develop.

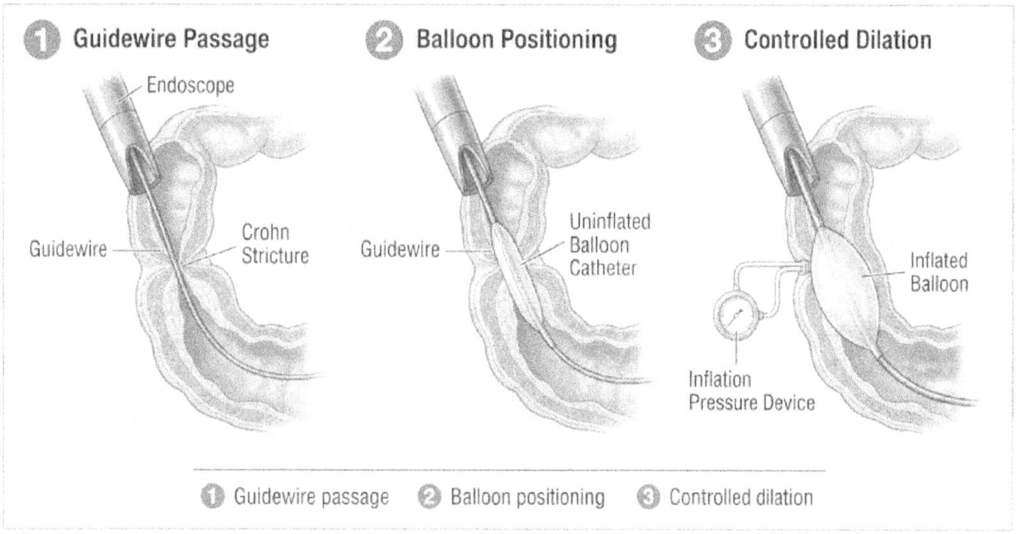

Figure 19.4 — Procedural Diagram: Endoscopic Balloon Dilation of Crohn Stricture.

KEY POINT: Prestenotic dilation exceeding approximately 3 centimeters suggests a hemodynamically significant, longstanding obstruction less likely to respond adequately to medical therapy alone; this measurement, together with stricture length and mural activity characterization, informs the choice between endoscopic dilation, strictureplasty, and segmental resection.

Clinical Case Presentations

Case 1. A 24-year-old man with a known history of ileal Crohn disease undergoes MR enterography for symptom flare, demonstrating mural hyperenhancement with a stratified pattern, restricted diffusion, and comb sign involving a 12-centimeter segment of terminal ileum. The radiologist categorizes the findings as active inflammatory disease and recommends escalation of biologic therapy, and the patient demonstrates clinical and, on follow-up imaging eight months later, radiologic improvement.

Case 2. A 31-year-old woman with longstanding Crohn disease and chronic partial small bowel obstruction symptoms undergoes MR enterography demonstrating a 4-centimeter segment of homogeneously, mildly enhancing terminal ileal wall thickening with low T2 signal, no diffusion restriction, and marked prestenotic dilation to 4.5 centimeters. The radiologist categorizes the findings as a fibrotic stricture and recommends surgical evaluation rather than medical therapy escalation, given the absence of active inflammatory features and the significant prestenotic dilation.

Case 3. A 27-year-old man with perianal drainage and pain undergoes dedicated pelvic MRI demonstrating a fistulous tract extending from the posterior midline anal crypt through both the internal and external anal sphincter into the ischioanal fossa, with a secondary horseshoe extension tracking to the contralateral ischioanal fossa and a small associated abscess. The radiologist categorizes the findings as a complex transsphincteric fistula with horseshoe extension and abscess, and the patient proceeds to staged seton placement and abscess drainage before definitive repair is considered.

Case 4. A 19-year-old woman with bloody diarrhea undergoes MR imaging demonstrating continuous mural thickening and mucosal hyperenhancement extending from the rectum through the descending colon without skip lesions, small bowel involvement, or perianal disease. The radiologist categorizes the pattern as consistent with ulcerative colitis rather than Crohn disease, correlating the continuous, rectum-originating distribution with the subsequent colonoscopic and histologic evaluation that confirms the diagnosis.

Case 5. A 35-year-old man with known Crohn disease presents with fever and right lower quadrant pain, and MR enterography demonstrates a rim-enhancing, diffusion-restricting fluid collection adjacent to a thickened terminal ileal segment, measuring 5 centimeters. The radiologist categorizes the findings as an intra-abdominal abscess and recommends percutaneous drainage before any consideration of surgical resection, given the substantially elevated anastomotic risk of proceeding directly to surgery in the setting of undrained active infection.

Case 6. A 29-year-old woman, two years following ileocecal resection for stricturing Crohn disease, undergoes surveillance MR enterography demonstrating new mural hyperenhancement with a stratified pattern and restricted diffusion confined to the neoterminal ileum immediately proximal to the surgical anastomosis, without evidence of stricture or fistula. The radiologist categorizes the findings as early postoperative recurrence, and the finding prompts endoscopic correlation and medical therapy optimization at a stage when the disease remains confined to a mild, purely inflammatory pattern rather than having progressed to structural complication.

THE SIGNAL-TO-CATEGORY DECISION SYSTEM — Inflammatory Bowel Disease Structural Arc

---

The Signal Pattern: This chapter's patterns span bowel wall and perianal characterization, from mural enhancement and diffusion assessment for Crohn disease activity, to complete fistula tract tracing for sphincter-relative classification.

Category Signature: Bowel wall segments are categorized active inflammatory, fibrotic, or mixed based on enhancement pattern and diffusion signal; perianal fistula tracts are categorized intersphincteric, transsphincteric, suprasphincteric, or extrasphincteric based on their course relative to the sphincter complex.

The Decision: Category assignment in this chapter ranges from medical therapy escalation for active inflammatory disease to endoscopic or surgical intervention for fibrotic stricture, and from simple fistulotomy for an intersphincteric tract to staged seton placement for a complex transsphincteric fistula.

The Trap Logic: Both patterns in this chapter share a common trap: relying on a single, incomplete feature, wall thickness alone or a partially traced fistula tract, rather than the complete characterization, enhancement kinetics plus diffusion, or the complete tract course including secondary extensions, that the framework requires.

Pattern Anchor: Characterize mural enhancement and diffusion together, and trace every fistula tract to its complete termination, before finalizing either category in this chapter; an incomplete assessment in either pattern risks a management decision the true underlying disease process does not support.

Summary and Key Concepts

MR enterography requires adequate oral contrast bowel distension and antiperistaltic agent administration to produce a diagnostically reliable examination.

Active Crohn disease shows stratified mural hyperenhancement, restricted diffusion, and the comb sign; fibrotic chronic disease shows homogeneous, mild, delayed enhancement with low T2 signal and no diffusion restriction.

The active-fibrotic distinction directly determines management: active disease supports medical escalation, while fibrotic stricture requires endoscopic dilation or surgical intervention.

Perianal fistula classification relative to the internal and external anal sphincter, intersphincteric through extrasphincteric, directly determines the surgical approach and requires tracing the complete tract including secondary extensions.

Ulcerative colitis demonstrates continuous, rectum-originating, mucosa-predominant inflammation without the skip lesions, small bowel involvement, or perianal fistulizing disease characteristic of Crohn disease.

Bowel stricture is confirmed by persistent narrowing across dynamic sequences with proportionate upstream dilation; prestenotic dilation exceeding approximately 3 centimeters suggests reduced likelihood of medical therapy response.

Intra-abdominal abscess generally requires drainage before surgical resection is undertaken, given the elevated anastomotic complication risk of operating in the setting of active, undrained infection.

CHAPTER 20: RECTAL CANCER STAGING AND PELVIC ONCOLOGIC IMAGING

Learning Objectives

1. Describe the dedicated high-resolution rectal MRI protocol and its relationship to total mesorectal excision surgical planning.
2. Apply T-staging criteria and assess mesorectal fascia involvement to determine circumferential resection margin status.
3. Recognize nodal staging criteria and extramural vascular invasion and their prognostic significance.
4. Apply the MRI tumor regression grading system to assess response following neoadjuvant chemoradiation.
5. Recognize anal canal carcinoma imaging features and other pelvic oncologic considerations relevant to rectal cancer staging.

Clinical Overview

Rectal cancer staging represents one of the more surgically consequential applications of body MRI, since the mesorectal fascia distance measurement discussed throughout this chapter directly determines whether a patient proceeds to upfront surgery or neoadjuvant chemoradiation, a treatment-pathway decision with substantial implications for both oncologic outcome and surgical morbidity. This chapter proceeds from rectal MRI technique and anatomy, through T-staging and mesorectal fascia assessment, nodal staging and extramural vascular invasion, neoadjuvant therapy response assessment, and closes with anal canal carcinoma and other pelvic oncologic considerations.

Two instances of the Signal-to-Category Decision System are applied in this chapter, the first to mesorectal fascia threat assessment at initial staging, and the second to post-neoadjuvant response categorization using the MRI tumor regression grading framework, reflecting the two most treatment-consequential categorization tasks in rectal cancer imaging.

Rectal MRI Technique and Anatomy

High-Resolution Protocol and Bowel Preparation

Dedicated rectal MRI relies fundamentally on high-resolution, small field-of-view T2-weighted imaging acquired in planes oriented perpendicular and parallel to the tumor's long axis, rather than the standard body-plane orientation used for most other pelvic imaging discussed throughout this book, since this tumor-specific oblique orientation provides the fine spatial resolution required to reliably assess the millimeter-scale distances that determine mesorectal fascia involvement, the single most surgically consequential measurement this chapter's framework addresses. Unlike the MR enterography protocol discussed in the preceding chapter, rectal MRI does not require oral contrast bowel distension, and antispasmodic agent administration, while used in some but not all protocols, plays a comparatively secondary role relative to the meticulous, tumor-oriented sequence planning that represents this protocol's defining technical requirement, underscoring why rectal MRI interpretation benefits substantially from radiologist-directed, real-time sequence planning at the scanner rather than a fully standardized, tumor-independent acquisition.

Mesorectal Anatomy and the Total Mesorectal Excision Concept

The mesorectum, the fatty, vascular, and lymphatic tissue envelope surrounding the rectum and bounded by the mesorectal fascia, represents the anatomic compartment that total mesorectal excision, the standard surgical technique for rectal cancer, aims to remove intact and unbreached, and the mesorectal fascia itself, corresponding to the surgical dissection plane targeted during this procedure, functions as the radiologic surrogate for the circumferential resection margin, the single most important predictor of local recurrence risk following rectal cancer surgery. This direct correspondence between the mesorectal fascia identified on MRI and the surgical circumferential resection margin is the conceptual foundation underlying this chapter's entire staging framework, since a preoperative MRI measurement of tumor distance from this fascia provides the surgical team with a reliable preoperative surrogate for a margin status that would otherwise only be definitively known following pathologic examination of the resected specimen, allowing preoperative treatment planning, whether upfront surgery or neoadjuvant therapy, to proceed with meaningful confidence regarding anticipated margin adequacy.

Peritoneal Reflection and Rectal Segment Localization

Precise localization of the tumor relative to the peritoneal reflection, the point at which the peritoneum transitions from covering the anterior and lateral upper rectum to becoming absent along the extraperitoneal lower rectum, carries direct staging and prognostic significance, since a tumor located below the peritoneal reflection lacks the serosal covering that would otherwise provide a natural anatomic barrier to local spread, making this specific segment of rectum, the lower and, to a variable degree, the middle third, the segment in which mesorectal fascia involvement carries its most direct oncologic consequence. Tumor distance from the anal verge, conventionally divided into lower rectum, within 5 centimeters, middle rectum, 5 to 10 centimeters, and upper rectum, 10 to 15 centimeters, similarly carries direct surgical planning relevance beyond staging alone, since this distance measurement directly informs the feasibility of sphincter-preserving low anterior resection versus abdominoperineal resection with permanent colostomy, making accurate localization, together with the mesorectal fascia and T-stage assessment discussed throughout this chapter, an essential component of the complete rectal MRI staging report.

Patient Education and Counseling for Rectal Cancer Staging

Communicating rectal cancer staging results to a patient benefits from clear explanation of why the mesorectal fascia distance measurement, a concept unfamiliar to most patients encountering this diagnosis for the first time, carries such direct influence over the recommended treatment pathway, since patients frequently arrive with an expectation that surgery represents the immediate, singular next step and can find a recommendation for neoadjuvant chemoradiation before surgery counterintuitive without this specific explanation of how the imaging findings inform sequencing. Discussion of anticipated treatment-related effects, including bowel, bladder, and sexual function changes following pelvic radiation and total mesorectal excision surgery, and, for a low rectal tumor, the specific possibility of permanent colostomy should abdominoperineal resection prove necessary, supports realistic patient expectations and informed treatment decision-making from the earliest stages of the diagnostic and staging process, and clear, empathetic communication of the watch-and-wait organ-preservation possibility, when genuinely applicable based on tumor location and stage, together with its associated surveillance commitment and salvage surgery contingency, allows a patient facing this diagnosis to meaningfully participate in a values-informed choice between organ preservation and standard surgical management.

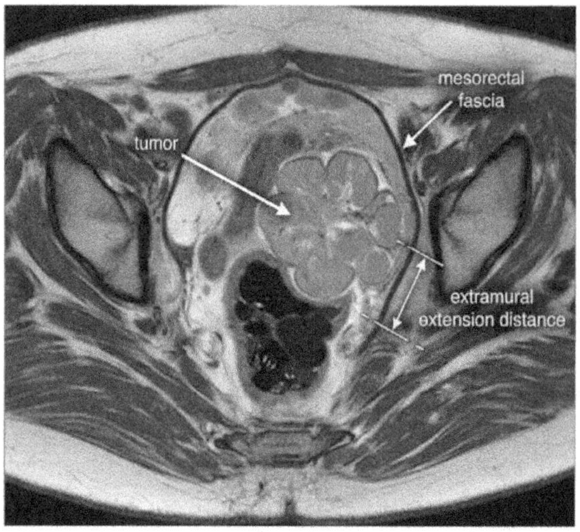

Figure 20.1

MRI Versus Endorectal Ultrasound and CT in Staging

Endorectal ultrasound, historically the primary modality for early-stage rectal tumor assessment given its excellent resolution for distinguishing the individual wall layers relevant to differentiating T1 from T2 disease, has been progressively supplanted by MRI as the primary staging modality for the great majority of rectal cancers, reflecting MRI's superior soft tissue contrast for mesorectal fascia distance assessment, the central staging determination this chapter's framework addresses, together with MRI's ability to comprehensively evaluate nodal status and extramural vascular invasion within the same examination, capabilities that endorectal ultrasound's limited field of view cannot adequately provide. Endorectal ultrasound retains a complementary role for the specific subset of very early, superficial tumors where the T1-versus-T2 distinction, determining candidacy for local excision rather than radical resection, benefits from ultrasound's superior layer-by-layer resolution at this fine level of detail, while CT, though inadequate for the local mesorectal fascia and nodal characterization this chapter emphasizes given its comparatively limited soft tissue contrast resolution, remains essential for distant metastatic staging, most commonly to the liver and lungs, complementing rather than substituting for the local staging role MRI provides throughout this chapter's discussion.

T-Staging and Mesorectal Fascia Assessment

Complications and Prognosis Following Total Mesorectal Excision

Total mesorectal excision surgery, while representing the standard curative-intent approach for staged rectal cancer discussed throughout this chapter, carries a recognized complication profile including anastomotic leak, a particularly consequential complication given its association with both increased perioperative morbidity and, in several studies, elevated long-term local recurrence risk, urinary and sexual dysfunction related to pelvic autonomic nerve injury during the mesorectal dissection, and, for a low anterior resection, low anterior resection syndrome, a constellation of altered bowel function including urgency, frequency, and incontinence that can substantially affect quality of life even following an oncologically successful resection. Anastomotic leak risk correlates with several identifiable factors, including anastomotic height, a lower anastomosis carrying elevated risk relative to a higher one, and preoperative radiation exposure, considerations that inform the surgical team's decision regarding diverting loop ileostomy, a temporary stoma protecting a lower or higher-risk anastomosis while healing occurs, before eventual stoma reversal once anastomotic integrity has been confirmed, typically through a contrast enema or similar imaging study performed several weeks following the index surgery. Overall prognosis following complete surgical resection with clear margins correlates strongly with the pathologic staging ultimately determined, itself substantially predicted by the preoperative MRI staging framework this chapter addresses, and five-year survival for early-stage, node-negative disease with a clear circumferential resection margin substantially exceeds that of more advanced, node-positive, or margin-involved disease, reinforcing the direct prognostic, in addition to purely treatment-planning, significance of the accurate preoperative staging this chapter's framework is designed to provide.

Epidemiology and Risk Factors for Rectal Cancer

Rectal cancer, together with colon cancer under the combined colorectal cancer designation, represents one of the most common malignancies affecting both men and women, with incidence rising with age though notably demonstrating a concerning increase in early-onset disease, presentation before age 50, over recent decades, a trend whose underlying cause remains an area of active investigation spanning proposed dietary, microbiome, and environmental contributing factors. A family history of colorectal cancer, hereditary syndromes including Lynch syndrome and familial adenomatous polyposis, personal history of inflammatory bowel disease discussed in the preceding chapter given its own recognized colorectal cancer risk elevation with longstanding, extensive disease, and modifiable lifestyle factors including diet, physical inactivity, obesity, and tobacco and alcohol use each contribute to an individual patient's overall risk, and this risk factor profile, together with the rising early-onset incidence trend noted above, has informed lowered population screening initiation age recommendations in several jurisdictions over recent years.

T-Stage Criteria and Layer-by-Layer Wall Assessment

T-staging on rectal MRI proceeds through systematic assessment of tumor depth relative to the rectal wall's distinct anatomic layers, visualized as a characteristic multilayered signal pattern on high-resolution T2-weighted imaging, with T1 and T2 tumors confined within the submucosa or muscularis propria respectively without extension beyond the outer muscularis border, T3 tumors demonstrating extension through the muscularis propria into the perirectal mesorectal fat, further subdivided by the depth of this extramural extension, and T4 tumors demonstrating invasion of an adjacent organ or structure or extension through the visceral peritoneum. This layer-by-layer assessment, while conceptually analogous to the wall-layer characterization discussed for other luminal organs throughout this book, carries particular technical demand in the rectal cancer context given the fine, millimeter-scale distinctions between T-stage subcategories that directly influence treatment pathway selection, reinforcing why the high-resolution, tumor-oriented sequence acquisition discussed in the preceding technique section represents a genuine technical prerequisite rather than an optional refinement for reliable T-staging.

Extramural Extension Depth and Mesorectal Fascia Distance

For a T3 tumor, the specific depth of extramural extension beyond the muscularis propria, measured in millimeters, provides meaningfully more staging and prognostic granularity than the T3 designation alone, with minimal extension, generally under 5 millimeters, carrying a more favorable prognosis than extensive extension, and this same extramural extension measurement feeds directly into the mesorectal fascia distance assessment central to this chapter's primary staging framework, since the shortest measured distance between the tumor's leading edge, whether the primary tumor itself, a tumor deposit, or an involved lymph node discussed in the following section, and the mesorectal fascia determines whether the circumferential resection margin is anticipated to be clear, threatened, or involved following surgery. A mesorectal fascia distance of 1 millimeter or less is generally considered involved, predicting a positive circumferential resection margin and correspondingly elevated local recurrence risk if surgery were performed without neoadjuvant therapy, while a distance exceeding this threshold, generally by a comfortable margin, supports a clear anticipated margin, and this specific distance measurement, rather than T-stage classification alone, represents the single most direct driver of the upfront-surgery-versus-neoadjuvant-therapy treatment pathway decision this chapter's framework addresses.

THE SIGNAL-TO-CATEGORY DECISION SYSTEM — Mesorectal Fascia Threat Assessment

The Signal Pattern: A rectal tumor is identified on high-resolution MRI, and the reader must measure the shortest distance from the tumor's leading edge, including any discrete tumor deposit or involved lymph node, to the mesorectal fascia.

Category Signature: A distance clearly exceeding the involved threshold is categorized as a clear anticipated circumferential resection margin; a distance approaching but not meeting the involved threshold is categorized as a threatened margin; a distance of 1 millimeter or less is categorized as an involved margin.

The Decision: A clear margin generally supports proceeding directly to total mesorectal excision surgery; a threatened or involved margin supports neoadjuvant chemoradiation before surgery, aiming to achieve tumor downstaging and a clear margin at the time of eventual resection.

Trap Logic: Peritumoral desmoplastic fibrotic reaction, a reactive fibrous response surrounding the tumor's true invasive margin, can mimic direct tumor extension on T2-weighted imaging given its similarly intermediate signal intensity, risking overstaging of both T-category and mesorectal fascia distance if the reader does not carefully distinguish this reactive fibrotic tissue from genuine tumor infiltration; the discriminating step is recognizing that desmoplastic reaction typically demonstrates a more irregular, spiculated morphology with signal characteristics distinct from the tumor's own bulk when both are carefully compared side by side.

Pattern Anchor: Measure the shortest tumor-to-mesorectal-fascia distance, including deposits and nodes, not tumor size or T-stage alone; distinguish peritumoral desmoplastic reaction from true tumor extension before finalizing this measurement.

Figure 20.2: Rectal Wall Layer Anatomy and Mesorectal Fascia

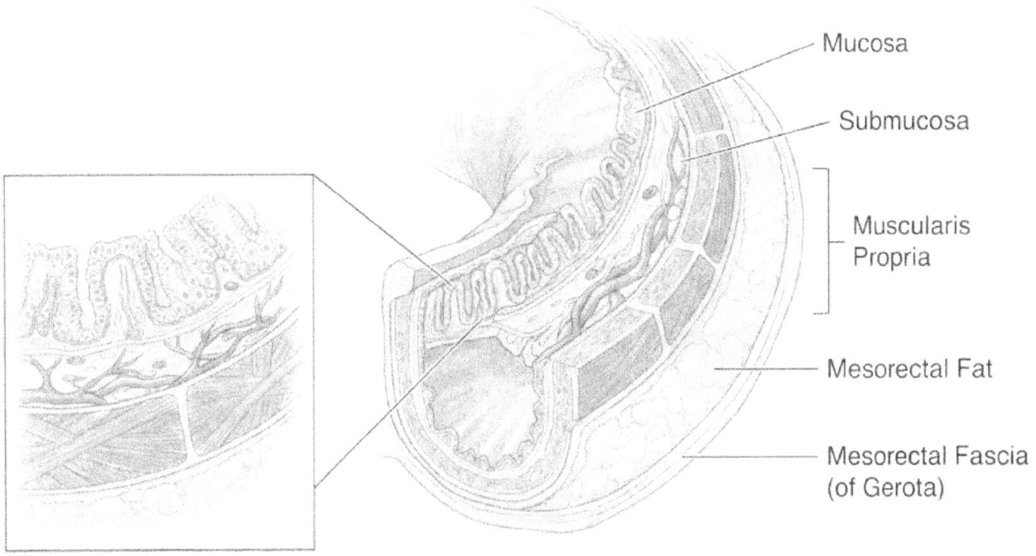

T-Stage	Depth of Invasion	Mesorectal Fascia Relevance
T1	Confined to submucosa	Generally not threatened
T2	Confined to muscularis propria	Generally not threatened
T3	Extension into mesorectal fat, subdivided by depth	Distance from fascia determines threat category
T4	Invasion of adjacent organ or peritoneal surface	Margin generally threatened or involved

CLINICAL PEARL: Report the mesorectal fascia distance in millimeters, not simply as a categorical clear-versus-threatened impression, since the surgical and radiation oncology team uses this specific measurement, together with its trend on any restaging examination, to guide both initial treatment selection and, following neoadjuvant therapy, the timing and extent of eventual surgery.

Nodal Staging and Extramural Vascular Invasion

Differential Diagnosis of a Rectal Mass

While adenocarcinoma accounts for the great majority of rectal masses encountered in clinical practice, several important mimics warrant consideration before definitive staging proceeds, including a large villous or tubulovillous adenoma, which can demonstrate substantial size and a correspondingly complex, folded morphology without necessarily harboring invasive malignancy, a diagnosis ultimately requiring histologic confirmation given the imaging overlap with a superficial, non-invasive early carcinoma, and gastrointestinal stromal tumor, a comparatively uncommon submucosal mesenchymal neoplasm distinguished from adenocarcinoma by its characteristic origin from the muscularis propria layer itself rather than the mucosal surface. Rectal lymphoma, though rare as a primary rectal malignancy, should be considered particularly in an immunocompromised patient or one with disproportionately bulky, circumferential wall thickening relative to the degree of luminal narrowing, a pattern distinct from the more focal, luminal-narrowing mass effect typical of adenocarcinoma, and metastatic disease to the rectum from an adjacent or distant primary, whether direct extension from a prostate, cervical, or bladder malignancy discussed elsewhere in this book, or hematogenous or peritoneal spread from a more distant primary, should be considered when the imaging morphology or clinical context does not fit the typical adenocarcinoma presentation this chapter's framework otherwise addresses.

Lymph Node Characterization Criteria

Lymph node staging on rectal MRI relies less heavily on the size-based criteria applied in many other oncologic imaging contexts and more heavily on morphologic features, irregular margin contour and heterogeneous internal signal intensity, since a substantial proportion of malignant mesorectal lymph nodes remain below the size threshold that would trigger suspicion under a size-alone approach, while a proportion of larger, reactive nodes remain entirely benign, making morphology-based assessment, evaluating each visualized node's border regularity and internal signal homogeneity rather than short-axis diameter alone, the more diagnostically reliable approach this chapter's framework emphasizes for mesorectal nodal staging specifically. Extramesorectal or lateral pelvic sidewall lymph nodes, distinct from the mesorectal nodes discussed above, carry particular staging and surgical planning significance when involved, since standard total mesorectal excision does not routinely clear this nodal basin, and identification of a suspicious lateral pelvic lymph node may prompt consideration of extended lateral pelvic lymph node dissection or inclusion of this nodal basin within the neoadjuvant radiation treatment field, a management implication distinct from mesorectal nodal involvement alone.

Extramural Vascular Invasion

Extramural vascular invasion, tumor infiltration into perirectal blood vessels beyond the muscularis propria, represents an independent, MRI-detectable adverse prognostic feature carrying elevated risk for both distant metastatic spread and local recurrence, recognized on high-resolution T2-weighted imaging as a tubular, vessel-shaped structure containing intermediate tumor-signal material expanding and distorting the normal vessel contour, distinct from a normal, thin-walled vascular structure of uniform low signal. Recognition of extramural vascular invasion carries treatment-planning significance independent of, and additive to, the T-stage and mesorectal fascia assessment discussed throughout this chapter, since its presence has been associated with reduced disease-free survival even among tumors otherwise categorized as having a clear anticipated circumferential resection margin, supporting a case for more assertive systemic and neoadjuvant treatment consideration in a tumor demonstrating this specific adverse feature regardless of its mesorectal fascia distance measurement in isolation.

Figure 20.3 — Procedural Diagram: Total Mesorectal Excision

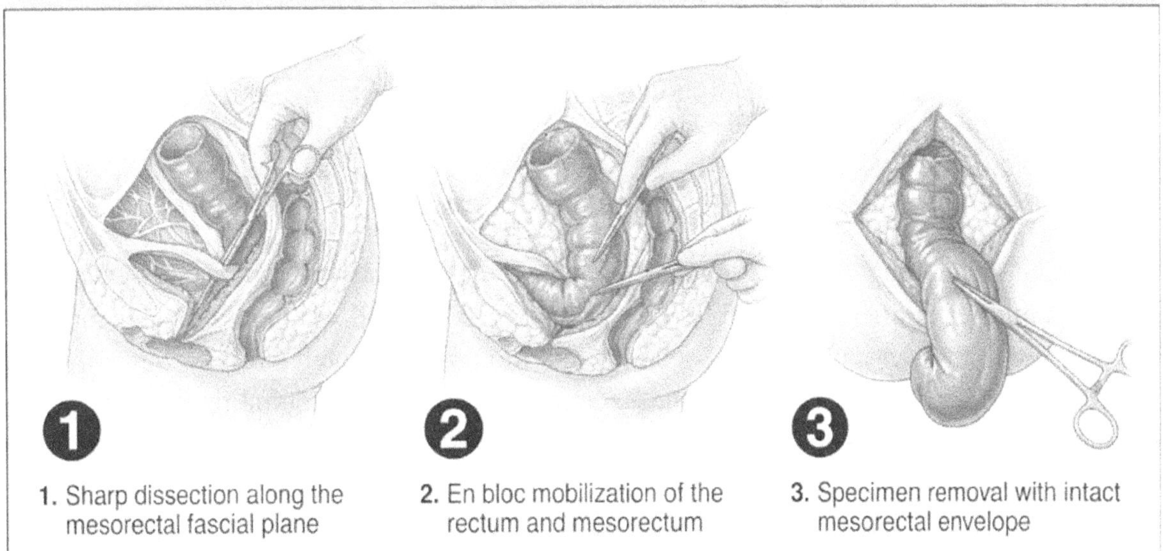

Figure 20.3 — Procedural Diagram: Total Mesorectal Excision

KEY POINT: Nodal characterization for mesorectal lymph nodes relies primarily on border irregularity and internal signal heterogeneity rather than short-axis size alone, since a substantial proportion of malignant mesorectal nodes fall below the size threshold that would trigger suspicion under a size-based approach used in other oncologic imaging contexts.

Neoadjuvant Therapy Response Assessment

MRI Tumor Regression Grading

Restaging MRI performed following neoadjuvant chemoradiation applies the MRI tumor regression grading system, assessing the relative proportion of residual intermediate-signal tumor tissue versus low-signal fibrotic scar tissue within the treated tumor bed, ranging from grade 1, complete radiologic response with fibrosis alone and no visible residual tumor signal, through grade 5, minimal or no evident fibrotic response with predominantly persistent tumor signal, and this grading framework, while conceptually parallel to the mural activity characterization applied to inflammatory bowel disease in the preceding chapter, in this oncologic context specifically distinguishes viable, treatment-resistant tumor from successfully treated, sterilized fibrotic tissue rather than distinguishing active from chronic inflammatory change. Diffusion-weighted imaging meaningfully complements the T2-weighted morphologic assessment underlying tumor regression grading, since densely fibrotic, successfully treated tissue characteristically demonstrates reduced or absent diffusion restriction given its markedly reduced cellularity, while persistent viable tumor tissue retains the restricted diffusion pattern characteristic of densely cellular malignancy, providing a complementary, cellularity-based confirmation that helps resolve genuinely ambiguous cases where T2 morphology alone leaves uncertainty between dense fibrosis and a small volume of residual viable tumor.

Complete Clinical Response and the Watch-and-Wait Strategy

A subset of patients achieving complete or near-complete radiologic response, corroborated by concordant endoscopic and digital rectal examination findings showing no residual visible or palpable tumor, are now increasingly offered a watch-and-wait, or organ-preservation, management strategy, deferring or entirely avoiding total mesorectal excision surgery and its associated morbidity, including permanent colostomy for a low rectal tumor, in favor of close, structured surveillance with the expectation of salvage surgery should local regrowth subsequently occur, an evolving management paradigm that has meaningfully elevated the clinical stakes and required diagnostic precision of the restaging MRI tumor regression assessment discussed throughout this section beyond its earlier role as a comparatively lower-stakes adjunct to standard surgical planning. This watch-and-wait strategy requires particularly rigorous, structured surveillance imaging at defined intervals following the initial complete response determination, since local regrowth, while occurring in only a minority of patients who achieve an initial complete response, remains a recognized risk requiring timely detection to preserve the salvage surgery option before regrowth progresses beyond a resectable, organ-preserving surgical window.

THE SIGNAL-TO-CATEGORY DECISION SYSTEM — Post-Neoadjuvant Response Categorization

---

The Signal Pattern: Restaging MRI is performed following completion of neoadjuvant chemoradiation, and the reader must characterize the relative proportion of residual tumor signal versus fibrotic scar tissue within the treated tumor bed, correlating T2 morphology with diffusion-weighted imaging.

Category Signature: Fibrosis alone without visible residual tumor signal or diffusion restriction is categorized as complete radiologic response; predominantly fibrotic tissue with a small residual focus of intermediate signal and diffusion restriction is categorized as good partial response; substantial persistent intermediate-signal tumor tissue with corresponding diffusion restriction is categorized as poor response.

The Decision: Complete radiologic response, when concordant with endoscopic and clinical examination, supports consideration of a watch-and-wait organ-preservation strategy with structured surveillance; good partial response generally supports proceeding to standard total mesorectal excision surgery; poor response prompts reconsideration of the treatment plan, potentially including additional systemic therapy before surgery.

Trap Logic: Dense post-radiation fibrosis can occasionally retain a degree of diffusion restriction related to its compact cellular and collagenous architecture even without genuine residual viable tumor, risking a falsely low regression grade if diffusion signal is interpreted in isolation without careful correlation to the corresponding T2 morphology and, where available, comparison with the pretreatment examination; the discriminating step is correlating diffusion findings with T2 morphology and pretreatment imaging rather than relying on diffusion restriction alone to identify residual tumor.

Pattern Anchor: Correlate T2 fibrosis morphology with diffusion-weighted signal, not either feature in isolation, before assigning tumor regression grade; a falsely elevated grade risks inappropriate surgery, while a falsely low grade risks missing a genuine candidate for organ-preserving watch-and-wait management.

EVIDENCE: Prospective watch-and-wait cohort studies have demonstrated organ preservation in a substantial majority of patients achieving a confirmed complete clinical response, with salvage surgery remaining a viable option for the minority who experience local regrowth during structured surveillance, findings that have meaningfully expanded organ-preservation candidacy beyond the highly selected populations initially considered for this strategy.

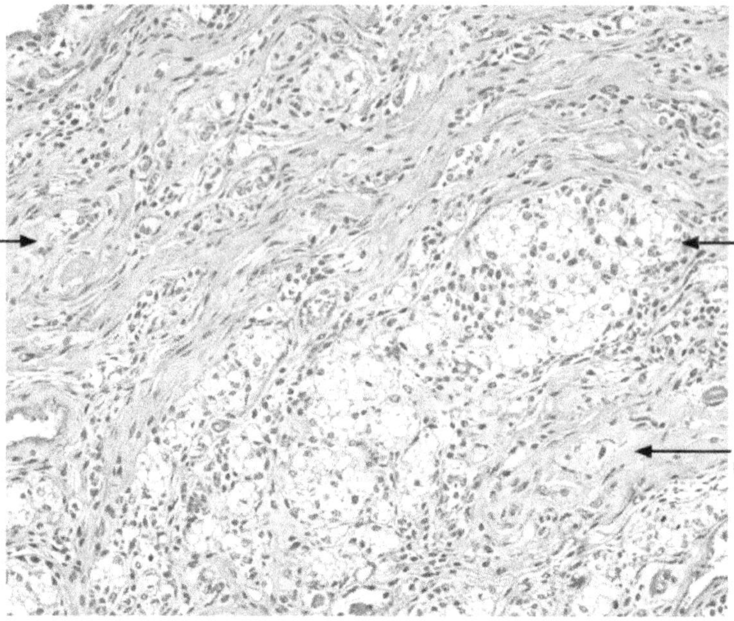

Anal Canal and Other Pelvic Oncologic Considerations

Rectal Cancer Risk and Surveillance in Inflammatory Bowel Disease

Patients with longstanding, extensive ulcerative colitis or Crohn colitis, discussed in the preceding chapter's inflammatory bowel disease discussion, carry elevated colorectal cancer risk relative to the general population, with risk rising with both disease duration and anatomic extent, and colitis-associated colorectal cancer follows a distinct pathway, often arising from flat or subtle dysplastic mucosal change rather than the more readily visible polypoid adenoma-to-carcinoma sequence characteristic of sporadic colorectal cancer discussed earlier in this chapter, a pathway that has informed dedicated chromoendoscopic and structured biopsy surveillance protocols distinct from standard average-risk colorectal cancer screening. When colitis-associated rectal cancer does develop, the same MRI staging framework and mesorectal fascia assessment discussed throughout this chapter apply directly, though the interpreting radiologist should anticipate a potentially more complex background of chronic mural thickening and fibrotic change from the underlying inflammatory bowel disease itself, a background that can complicate the tumor-versus-background-inflammation distinction in a way not typically encountered when staging a sporadic rectal cancer arising in an otherwise normal rectum, reinforcing the value of correlating any staging MRI findings with the patient's known inflammatory bowel disease distribution and activity history from prior examinations.

CAUTION: A rectal mass arising in a patient with longstanding inflammatory bowel disease may be superimposed upon a background of chronic mural thickening and fibrosis from the underlying colitis itself; correlating staging findings with the patient's known disease distribution and activity history supports accurate distinction between tumor and background inflammatory change.

Anal Canal Carcinoma Imaging Features

Anal canal carcinoma, most commonly squamous cell carcinoma and strongly associated with human papillomavirus infection, is staged and managed distinctly from rectal adenocarcinoma discussed throughout this chapter, with primary chemoradiation, rather than upfront surgical resection, representing standard initial therapy for the great majority of cases, reflecting anal squamous cell carcinoma's characteristically favorable radiosensitivity, and MRI staging for anal canal carcinoma emphasizes tumor size, depth of sphincter complex invasion, and inguinal as well as mesorectal and pelvic sidewall nodal involvement, given the anal canal's distinct lymphatic drainage pattern extending to the inguinal nodal basin in addition to the pelvic nodal stations relevant to rectal cancer. Distinguishing a distal rectal tumor extending into the anal canal from a primary anal canal carcinoma extending proximally can occasionally present genuine diagnostic ambiguity, and this distinction carries direct management significance given the substantially different standard treatment pathways, primary chemoradiation for anal carcinoma versus the surgery-centered or neoadjuvant-therapy-then-surgery pathway for rectal adenocarcinoma discussed throughout this chapter, making histologic confirmation, together with careful attention to the tumor's epicenter and any macroscopic association with the dentate line, essential to accurate management pathway assignment in a genuinely borderline case.

Special Populations and Long-Term Survivorship Considerations

Rectal cancer increasingly affects younger patients given the early-onset incidence trend discussed earlier in this chapter, and treatment planning in this population carries distinct considerations beyond the staging framework this chapter otherwise emphasizes, including fertility preservation counseling before pelvic radiation, given radiation's recognized gonadal toxicity, and heightened attention to long-term survivorship quality of life given the substantially longer anticipated post-treatment lifespan in a younger patient relative to the historically older typical rectal cancer population, considerations that support multidisciplinary counseling extending beyond the purely oncologic staging and treatment-pathway determinations addressed throughout the remainder of this chapter. Long-term surveillance following completed treatment, whether standard surgery or watch-and-wait organ preservation discussed earlier in this chapter, follows a structured, guideline-directed imaging and clinical examination schedule extending several years beyond initial treatment completion, reflecting the recognized, though gradually diminishing, local and distant recurrence risk window characteristic of treated rectal cancer, and the interpreting radiologist's familiarity with expected posttreatment anatomic change, whether postsurgical or the fibrotic tumor bed changes discussed in this chapter's response assessment section, remains essential to confidently distinguishing genuine recurrence from expected treatment-related change throughout this extended surveillance period.

Locally Recurrent Rectal Cancer and Pelvic Exenteration

Locally recurrent rectal cancer, occurring in a minority of patients despite optimal initial staging and treatment, presents distinct imaging challenges given the frequently distorted, fibrotic postsurgical anatomy within which recurrence must be identified, and MRI, applying the same T2 morphology and diffusion-weighted correlation principles discussed throughout this chapter's response assessment section, remains the primary imaging modality for characterizing suspected recurrence and, critically, for determining resectability, specifically whether adjacent pelvic sidewall, sacral, or other structures are involved in a pattern that would require pelvic exenteration, an extensive multi-organ resection, rather than a more limited local re-resection. Pelvic exenteration, encompassing en bloc resection of the rectum together with adjacent involved pelvic organs, whether bladder, prostate or uterus and vagina, and, for posterior sacral involvement, a component of the sacrum itself, represents a technically demanding but potentially curative option for carefully selected patients with locally recurrent or locally advanced primary disease without distant metastasis, and comprehensive preoperative MRI mapping of the precise structures involved, applying the same systematic, compartment-based search discipline emphasized throughout this book's pelvic oncologic imaging chapters, is essential to appropriate patient selection and surgical planning for this major undertaking given the substantial associated morbidity that must be weighed against the potential for cure in this specific patient population.

Clinical Case Presentations

Case 1. A 58-year-old man with rectal bleeding undergoes high-resolution rectal MRI demonstrating a mid-rectal tumor with extramural extension measuring 8 millimeters beyond the muscularis propria and a shortest measured distance of 4 millimeters from the mesorectal fascia. The radiologist categorizes the findings as a threatened circumferential resection margin and recommends neoadjuvant chemoradiation before surgery, given the elevated local recurrence risk that upfront surgery would carry with this margin distance.

Case 2. A 45-year-old woman with a low rectal tumor undergoes staging MRI demonstrating tumor confined to the muscularis propria without extramural extension, a clear mesorectal fascia distance, and no suspicious mesorectal lymph nodes. The radiologist categorizes the findings as T2N0 disease with a clear anticipated margin and recommends proceeding directly to total mesorectal excision without neoadjuvant therapy, given the favorable staging profile.

Case 3. A 62-year-old man completes neoadjuvant chemoradiation for a threatened-margin mid-rectal tumor, and restaging MRI demonstrates near-complete replacement of the original tumor bed with low T2 signal fibrotic tissue and no corresponding diffusion restriction, concordant with a complete clinical response on subsequent endoscopic and digital examination. The radiologist categorizes the findings as a complete radiologic response, and the patient, after informed discussion of the alternatives, elects to pursue a watch-and-wait organ-preservation strategy with structured surveillance.

Case 4. A 51-year-old woman with a mid-rectal tumor undergoes staging MRI demonstrating a tubular structure adjacent to the tumor containing intermediate tumor-signal material with an expanded, distorted contour relative to the normal vascular caliber elsewhere. The radiologist categorizes the finding as extramural vascular invasion and includes this adverse prognostic feature in the staging report, supporting the multidisciplinary team's discussion of more assertive systemic treatment consideration despite an otherwise clear mesorectal fascia margin.

Case 5. A 47-year-old man with anal pain and a palpable mass undergoes pelvic MRI demonstrating a tumor centered at the anal canal with sphincter complex invasion and bilateral inguinal as well as mesorectal lymphadenopathy. Given the epicenter and pattern of nodal involvement, the radiologist favors primary anal squamous cell carcinoma over a distal rectal primary, a distinction confirmed on subsequent biopsy, and the patient proceeds to primary chemoradiation rather than upfront surgical resection.

Case 6. A 55-year-old woman, three years following total mesorectal excision for rectal cancer, presents with new pelvic pain, and MRI demonstrates an intermediate-signal, diffusion-restricting mass within the presacral space extending to abut but not clearly invade the anterior sacrum, distinct from the expected postsurgical fibrotic scar tissue seen on her prior surveillance examinations. The radiologist categorizes the findings as locally recurrent disease and, given the presacral location and proximity to but uncertain invasion of the sacrum, recommends multidisciplinary discussion of resectability and potential pelvic exenteration planning.

THE SIGNAL-TO-CATEGORY DECISION SYSTEM — Rectal Cancer Treatment Pathway Arc

The Signal Pattern: This chapter's patterns span the rectal cancer treatment timeline, from mesorectal fascia distance measurement at initial staging to tumor regression grading following neoadjuvant chemoradiation.

Category Signature: Initial staging categorizes the anticipated circumferential resection margin as clear, threatened, or involved based on measured distance; restaging categorizes treatment response as complete, good partial, or poor based on correlated T2 morphology and diffusion signal.

The Decision: Category assignment in this chapter ranges from upfront surgery for a clear margin to neoadjuvant chemoradiation for a threatened or involved margin, and from watch-and-wait organ preservation for a complete response to standard surgery for a partial or poor response.

The Trap Logic: Both patterns in this chapter share a common trap: a reactive or treatment-related tissue change, peritumoral desmoplastic fibrosis or dense post-radiation fibrosis, that can mimic or obscure the true underlying tumor status if a single imaging feature is relied upon in isolation.

Pattern Anchor: Distinguish reactive or treatment-related fibrotic change from true tumor extension or residual viable tumor in both patterns this chapter describes, correlating multiple imaging features rather than relying on any single feature alone before committing to a category that will directly determine the treatment pathway.

Summary and Key Concepts

Dedicated rectal MRI uses high-resolution, tumor-oriented T2-weighted imaging to assess mesorectal fascia distance, the radiologic surrogate for the surgical circumferential resection margin.

T-staging assesses tumor depth relative to the rectal wall layers; for T3 tumors, the specific depth of extramural extension and mesorectal fascia distance provide greater prognostic granularity than T-stage alone.

A mesorectal fascia distance of 1 millimeter or less is categorized as an involved margin; this measurement directly determines the choice between upfront surgery and neoadjuvant chemoradiation.

Mesorectal lymph node staging relies on morphologic criteria, irregular border and heterogeneous signal, rather than size alone; extramural vascular invasion is an independent adverse prognostic feature.

MRI tumor regression grading following neoadjuvant chemoradiation correlates T2 fibrosis morphology with diffusion-weighted signal to distinguish complete response from residual viable tumor.

A confirmed complete radiologic response, concordant with clinical and endoscopic findings, increasingly supports a watch-and-wait organ-preservation strategy with structured surveillance.

Anal canal carcinoma is staged and managed distinctly from rectal adenocarcinoma, with primary chemoradiation as standard therapy and a distinct nodal drainage pattern extending to the inguinal basin.

CHAPTER 21: MESENTERIC AND PERITONEAL DISEASE

Learning Objectives

1. Describe the peritoneal cavity anatomy and MRI technique used for peritoneal disease evaluation.
2. Apply the peritoneal cancer index to characterize peritoneal carcinomatosis and inform cytoreductive surgery candidacy.
3. Recognize mesenteric masses, including desmoid tumor and mesenteric lymphoma, and their distinguishing imaging features.
4. Assess mesenteric ischemia and bowel viability based on vessel involvement and mural enhancement pattern.
5. Recognize peritoneal infectious and inflammatory conditions and distinguish them from peritoneal malignancy.

Clinical Overview

Mesenteric and peritoneal disease imaging draws together threads from throughout this book, since peritoneal carcinomatosis represents the endpoint of transcoelomic spread discussed in the context of high-grade serous ovarian carcinoma several chapters earlier, and mesenteric vascular disease shares fundamental pathophysiologic principles with the vascular assessment framework applied throughout the abdominal organ chapters. This chapter proceeds from peritoneal anatomy and MRI technique, through peritoneal carcinomatosis and the peritoneal cancer index, mesenteric masses including desmoid tumor, mesenteric ischemia, and closes with peritoneal infectious and inflammatory conditions.

Two instances of the Signal-to-Category Decision System are applied in this chapter, the first to peritoneal cancer index regional scoring for carcinomatosis, and the second to mesenteric ischemia vascular territory and bowel viability assessment, reflecting this chapter's two most surgically time-critical categorization tasks.

Peritoneal Anatomy and MRI Technique for Peritoneal Disease

Peritoneal Cavity Compartments and Ligamentous Anatomy

The peritoneal cavity is subdivided by mesenteric and ligamentous attachments into a series of interconnected compartments and recesses, including the supramesocolic and inframesocolic compartments separated by the transverse mesocolon, the paracolic gutters providing longitudinal communication pathways along the ascending and descending colon, and the pelvic peritoneal recesses discussed in the preceding gynecologic and rectal cancer chapters, and familiarity with this compartmental anatomy directly informs interpretation of fluid and tumor spread patterns throughout the peritoneal cavity, since malignant ascites and peritoneal tumor deposits characteristically follow these same anatomic pathways and dependent recesses that govern normal peritoneal fluid circulation. The greater and lesser omentum, mesenteric fat-containing structures suspending and connecting the stomach, transverse colon, and small bowel, represent particularly common sites of peritoneal tumor deposit accumulation given their extensive peritoneal surface area and relatively fixed anatomic position within the peritoneal cavity's overall fluid circulation pattern, a predilection directly relevant to the systematic peritoneal surface assessment discussed throughout this chapter.

MRI Protocol for Peritoneal Disease Evaluation

A dedicated peritoneal MRI protocol incorporates high-resolution T2-weighted imaging in multiple planes for detailed peritoneal surface and mesenteric assessment, diffusion-weighted imaging, which has assumed a particularly valuable role in peritoneal carcinomatosis detection given small-volume peritoneal deposits' characteristic diffusion restriction that can be more conspicuous against the surrounding low-signal peritoneal fat background than on T2-weighted imaging alone, and dynamic contrast-enhanced imaging to characterize the enhancement pattern of identified peritoneal nodularity or masses. Whole-body or extended field-of-view coverage, encompassing the entire abdomen and pelvis rather than a more limited, organ-focused field of view, represents an essential technical requirement given peritoneal disease's characteristic diffuse or multifocal distribution pattern, and this comprehensive coverage requirement, together with the specific diffusion-weighted emphasis discussed above, together distinguish a genuine peritoneal-disease-optimized protocol from a standard abdominal MRI performed without these specific technical considerations in mind.

Peritoneal Cancer Index Region Score	Lesion Size	Description
0	No visible disease	Region free of tumor deposits
1	Up to 0.5 cm	Punctate or thin nodular deposits
2	0.5 to 5 cm	Discrete nodular or plaque-like deposits
3	Greater than 5 cm, or confluent	Bulky or confluent tumor deposits

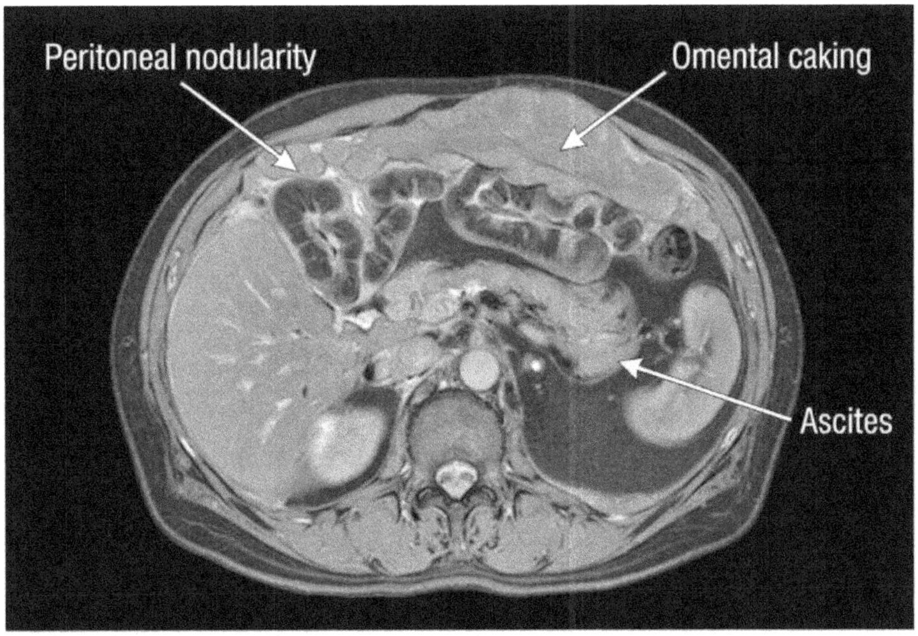

Figure 21.1: Peritoneal Carcinomatosis with Omental Caking

Peritoneal Carcinomatosis and the Peritoneal Cancer Index

Epidemiology and Sources of Peritoneal Carcinomatosis

Peritoneal carcinomatosis, diffuse malignant seeding of the peritoneal surfaces, most commonly arises from ovarian carcinoma, discussed in detail in the adnexal masses chapter earlier in this book, gastric and colorectal adenocarcinoma, and, as a distinct primary peritoneal malignancy, malignant mesothelioma, and the specific primary source carries direct relevance to expected distribution pattern and treatment approach, with ovarian carcinoma-related carcinomatosis, for instance, generally demonstrating a more diffuse, small-volume miliary pattern relative to the comparatively larger, more discrete deposits sometimes characteristic of gastrointestinal primary-related carcinomatosis. Pseudomyxoma peritonei, a distinct clinical and imaging entity characterized by diffuse mucinous ascites and peritoneal implants, most commonly arising from a ruptured or perforated appendiceal mucinous neoplasm, produces a characteristic scalloped appearance along the liver and spleen margins from the gelatinous mucinous material's mass effect on these solid organ surfaces, a distinctive pattern that should prompt specific consideration of this entity and its associated appendiceal primary given the entity's distinct management pathway relative to more typical carcinomatosis.

Peritoneal Cancer Index Scoring Methodology

The peritoneal cancer index provides a standardized, reproducible quantitative framework for peritoneal disease burden assessment, dividing the abdomen and pelvis into thirteen defined regions, nine abdominopelvic quadrant-based regions and four small bowel-specific regions, and assigning each region a lesion size score from zero, no visible disease, through three, a lesion or confluent lesions exceeding 5 centimeters, with the sum of all thirteen regional scores yielding a composite index directly correlating with both surgical cytoreductive complexity and expected completeness of cytoreduction. This composite index has become the standard preoperative and intraoperative common language between the radiologist and surgical oncology team specifically evaluating candidacy for cytoreductive surgery with hyperthermic intraperitoneal chemotherapy, an aggressive combined surgical and regional chemotherapy approach reserved for carefully selected patients with peritoneal carcinomatosis, since a lower index score generally correlates with a higher likelihood of achieving complete or near-complete cytoreduction, the single strongest predictor of favorable long-term outcome following this procedure, while a markedly elevated index score may indicate disease too extensive for complete surgical clearance, favoring a systemic, non-surgical treatment approach instead.

Small Bowel and Mesenteric Region Assessment

The four small bowel-specific regions within the peritoneal cancer index framework, encompassing the small bowel itself and its mesentery, warrant particular interpretive attention given this region's disproportionate contribution to imaging-surgical discordance relative to the abdominopelvic quadrant regions, since small-volume serosal and mesenteric tumor deposits studding the small bowel surface can be considerably more difficult to detect on preoperative imaging than the comparatively more conspicuous omental and parietal peritoneal deposits discussed elsewhere in this chapter, given the small bowel's complex, folded, and mobile anatomic configuration relative to the more fixed, readily surveyed peritoneal surfaces. This recognized imaging limitation for small bowel and mesenteric disease burden carries direct clinical significance, since extensive small bowel serosal involvement, even when incompletely appreciated on preoperative imaging, can preclude complete cytoreduction at the time of surgery regardless of an otherwise favorable overall peritoneal cancer index score based on the more readily visualized regions, making deliberate, careful scrutiny of the small bowel and mesenteric regions, together with transparent communication of this modality-specific limitation to the surgical team, an essential component of the complete peritoneal carcinomatosis staging report.

THE SIGNAL-TO-CATEGORY DECISION SYSTEM — Peritoneal Cancer Index Regional Scoring

---

The Signal Pattern: Diffuse-coverage MRI is performed for suspected or known peritoneal carcinomatosis, and the reader must systematically score each of the thirteen defined peritoneal cancer index regions, including the four small bowel-specific regions, by lesion size.

Category Signature: No visible disease in a region scores zero; a lesion up to 0.5 centimeters scores one; a lesion 0.5 to 5 centimeters scores two; a lesion or confluent lesions exceeding 5 centimeters scores three, with the sum across all thirteen regions yielding the composite index.

The Decision: A lower composite index generally supports consideration for cytoreductive surgery with hyperthermic intraperitoneal chemotherapy, given the higher associated likelihood of complete cytoreduction; a markedly elevated composite index, particularly with extensive small bowel or mesenteric involvement, favors systemic, non-surgical treatment given the reduced likelihood of achieving surgical benefit.

Trap Logic: Small bowel and mesenteric serosal deposits are disproportionately prone to imaging underestimation relative to intraoperative findings given this region's complex, mobile anatomy, risking a falsely favorable composite index that does not reflect the true disease burden the surgical team will encounter; the discriminating step is applying particular scrutiny to the small bowel-specific regions and explicitly communicating this modality-specific limitation rather than presenting the composite index as a fully precise, surgery-equivalent measurement.

Pattern Anchor: Score all thirteen regions systematically, applying particular scrutiny to the small bowel and mesenteric regions given their recognized imaging-surgical discordance risk; communicate this limitation explicitly rather than presenting the index as a precise surrogate for intraoperative findings.

Figure 21.2: Peritoneal Cavity Compartment Anatomy

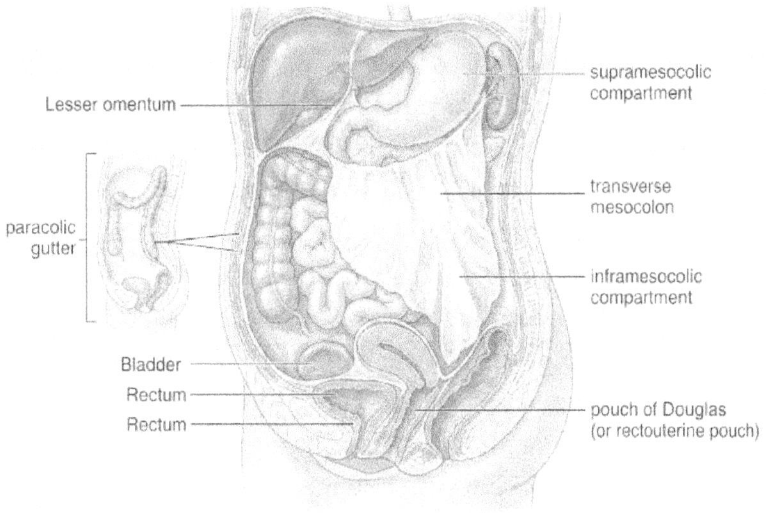

CLINICAL PEARL: A scalloped hepatic and splenic surface contour from adjacent gelatinous mucinous ascites, rather than the more mobile, freely layering simple ascites typical of other causes, is a specific and helpful sign of pseudomyxoma peritonei and should prompt search for an underlying appendiceal mucinous neoplasm.

Patient Education and Counseling for Peritoneal Carcinomatosis Staging

Communicating a peritoneal carcinomatosis staging result to a patient benefits from careful framing given the substantial emotional weight this diagnosis carries, and explaining the composite peritoneal cancer index in accessible terms, a measure of how much of the abdominal lining is affected, used to help the surgical team decide whether extensive surgery is likely to be able to remove all visible disease, supports patient understanding of why a treatment recommendation, whether aggressive cytoreductive surgery or a more systemic, non-surgical approach, has been made, and clear acknowledgment of the small bowel and mesenteric imaging limitation discussed throughout this section, that the true extent of disease may only become fully apparent at the time of surgery itself, supports realistic expectations about the possibility that a planned complete cytoreduction may prove incomplete once surgical exploration begins. For a patient being considered for the observation-based desmoid tumor management strategy discussed in this chapter's mesenteric mass section, counseling that emphasizes the meaningful possibility of spontaneous stabilization or regression, together with clear expectations regarding the structured serial imaging surveillance this observation approach requires, supports informed acceptance of this less immediately interventional management pathway relative to a more familiar, surgery-first expectation many patients bring to a new mass diagnosis.

Complications and Prognosis of Cytoreductive Surgery With Hyperthermic Intraperitoneal Chemotherapy

Cytoreductive surgery with hyperthermic intraperitoneal chemotherapy represents a technically extensive procedure carrying a substantial associated morbidity profile, including anastomotic leak from the multiple bowel resections often required to clear peritoneal disease from the small bowel and colon, prolonged ileus, and the systemic toxicity associated with the intraperitoneal chemotherapy perfusion itself, considerations that reinforce why this procedure is generally reserved for carefully selected patients at experienced, high-volume centers with the multidisciplinary infrastructure to manage this recognized complication profile. Long-term prognosis following cytoreductive surgery with hyperthermic intraperitoneal chemotherapy correlates strongly with the completeness of cytoreduction achieved, with patients achieving complete or near-complete macroscopic tumor clearance demonstrating substantially improved survival relative to those with residual gross disease following surgery, a completeness-outcome relationship that further reinforces the direct clinical significance of the accurate preoperative peritoneal cancer index scoring this chapter's framework addresses, since a preoperative score suggesting a high likelihood of achievable complete cytoreduction directly supports the case for proceeding with this extensive procedure over a more conservative systemic therapy approach.

Mesenteric Masses and Desmoid Tumor

Desmoid Tumor: Imaging Features and Association With Familial Adenomatous Polyposis

Desmoid tumor, a locally aggressive but non-metastasizing mesenchymal neoplasm arising from mesenteric or abdominal wall fibroblastic tissue, demonstrates a characteristic infiltrative, spiculated margin with variable, often heterogeneously low T2 signal reflecting the tumor's dense collagenous composition, a signal pattern distinguishing it from the more homogeneously intermediate signal characteristic of most other mesenteric masses discussed throughout this section, and desmoid tumor carries a strong, well-recognized association with familial adenomatous polyposis, discussed in the preceding chapter's colorectal cancer risk factor context, occurring with substantially elevated frequency in this population, often following colectomy performed for the polyposis itself, a temporal association that has generated ongoing investigation into the surgical trauma-related and hormonal contributing mechanisms underlying this specific association. Management of desmoid tumor has shifted over recent years toward an initial observation-based approach for many patients, reflecting recognition that a meaningful proportion of desmoid tumors demonstrate spontaneous stabilization or even regression without intervention, reserving more assertive treatment, whether systemic therapy or surgical resection, for a tumor demonstrating clear growth or causing mass effect on adjacent structures such as bowel or ureter, and serial MRI, applying the same size and morphology comparison principles discussed throughout this book's oncologic surveillance contexts, provides the primary tool for this observation-based monitoring strategy.

Differential Diagnosis of a Mesenteric Mass

Beyond desmoid tumor and lymphoma discussed throughout this section, the mesenteric mass differential extends to include carcinoid tumor, most commonly arising from a small bowel primary and characteristically producing a spiculated, calcified mesenteric mass with radiating soft tissue strands, a distinctive appearance reflecting this tumor's characteristic intense desmoplastic reaction, generally more pronounced than the desmoplastic response typically associated with adenocarcinoma metastasis, gastrointestinal stromal tumor metastasis, which, unlike the more common hepatic and peritoneal surface metastatic pattern of most gastrointestinal malignancies, can present as a discrete, often necrotic or cystic mesenteric mass distinct from the more infiltrative pattern of the entities discussed elsewhere in this section, and mesenteric fibromatosis-adjacent benign entities including mesenteric cyst and lymphangioma, generally demonstrating simple or septated fluid signal without the solid, enhancing components that would suggest a neoplastic process. Correlating the specific morphology, infiltrative and spiculated versus discrete and encapsulated, the enhancement pattern, and the clinical context, including any known primary malignancy history or carcinoid syndrome symptoms such as flushing and diarrhea, supports accurate categorization within this broad differential, and, as with several other differential diagnosis discussions throughout this book, definitive distinction in a genuinely ambiguous case ultimately relies on image-guided or surgical biopsy for histologic confirmation.

Mesenteric Lymphoma and Other Mesenteric Masses

Mesenteric lymphoma, most commonly non-Hodgkin lymphoma, characteristically presents as bulky, confluent mesenteric lymphadenopathy encasing but, notably, not typically invading or obstructing the mesenteric vasculature, producing the classically described sandwich sign in which mesenteric vessels and fat remain visible coursing between anterior and posterior lymphomatous masses, a distinguishing pattern from the more infiltrative, vessel-obliterating growth typically characteristic of carcinomatosis or an aggressive mesenteric sarcoma. Mesenteric panniculitis, an inflammatory and fibrosing condition of mesenteric fat of uncertain but likely multifactorial etiology, produces a distinctive misty mesentery appearance with mesenteric fat haziness, often surrounding a central, comparatively preserved fatty halo around individual mesenteric vessels and lymph nodes, termed the fat ring sign, a pattern generally considered a benign, often incidental finding not requiring specific treatment beyond addressing any associated symptoms, though careful correlation with clinical context remains warranted given some reported associations between mesenteric panniculitis and an underlying malignancy in a subset of cases.

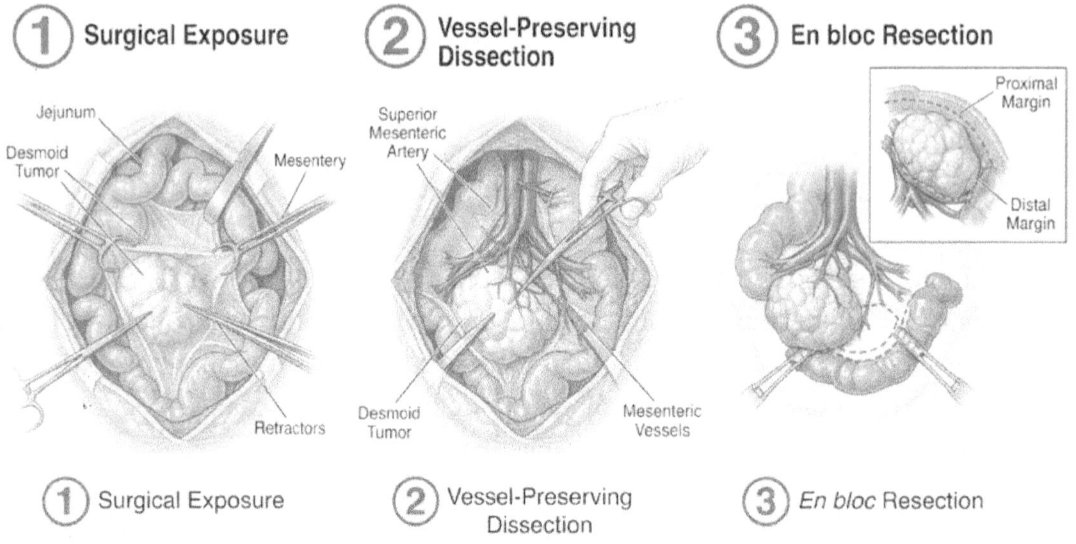

Figure 21.3: Surgical Resection of Mesenteric Desmoid Tumor.

Mesenteric Ischemia and Vascular Disease

Epidemiology and Risk Factors for Mesenteric Ischemia

Acute mesenteric ischemia disproportionately affects older patients with underlying cardiovascular risk factors, atrial fibrillation representing the dominant risk factor for the embolic subtype given its propensity for left atrial thrombus formation and subsequent systemic embolization, and generalized atherosclerotic disease, often with concurrent coronary or peripheral arterial disease, representing the dominant risk factor for the thrombotic subtype, typically superimposed upon a preexisting chronic mesenteric arterial stenosis discussed further in the following section. Mesenteric venous thrombosis, a distinct and generally more indolent mechanism relative to the arterial etiologies discussed above, is associated with hypercoagulable states, whether inherited thrombophilia, malignancy-associated hypercoagulability, or, less commonly, local factors including intra-abdominal infection or inflammatory conditions producing regional venous stasis and endothelial injury, and non-occlusive mesenteric ischemia, occurring in the absence of a discrete vascular occlusion, is instead related to severe systemic hypoperfusion, whether from cardiogenic shock, sepsis, or vasopressor-related mesenteric vasoconstriction, in a critically ill patient, a mechanism that requires the interpreting radiologist to consider this specific ischemic etiology even in the absence of a clearly identifiable vascular occlusion when the clinical context, a hemodynamically unstable, critically ill patient, is compatible.

Chronic Mesenteric Ischemia

Chronic mesenteric ischemia, distinct from the acute presentations discussed throughout this section, results from progressive atherosclerotic narrowing of the mesenteric vessels, classically producing postprandial abdominal pain, colloquially termed intestinal angina, related to the mismatch between increased postprandial mesenteric blood flow demand and the fixed, inadequate supply through the stenotic vessels, together with associated food aversion and unintentional weight loss as patients learn to avoid the pain-triggering postprandial state. Given the mesenteric circulation's extensive collateral network, discussed in this chapter's rhythm framework, chronic mesenteric ischemia typically requires significant, multivessel stenosis or occlusion, often involving at least two of the three major mesenteric vessels, celiac, superior mesenteric, and inferior mesenteric artery, before becoming clinically symptomatic, reflecting the substantial compensatory capacity these collateral pathways provide when only a single vessel is affected, and this multivessel involvement threshold, together with the characteristic postprandial symptom pattern, should prompt MR angiography evaluation in an appropriately aged patient with vascular risk factors and this compatible clinical presentation.

Acute Mesenteric Ischemia: Etiology and Vascular Territories

Acute mesenteric ischemia, a time-critical emergency carrying substantial mortality risk when diagnosis and treatment are delayed, arises from arterial embolism, most commonly to the superior mesenteric artery given its comparatively wide caliber and favorable takeoff angle from the aorta relative to the celiac and inferior mesenteric arteries, arterial thrombosis, typically occurring at a site of preexisting atherosclerotic stenosis, or, less commonly, mesenteric venous thrombosis or non-occlusive mesenteric ischemia related to severe systemic hypoperfusion in a critically ill patient without a discrete identifiable vascular occlusion. MR angiography provides direct visualization of the mesenteric vasculature, identifying the specific occluded or severely stenotic vessel and its territory, and this direct vascular assessment, together with the bowel wall viability characterization discussed in the following section, together determine both the underlying mechanism, informing whether embolectomy, thrombolysis, or anticoagulation represents the appropriate vascular intervention, and the urgency of any accompanying surgical bowel assessment.

Bowel Wall Viability Assessment

Bowel wall enhancement pattern following intravenous contrast administration provides the most direct and clinically actionable indicator of bowel viability in the setting of mesenteric ischemia, with preserved, even if diminished, mural enhancement suggesting viable, potentially salvageable bowel that may respond to vascular intervention alone without requiring bowel resection, while absent mural enhancement indicates non-viable, infarcted bowel requiring surgical resection regardless of any vascular intervention performed, since restoring blood flow to already-infarcted bowel does not restore tissue viability and instead risks reperfusion-related complications including systemic inflammatory response. Pneumatosis intestinalis, gas within the bowel wall itself, and portal venous gas, when present together with the clinical and vascular findings of mesenteric ischemia, represent ominous findings suggesting transmural bowel wall necrosis with gas-forming bacterial translocation into the compromised wall and portal circulation, though the interpreting radiologist should recognize that pneumatosis can occasionally represent a benign, incidental finding in other specific clinical contexts, including certain medications, and correlating this finding with the overall clinical presentation and the vascular and mural enhancement findings discussed throughout this section, rather than treating pneumatosis as a universally ominous finding in isolation, supports accurate risk stratification.

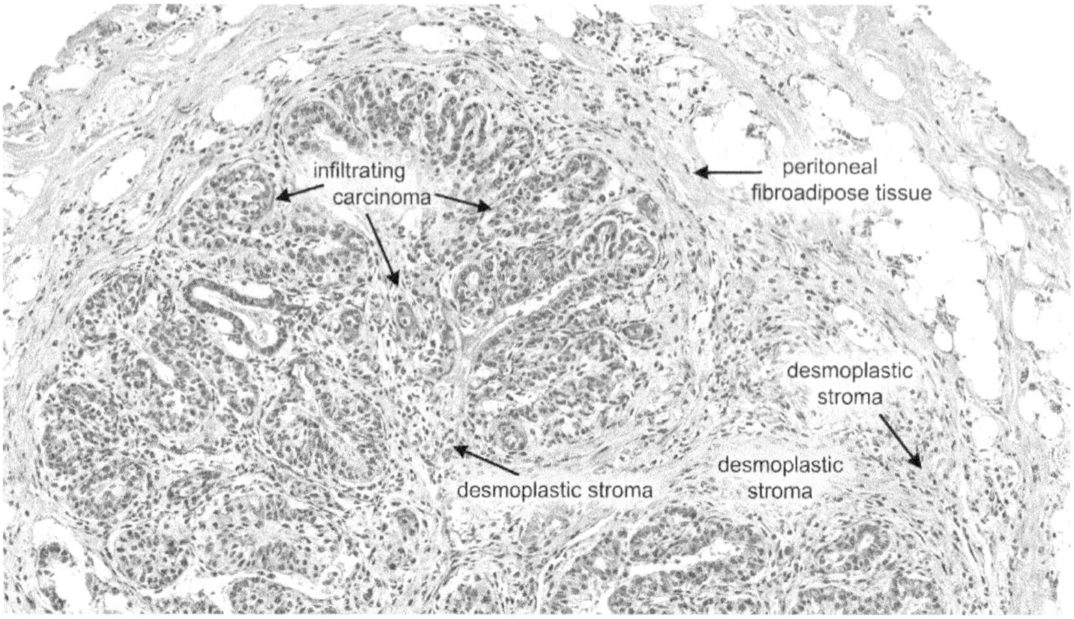

THE SIGNAL-TO-CATEGORY DECISION SYSTEM — Mesenteric Ischemia Vascular Territory Assessment

The Signal Pattern: A patient with acute abdominal pain undergoes MR angiography and MRI, and the reader must identify the occluded or stenotic mesenteric vessel and assess the corresponding bowel segment's mural enhancement pattern.

Category Signature: A stenotic or occluded vessel with preserved, even if diminished, downstream mural enhancement is categorized as ischemic but potentially viable bowel; a stenotic or occluded vessel with absent downstream mural enhancement, particularly with associated pneumatosis or portal venous gas, is categorized as non-viable, infarcted bowel.

The Decision: Viable bowel supports vascular intervention, whether endovascular or surgical revascularization, potentially without bowel resection; non-viable bowel requires urgent surgical resection of the infarcted segment regardless of the vascular intervention performed, given that restored perfusion cannot reverse established tissue necrosis.

Trap Logic: Chronic mesenteric ischemia with well-developed collateral vascular pathways can produce a deceptively preserved bowel wall enhancement pattern despite severe, high-grade stenosis of the primary mesenteric vessels, potentially understating the hemodynamic significance of the underlying vascular disease if collateral flow is not specifically recognized and accounted for; the discriminating step is assessing the full collateral vascular network, not vessel stenosis severity in isolation, when characterizing chronic ischemic risk.

Pattern Anchor: Correlate bowel wall enhancement with vessel patency and collateral status, not stenosis severity in isolation, to determine bowel viability and surgical urgency; absent enhancement mandates surgical resection regardless of subsequent vascular intervention.

CAUTION: Absent bowel wall enhancement in the setting of acute mesenteric ischemia indicates non-viable bowel requiring surgical resection; restoring vascular flow through embolectomy or thrombolysis alone does not reverse established transmural necrosis and should not delay surgical evaluation in a patient with this finding.

Differential Diagnosis of Ascites

Ascites, fluid accumulation within the peritoneal cavity, carries a broad differential extending well beyond the malignant carcinomatosis-related ascites emphasized throughout this chapter, including cirrhotic ascites from portal hypertension, the most common cause of ascites overall in most clinical populations, cardiac ascites from right heart failure and systemic venous congestion, and, less commonly, ascites related to nephrotic syndrome, tuberculous peritonitis discussed further below, or, distinctly, chylous ascites from lymphatic obstruction or disruption, and distinguishing among these etiologies relies on a combination of clinical context, ascites imaging characteristics, including signal intensity and any associated peritoneal nodularity or thickening, and, when genuinely ambiguous, diagnostic paracentesis with fluid analysis. Simple, transudative ascites, characteristic of cirrhotic and cardiac etiologies, generally demonstrates uniform, simple fluid signal without associated peritoneal nodularity or thickening, in contrast to the peritoneal nodularity, omental caking, and other malignancy-associated findings emphasized throughout this chapter's carcinomatosis discussion, making the presence or absence of these specific associated peritoneal findings, rather than ascites volume alone, the key imaging discriminator supporting further malignancy-focused workup versus a more straightforward hepatic or cardiac etiology evaluation.

Peritoneal Infection and Inflammatory Conditions

Peritoneal Abscess and Intra-Abdominal Infection

Intra-abdominal and peritoneal abscess, most commonly arising as a complication of appendicitis, diverticulitis, or postoperative anastomotic leak, appears as a rim-enhancing fluid collection with internal diffusion restriction reflecting purulent content, a pattern directly analogous to the tubo-ovarian and other abscess presentations discussed in earlier chapters of this book, and distinguishing a peritoneal abscess from a peritoneal malignant deposit or loculated ascites relies on this combination of rim enhancement, diffusion restriction, and compatible clinical presentation, fever, leukocytosis, and localizing pain, together supporting the infectious diagnosis over a malignant or purely inflammatory alternative. Percutaneous image-guided drainage represents the primary management approach for a well-localized, accessible peritoneal abscess, generally combined with targeted antibiotic therapy, and this drainage approach has substantially reduced the need for immediate surgical intervention in many presentations, reserving surgery for a collection not amenable to percutaneous access or for a patient with diffuse peritonitis or another indication for urgent surgical source control beyond what image-guided drainage alone can address.

Tuberculous Peritonitis and Other Granulomatous Conditions

Tuberculous peritonitis, while comparatively uncommon in regions of low tuberculosis prevalence, warrants specific consideration given its imaging overlap with peritoneal carcinomatosis, both conditions capable of producing diffuse peritoneal nodularity, thickening, and ascites, and distinguishing features favoring tuberculous peritonitis over carcinomatosis include high-attenuation or high-signal ascites reflecting its proteinaceous, cellular content, smooth rather than nodular peritoneal thickening in many though not all cases, and a compatible clinical and epidemiologic context including known tuberculosis exposure or endemic region residence, though genuinely ambiguous cases not infrequently require peritoneal biopsy for definitive histologic and microbiologic distinction given the substantial imaging overlap and the very different management pathways, antituberculous therapy versus oncologic treatment, that each diagnosis demands. Sclerosing peritonitis, a rare but clinically significant fibrosing condition most classically associated with long-term peritoneal dialysis, produces progressive peritoneal thickening and calcification that can encase and functionally obstruct bowel loops, a distinct entity from the malignant and infectious peritoneal processes discussed throughout this chapter, and recognition of this specific association, together with a compatible peritoneal dialysis history, supports accurate diagnosis in a patient presenting with the resulting bowel obstruction symptoms this condition characteristically produces.

Special Populations: Peritoneal Disease in the Postoperative and Peritoneal Dialysis Patient

Peritoneal imaging interpretation in the early postoperative patient requires careful consideration of expected postsurgical change, including a degree of peritoneal fluid, reactive peritoneal enhancement, and localized fat stranding near the surgical bed, each of which can be mistaken for infection, malignant recurrence, or a genuinely pathologic process if the recent surgical history is not carefully incorporated into the interpretation, making direct comparison with the operative report and, when available, a baseline early postoperative examination valuable context for confidently distinguishing expected postsurgical change from a genuinely new, actionable finding. The peritoneal dialysis patient represents a further distinct population warranting specific consideration, given both this population's elevated risk for the sclerosing peritonitis entity discussed earlier in this chapter and the general expectation of some baseline peritoneal thickening and enhancement related to the dialysis process itself, considerations that should inform a measured, clinically correlated interpretive approach rather than over-calling every degree of peritoneal thickening as pathologic in a patient with this specific dialysis history, while still maintaining appropriate vigilance for the genuinely concerning sclerosing peritonitis pattern, progressive thickening with calcification and bowel encasement, that does warrant specific identification and communication given its distinct management implications.

Clinical Case Presentations

Case 1. A 61-year-old woman with a history of high-grade serous ovarian carcinoma undergoes restaging MRI demonstrating omental caking, scattered peritoneal nodularity across multiple abdominopelvic regions, and small bowel serosal studding, with a composite peritoneal cancer index score of 14. Given the moderate composite score and the surgical oncology team's assessment of achievable complete cytoreduction, the patient proceeds to cytoreductive surgery with hyperthermic intraperitoneal chemotherapy.

Case 2. A 44-year-old man with a history of familial adenomatous polyposis and prior colectomy presents with a palpable abdominal mass, and MRI demonstrates a 6-centimeter infiltrative, spiculated, heterogeneously low T2 signal mesenteric mass without evidence of bowel obstruction or ureteral involvement. The radiologist categorizes the findings as consistent with desmoid tumor and, given the absence of mass effect on adjacent structures, recommends initial observation with serial MRI rather than immediate intervention.

Case 3. A 72-year-old man with atrial fibrillation presents with acute, severe abdominal pain out of proportion to physical examination findings, and MR angiography demonstrates abrupt cutoff of the proximal superior mesenteric artery with absent enhancement of the corresponding jejunal and ileal loops, together with associated pneumatosis intestinalis. The radiologist categorizes the findings as acute superior mesenteric artery embolism with non-viable bowel, prompting urgent surgical exploration and resection rather than endovascular intervention alone.

Case 4. A 55-year-old man with vague abdominal discomfort undergoes incidental MRI demonstrating mesenteric fat haziness with a preserved fatty halo surrounding the mesenteric vessels and lymph nodes, without discrete mass or lymphadenopathy. The radiologist categorizes the findings as mesenteric panniculitis, a benign finding, and recommends no specific intervention beyond routine clinical follow-up given the absence of any additional concerning feature.

Case 5. A 38-year-old man with fever and localized abdominal pain following recent appendectomy undergoes MRI demonstrating a rim-enhancing, diffusion-restricting fluid collection in the right lower quadrant adjacent to the surgical bed. The radiologist categorizes the findings as a postoperative abscess and recommends percutaneous image-guided drainage together with targeted antibiotic therapy rather than immediate surgical re-exploration.

Case 6. A 68-year-old woman with known atherosclerotic disease reports several months of postprandial abdominal pain and 8 kilograms of unintentional weight loss, and MR angiography demonstrates high-grade stenosis of both the celiac and superior mesenteric arteries with a patent but diminutive inferior mesenteric artery providing collateral flow. The radiologist categorizes the findings as chronic mesenteric ischemia from multivessel disease and recommends vascular surgery referral for revascularization, correlating the imaging findings with her classic postprandial pain and food-avoidance pattern.

Case 7. A 49-year-old man with a known hypercoagulable disorder presents with several days of vague, poorly localized abdominal pain, and MRI demonstrates thrombus within the superior mesenteric vein with associated bowel wall thickening but preserved mural enhancement and no pneumatosis. The radiologist categorizes the findings as mesenteric venous thrombosis with viable bowel and recommends anticoagulation with close clinical monitoring rather than surgical exploration, given the preserved enhancement and absence of transmural necrosis features.

THE SIGNAL-TO-CATEGORY DECISION SYSTEM — Mesenteric and Peritoneal Triage Arc

The Signal Pattern: This chapter's patterns span both oncologic and vascular peritoneal disease, from systematic regional scoring for peritoneal carcinomatosis to vessel-and-viability assessment for mesenteric ischemia.

Category Signature: Peritoneal carcinomatosis is categorized by composite peritoneal cancer index score summed across thirteen regions; mesenteric ischemia is categorized by vessel patency and bowel wall enhancement as viable or non-viable.

The Decision: Category assignment in this chapter ranges from cytoreductive surgery candidacy for a lower peritoneal cancer index to systemic therapy for extensive disease, and from vascular intervention alone for viable ischemic bowel to urgent surgical resection for non-viable bowel.

The Trap Logic: Both patterns in this chapter share a common trap: an incompletely assessed region or vessel territory, underestimated small bowel and mesenteric disease burden, or collateral flow masking severe stenosis, that produces a category assignment not reflecting the true underlying disease extent.

Pattern Anchor: Apply particular scrutiny to the small bowel and mesenteric regions in carcinomatosis scoring, and to collateral vascular status in ischemia assessment, before finalizing either category in this chapter; both patterns carry a recognized risk of imaging underestimation that the reader must explicitly account for.

Summary and Key Concepts

The peritoneal cavity's compartmental anatomy, supramesocolic and inframesocolic spaces, paracolic gutters, and omentum, governs the characteristic distribution pattern of malignant ascites and peritoneal tumor deposits.

The peritoneal cancer index scores thirteen regions, including four small bowel-specific regions, by lesion size to produce a composite score guiding cytoreductive surgery candidacy.

Small bowel and mesenteric peritoneal disease is disproportionately prone to imaging underestimation relative to intraoperative findings, warranting particular interpretive scrutiny.

Desmoid tumor shows an infiltrative, spiculated, low T2 signal mass and carries a strong association with familial adenomatous polyposis; many cases are now managed with initial observation.

Bowel wall enhancement, not vessel stenosis severity alone, determines bowel viability in mesenteric ischemia; absent enhancement mandates surgical resection regardless of vascular intervention.

Pneumatosis intestinalis and portal venous gas suggest transmural bowel necrosis in the appropriate clinical context but can rarely represent benign findings requiring careful clinical correlation.

Tuberculous peritonitis and sclerosing peritonitis each carry imaging overlap with more common peritoneal processes and require specific clinical context recognition for accurate diagnosis.

CHAPTER 22: WHOLE-BODY MRI FOR ONCOLOGIC STAGING AND SURVEILLANCE

Learning Objectives

1. Describe the whole-body MRI protocol, including diffusion-weighted whole-body imaging with background suppression.
2. Apply whole-body MRI to multiple myeloma staging and skeletal survey applications.
3. Apply structured surveillance protocols for cancer predisposition syndromes and categorize incidental findings.
4. Recognize the role of whole-body MRI in metastatic disease staging and treatment response assessment.
5. Compare whole-body MRI and PET-CT strengths and limitations for oncologic staging applications.

Clinical Overview

Whole-body MRI has matured from a research curiosity into a genuinely established clinical tool for several specific oncologic applications, most notably multiple myeloma staging, cancer predisposition syndrome surveillance, and, increasingly, metastatic disease staging where its radiation-free, comprehensive skeletal and soft tissue coverage offers meaningful advantages over conventional staging approaches for carefully selected clinical scenarios. This chapter proceeds from whole-body MRI technique, through multiple myeloma and skeletal survey applications, cancer predisposition syndrome surveillance, metastatic disease staging and response assessment, and closes with a comparison of whole-body MRI and PET-CT.

Two instances of the Signal-to-Category Decision System are applied in this chapter, the first to diffusion whole-body lesion categorization distinguishing benign marrow change from metastatic infiltration, and the second to cancer predisposition syndrome surveillance finding categorization, reflecting this chapter's two most consequential whole-body interpretive tasks.

Whole-Body MRI Technique and Diffusion-Weighted Whole-Body Imaging

Protocol Design and Coverage

A comprehensive whole-body MRI protocol acquires sequential stations from the skull vertex through the mid-thigh or, for a full skeletal survey application, through the feet, combining these stations into a single, seamless composite dataset for review, and the core sequence combination anchoring this protocol includes coronal and axial T1-weighted imaging, providing excellent anatomic detail and bone marrow fat content assessment, short tau inversion recovery or Dixon-based fat-suppressed T2-weighted imaging for fluid-sensitive lesion detection, and diffusion-weighted imaging with background body signal suppression, discussed in greater technical detail in the following section, which has become the single most influential sequence addition driving whole-body MRI's expanding oncologic role over recent years. Total examination time, while historically a limiting factor relative to the comparatively rapid PET-CT acquisition discussed later in this chapter, has been substantially reduced through parallel imaging and simultaneous multi-slice acceleration techniques, bringing many contemporary whole-body protocols within a clinically practical duration that supports broader adoption for the specific indications this chapter addresses.

Diffusion-Weighted Whole-Body Imaging With Background Suppression

Diffusion-weighted whole-body imaging with background suppression, often referenced by the acronym describing its combination of fat suppression, diffusion weighting, and inversion recovery-based background signal nulling, produces a composite, inverted-grayscale image format that intentionally visually resembles a PET-CT maximum intensity projection, a deliberate design choice supporting rapid visual pattern recognition of diffusion-restricting lesions against a suppressed, low-signal normal background across the entire imaged body region. This sequence's exceptional sensitivity for detecting diffusion-restricting lesions, whether skeletal, nodal, or soft tissue, represents both its principal strength and its principal interpretive challenge, since a wide range of both malignant and entirely benign processes can demonstrate diffusion restriction, making correlation with the conventional T1 and T2-weighted anatomic sequences discussed above, rather than diffusion-weighted imaging interpreted in isolation, essential to distinguishing genuinely concerning findings from the numerous benign diffusion-restricting mimics this chapter's framework addresses throughout the following sections.

Apparent Diffusion Coefficient Mapping and Quantitative Assessment

Apparent diffusion coefficient mapping, generated from the diffusion-weighted acquisition's multiple b-value dataset, provides a quantitative measure of water diffusion restriction complementing the qualitative visual assessment discussed above, with a lower apparent diffusion coefficient value generally corresponding to greater diffusion restriction and, in the appropriate clinical and morphologic context, a higher likelihood of dense, hypercellular tumor tissue relative to a higher apparent diffusion coefficient value more characteristic of edematous, inflammatory, or less cellular tissue, though this quantitative value functions as a supportive, corroborating data point within the complete interpretive framework rather than a fully independent, standalone diagnostic threshold given the substantial overlap in apparent diffusion coefficient values between benign and malignant processes across the diverse tissue types whole-body imaging encompasses. Serial apparent diffusion coefficient measurement across sequential examinations provides a particularly valuable, quantitative treatment response assessment tool, discussed further in this chapter's metastatic disease response assessment section, since a rising apparent diffusion coefficient value in a previously identified lesion following treatment initiation generally correlates with decreasing cellularity and treatment response, complementing the more traditional size-based response assessment criteria applied throughout oncologic imaging.

Practical Considerations: Patient Tolerance and Examination Duration

Whole-body MRI examination duration, even with the acceleration techniques discussed above, generally exceeds that of a focused, single-region MRI examination or a comparable PET-CT acquisition, a practical consideration carrying direct relevance to patient tolerance, particularly for a patient with claustrophobia, chronic pain limiting prolonged immobility, or, in the pediatric population discussed in the following chapter, a limited capacity for sustained cooperation, and clear pre-examination patient preparation and coaching, together with judicious use of anxiolytic premedication or, for a younger child, sedation when genuinely necessary, support successful examination completion without motion-degraded image quality that would otherwise compromise the diagnostic reliability this chapter's interpretive framework depends upon. Coil positioning and repositioning between sequential imaging stations, together with the multiple distinct breath-hold or free-breathing sequence combinations often required across different body regions within a single comprehensive protocol, further extend total table time relative to a single-region examination, and technologist familiarity with an efficient, well-rehearsed whole-body workflow meaningfully reduces both total examination time and the patient discomfort and motion risk that a prolonged, inefficiently sequenced examination would otherwise introduce.

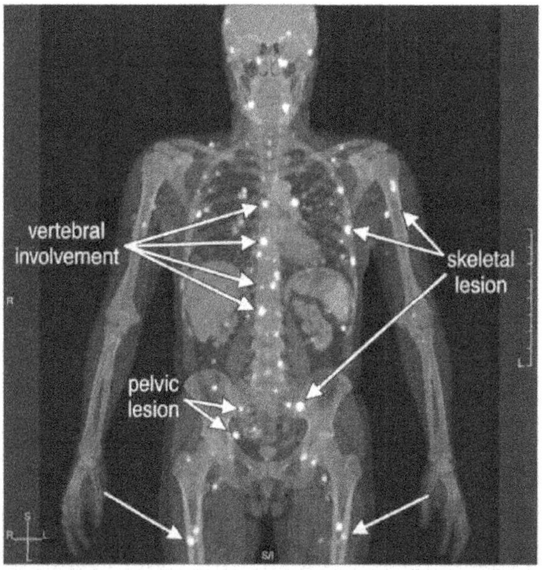

Figure 22.1 — Diagnostic Imaging: Whole-Body Diffusion-Weighted MRI

Multiple Myeloma and Skeletal Survey Applications

Special Populations: Whole-Body MRI Considerations in Pregnancy

Whole-body MRI performed during pregnancy, whether for a pregnant patient with known cancer predisposition syndrome surveillance needs or, more commonly, for staging evaluation of a malignancy newly diagnosed during pregnancy, carries the same gadolinium contrast avoidance considerations discussed throughout earlier chapters of this book, favoring a non-contrast protocol relying predominantly on the T1, T2, and diffusion-weighted sequences that anchor the core whole-body technique discussed throughout this chapter, sequences that retain substantial diagnostic value for both marrow-based and soft tissue disease detection even without the contrast-enhanced component that would otherwise be included in a comprehensive non-pregnant staging examination. Whole-body MRI's radiation-free nature carries particular value in this specific clinical scenario, since it allows comprehensive oncologic staging without the fetal radiation exposure that CT-based or scintigraphic staging alternatives would impose, and this radiation avoidance advantage, combined with careful multidisciplinary coordination between the radiology, oncology, and maternal-fetal medicine teams regarding examination timing and any medically necessary treatment initiation, supports a staging approach that appropriately balances maternal oncologic care needs against fetal safety considerations throughout the pregnancy.

Epidemiology and Diagnostic Criteria for Multiple Myeloma

Multiple myeloma, a plasma cell neoplasm predominantly affecting older adults, has undergone a substantial evolution in diagnostic criteria over recent years, with whole-body MRI, together with low-dose whole-body CT, now supplanting the historical skeletal radiographic survey given cross-sectional imaging's substantially superior sensitivity for detecting the marrow-infiltrating lesions and early osteolytic disease that radiographic skeletal survey characteristically underestimates or entirely misses given radiography's comparatively limited sensitivity for marrow-based disease before substantial cortical bone destruction has occurred. Contemporary diagnostic criteria specifically recognize a defined threshold number of focal marrow lesions on MRI as itself sufficient to establish a diagnosis of symptomatic multiple myeloma requiring treatment, even in a patient who might otherwise be categorized as having the earlier, asymptomatic smoldering myeloma stage based on laboratory criteria alone, reflecting the substantial prognostic and treatment-triggering significance whole-body MRI-detected marrow involvement now carries within the contemporary diagnostic framework.

Marrow Infiltration Patterns and Response Assessment

Multiple myeloma marrow involvement demonstrates several recognized infiltration patterns on whole-body MRI, including a normal, unaffected marrow appearance in early or minimal disease, a focal pattern with discrete, diffusion-restricting lesions against otherwise normal background marrow, a diffuse pattern with homogeneous marrow signal replacement throughout the imaged skeleton, and a variegated or salt-and-pepper pattern combining features of both focal and diffuse involvement, and this pattern classification carries direct prognostic significance, with diffuse involvement generally associated with higher disease burden and less favorable prognosis relative to a purely focal pattern with limited lesion number. Post-treatment response assessment on whole-body MRI applies both the visual resolution or persistence of previously identified diffusion-restricting lesions and the apparent diffusion coefficient trend discussed in the preceding technique section, with a notable and clinically important caveat that focal lesions can persist as low-signal, non-enhancing, non-diffusion-restricting residual marrow change even following successful treatment and genuine complete hematologic response, reflecting residual fibrotic or fatty marrow change rather than persistent viable disease, making this specific residual imaging appearance an important recognized pattern the interpreting radiologist should not misinterpret as treatment failure when the diffusion and enhancement characteristics no longer suggest active disease.

Complications and Prognosis in Multiple Myeloma

Multiple myeloma carries a recognized complication profile directly related to the marrow infiltration and associated skeletal disease this chapter's imaging framework characterizes, including pathologic fracture at a site of focal lytic disease, spinal cord or nerve root compression from vertebral involvement with associated epidural extension, a finding requiring urgent recognition and communication given its time-critical neurologic implications directly analogous to the malignant spinal cord compression considerations addressed in earlier chapters of this book, and hypercalcemia related to osteoclastic bone resorption from the disease process itself, a metabolic complication carrying its own distinct acute management urgency. Overall prognosis in multiple myeloma has improved substantially with the introduction of novel therapeutic agents over recent years, though the disease generally remains understood as a chronic, relapsing-remitting condition rather than a curable malignancy for the great majority of patients, and the whole-body MRI-based marrow infiltration pattern discussed throughout this chapter, together with standard laboratory and cytogenetic risk stratification, contributes to the overall prognostic assessment informing both initial treatment intensity selection and the anticipated surveillance interval for detecting eventual disease relapse or progression over the patient's long-term disease course.

Figure 22.2: Axial and Appendicular Skeletal Marrow Anatomy

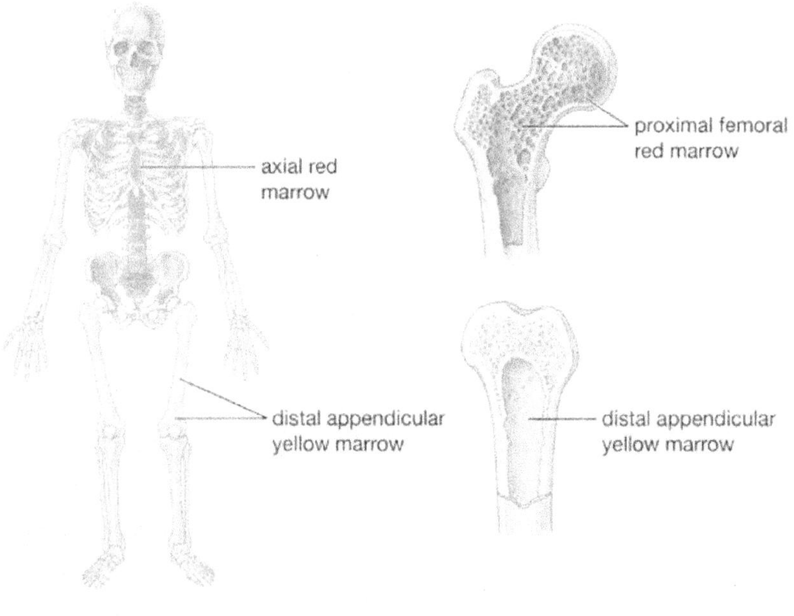

THE SIGNAL-TO-CATEGORY DECISION SYSTEM — Diffusion Whole-Body Lesion Categorization

---

The Signal Pattern: A diffusion-restricting marrow or soft tissue lesion is identified on whole-body MRI, and the reader must correlate this diffusion finding with T1-weighted signal and, where available, Dixon fat fraction or in-and-out-of-phase imaging.

Category Signature: Diffuse or patchy diffusion restriction with preserved or only mildly reduced T1 marrow fat signal in an expected red marrow distribution is categorized as benign red marrow reconversion; a discrete, focal diffusion-restricting lesion with markedly reduced T1 signal replacing normal marrow fat is categorized as suspicious for focal tumor infiltration.

The Decision: Benign red marrow reconversion, particularly with a compatible clinical context such as anemia, recent chemotherapy, or an endurance athlete, generally requires no further workup beyond documentation; suspicious focal marrow infiltration supports further characterization, whether additional imaging, laboratory correlation, or biopsy, depending on the clinical context and whether a known malignancy diagnosis is already established.

Trap Logic: Red marrow reconversion, physiologic expansion of hematopoietically active marrow in response to increased demand from anemia, chemotherapy, or heavy athletic training, produces genuine diffusion restriction that can closely mimic diffuse marrow infiltrative disease if the reader relies on diffusion signal alone without correlating T1 fat signal and overall distribution pattern; the discriminating step is recognizing that reconverted red marrow typically preserves a recognizable, if diminished, fat signal and follows the expected proximal-to-distal reconversion distribution pattern, in contrast to the more complete fat signal replacement and often less anatomically predictable distribution of true marrow infiltrative disease.

Pattern Anchor: Correlate diffusion restriction with T1 fat signal and marrow distribution pattern before categorizing a whole-body finding as suspicious; benign red marrow reconversion is a common and important mimic of diffuse marrow infiltrative disease.

CLINICAL PEARL: A persistent, non-enhancing, non-diffusion-restricting focal marrow lesion following successful multiple myeloma treatment represents residual fibrotic or fatty change rather than treatment failure; the absence of active diffusion restriction and enhancement, not the persistence of a visible focal abnormality alone, indicates genuine treatment response.

Differential Diagnosis of Diffuse Marrow Signal Abnormality

Beyond multiple myeloma and metastatic infiltration discussed throughout this chapter, diffuse marrow signal abnormality on whole-body MRI carries a broad differential extending to include the benign red marrow reconversion discussed in this chapter's rhythm framework, myelofibrosis, a bone marrow stromal disorder producing progressive fibrotic marrow replacement with a corresponding diffusely abnormal, low T1 signal appearance that can superficially resemble diffuse infiltrative marrow disease, and, in an appropriate clinical context, diffuse marrow edema-like signal related to a systemic inflammatory or rheumatologic condition rather than a primary hematologic or metastatic process. Distinguishing among these entities relies substantially on clinical and laboratory correlation, since the imaging appearance alone, particularly for the diffuse infiltrative patterns discussed throughout this differential, frequently demonstrates genuine overlap between entities, and a compatible peripheral blood count abnormality, known hematologic diagnosis, or systemic inflammatory condition history provides essential context that the interpreting radiologist should actively seek when a diffuse marrow signal abnormality is identified without a more specific, discriminating morphologic feature favoring one specific diagnosis over the others within this differential.

Cancer Predisposition Syndrome Surveillance

PATIENT EDUCATION: Whole-body MRI surveillance for a hereditary cancer predisposition syndrome involves no ionizing radiation and no intravenous contrast in many protocols, making it suitable for the repeated, often annual, lifelong surveillance this population requires; most patients tolerate the examination well, though the longer duration relative to a single-region MRI is worth anticipating and discussing beforehand.

Li-Fraumeni Syndrome and Other High-Risk Surveillance Populations

Li-Fraumeni syndrome, a hereditary cancer predisposition condition related to germline TP53 mutation and carrying a markedly elevated lifetime risk across a broad range of malignancies including sarcoma, breast carcinoma, brain tumor, and adrenocortical carcinoma, represents the archetypal indication for structured whole-body MRI surveillance, given both the radiation-free imaging approach's particular importance in a population with an underlying genetic predisposition toward radiation-induced secondary malignancy and the broad, multi-organ surveillance scope this specific syndrome's diverse tumor spectrum requires. Additional cancer predisposition syndromes benefiting from structured whole-body MRI surveillance include neurofibromatosis type 1, given this population's elevated risk for malignant peripheral nerve sheath tumor arising from a preexisting neurofibroma, and certain other hereditary syndromes with broad or multi-organ tumor predisposition, and the specific surveillance protocol applied, encompassing scan frequency and additional organ-specific sequences beyond the core whole-body protocol, is generally tailored to each syndrome's specific, characteristic tumor spectrum and typical age of onset for the component malignancies.

Structured Reporting and Incidental Finding Management

Whole-body MRI surveillance in an asymptomatic, high-risk population characteristically generates a substantial volume of incidental findings, given the comprehensive anatomic coverage this protocol provides, and structured, standardized reporting frameworks categorizing each identified finding as definitely benign requiring no further action, probably benign but warranting routine-interval follow-up, or indeterminate or suspicious warranting focused additional workup, have become essential to this surveillance application's practical sustainability, preventing both the clinical and psychological burden of reflexive additional workup for every minor incidental finding and the opposite risk of a genuinely significant finding being overlooked within a high volume of benign incidental observations. This structured categorization approach, directly paralleling the standardized reporting frameworks, LI-RADS, O-RADS, and PI-RADS, discussed throughout earlier chapters of this book, reflects a broader trend across body MRI toward standardized, reproducible interpretive frameworks specifically designed to support consistent, appropriately calibrated downstream management recommendations rather than a purely individualized, narrative interpretive approach that would introduce unacceptable variability into a surveillance program requiring consistency across repeated examinations and, often, multiple interpreting radiologists over a patient's lifetime of surveillance.

Figure 22.3: Whole-Body MRI Surveillance Scan Sequence

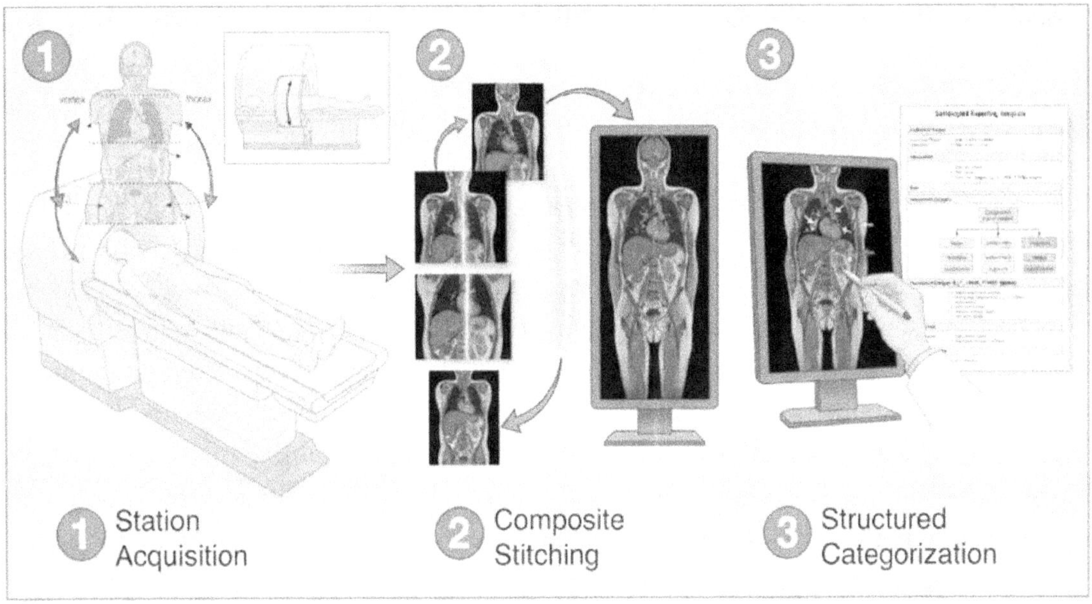

THE SIGNAL-TO-CATEGORY DECISION SYSTEM — Cancer Predisposition Surveillance Finding Categorization

The Signal Pattern: An asymptomatic patient with a known cancer predisposition syndrome undergoes structured whole-body MRI surveillance, and the reader must categorize every identified finding, expected and incidental alike, using a standardized reporting framework.

Category Signature: A finding with definitively benign imaging characteristics, such as a simple cyst or classic lipoma, is categorized as benign, no follow-up needed; a finding with nonspecific but likely benign characteristics is categorized as probably benign, routine-interval follow-up; a finding with morphology atypical for a benign process or inconsistent with the patient's known syndrome-associated risk pattern is categorized as indeterminate or suspicious, focused additional workup warranted.

The Decision: Benign findings require no further action beyond routine documentation; probably benign findings are incorporated into the standard surveillance interval for reassessment; indeterminate or suspicious findings prompt dedicated, focused additional imaging or biopsy outside the standard whole-body surveillance pathway.

Trap Logic: The sheer volume of incidental findings characteristic of whole-body surveillance in this population creates genuine risk of both under-triage, a clinically significant finding lost among numerous benign observations, and over-triage, reflexive additional workup for every minor incidental finding driving unsustainable patient anxiety and healthcare resource utilization; the discriminating step is applying the structured categorization framework consistently to every finding rather than allowing either extreme to dominate the interpretive approach.

Pattern Anchor: Apply the structured, standardized categorization framework to every finding, expected and incidental, rather than a purely individualized narrative approach; consistency across the surveillance program depends on this structured discipline being applied uniformly.

Metastatic Disease Staging and Response Assessment

Whole-Body MRI for Lymphoma Staging and Response Assessment

Lymphoma staging and response assessment has traditionally relied on PET-CT given fluorodeoxyglucose-avid lymphoma's excellent metabolic conspicuity, but whole-body MRI has gained increasing recognition as a radiation-free alternative particularly valuable for pediatric and young adult lymphoma patients, discussed further in the following chapter's pediatric oncologic imaging context, given this population's heightened cumulative radiation exposure sensitivity over an anticipated long survivorship period, with diffusion-weighted whole-body imaging providing comparable nodal and extranodal disease detection sensitivity to PET-CT for the great majority of lymphoma subtypes and treatment response patterns. Response assessment criteria adapted specifically for whole-body MRI in lymphoma, correlating diffusion restriction and apparent diffusion coefficient trend with nodal and extranodal lesion size change, parallel the standardized PET-based Deauville response criteria used in conventional lymphoma response assessment, and this MRI-based response framework has demonstrated meaningful concordance with PET-CT-based assessment in comparative studies, supporting its growing adoption as a genuine alternative rather than merely a supplementary tool for the specific patient populations, particularly pediatric and young adult patients, radiation avoidance benefits most.

Whole-Body MRI for Skeletal Metastatic Staging

Whole-body MRI's exceptional sensitivity for marrow-based disease, discussed throughout this chapter's multiple myeloma section, extends directly to skeletal metastatic staging for solid tumors with a recognized predilection for bone metastasis, most notably breast and prostate carcinoma, with diffusion-weighted whole-body imaging detecting marrow-infiltrating metastatic deposits at a comparably early stage to its myeloma detection capability, often before the degree of cortical bone destruction required for confident detection on conventional radiographic or CT-based skeletal assessment, or, alternatively, before the metabolic activity threshold required for confident detection on the bone scintigraphy traditionally used for this staging application. This capability has positioned whole-body MRI as a genuinely competitive, and in some specific clinical contexts preferred, alternative to bone scintigraphy for skeletal metastatic staging, particularly in prostate cancer, where whole-body MRI's combined skeletal and pelvic nodal and local staging capability within a single radiation-free examination offers a meaningfully comprehensive staging solution relative to the combination of separate bone scintigraphy and dedicated pelvic imaging examinations that would otherwise be required.

Treatment Response Assessment in Skeletal Metastatic Disease

Treatment response assessment for skeletal metastatic disease presents a distinct interpretive challenge relative to the more straightforward size-based response criteria applied to soft tissue metastatic disease elsewhere in the body, since a successfully treated skeletal metastasis characteristically demonstrates sclerotic, densifying change on conventional imaging, an appearance that can be misinterpreted as disease progression if the reader is unfamiliar with this expected treatment-related pattern, sometimes termed a flare response, in which a temporarily worsening-appearing sclerotic pattern actually reflects a favorable healing response rather than genuine progressive disease. Whole-body MRI's combined morphologic and diffusion-weighted assessment, together with apparent diffusion coefficient trend analysis discussed earlier in this chapter, provides a valuable complementary tool for resolving this specific interpretive ambiguity, since a treated lesion demonstrating resolving diffusion restriction and rising apparent diffusion coefficient values, even in the setting of increasing sclerotic change on conventional sequences, supports a genuine treatment response interpretation over disease progression, a distinction carrying direct and substantial treatment continuation-versus-change management implications for the treating oncology team.

Whole-Body MRI Versus PET-CT

Limitations and Practical Barriers to Adoption

Whole-body MRI's clinical adoption, despite its genuine and growing evidence base for the applications discussed throughout this chapter, continues to face several practical barriers beyond the examination duration considerations discussed earlier in this chapter, including the substantial interpretive expertise and dedicated interpretation time this comprehensive, multi-station examination requires relative to a more limited, single-region examination, variable reimbursement recognition for this comparatively newer application relative to the more established bone scintigraphy and PET-CT alternatives, and, importantly, the technical standardization challenges inherent in ensuring reproducible apparent diffusion coefficient measurements and consistent protocol quality across different scanner vendors and field strengths, a standardization challenge that has generated ongoing collaborative professional society efforts toward consensus protocol and reporting recommendations. These practical barriers, while not undermining the genuine clinical value whole-body MRI provides for its established indications, appropriately temper expectations regarding this technique's near-term capacity to fully supplant PET-CT or bone scintigraphy across the broader range of oncologic staging applications where those more established modalities continue to demonstrate a more mature, standardized evidence base and clinical infrastructure.

Feature	Whole-Body MRI	PET-CT
Ionizing radiation	None	Present, from both radiotracer and CT component
Marrow-based disease sensitivity	Excellent, particularly for myeloma	Variable, dependent on tumor metabolic avidity
Nodal and metabolic disease sensitivity	Good but generally inferior to PET-CT	Excellent, based on functional metabolic activity
Examination duration	Generally longer	Generally shorter
Preferred applications	Myeloma, predisposition surveillance, pediatric staging	Most solid tumor whole-body metabolic staging

Complementary Strengths and Modality Selection

Whole-body MRI and PET-CT, while both providing comprehensive whole-body oncologic assessment capability, carry distinct and, in several respects, genuinely complementary strengths rather than representing simple interchangeable alternatives, with PET-CT's metabolic activity assessment providing superior sensitivity for detecting disease based on functional, metabolic activity independent of anatomic size or morphology, a particular advantage for detecting small-volume nodal or soft tissue disease with elevated metabolic activity, while whole-body MRI's superior soft tissue contrast resolution provides advantages for detailed local anatomic staging, particularly within the brain, liver, and marrow-based disease discussed throughout this chapter, applications where PET-CT's comparatively limited spatial and soft tissue contrast resolution can prove genuinely limiting. Modality selection in contemporary oncologic practice increasingly reflects this complementary strength recognition, with PET-CT generally preferred for whole-body metabolic staging of most solid tumor malignancies given its superior nodal and distant metastatic detection sensitivity, while whole-body MRI is generally preferred for the specific applications this chapter has emphasized, multiple myeloma and marrow-based disease, radiation-avoidant cancer predisposition syndrome surveillance, and pediatric oncologic staging discussed in the following chapter, where radiation avoidance carries particular importance given this population's greater cumulative lifetime radiation exposure risk and radiation sensitivity relative to an older adult population.

KEY POINT: Whole-body MRI and PET-CT represent complementary rather than interchangeable modalities; PET-CT generally provides superior whole-body metabolic staging sensitivity for most solid tumors, while whole-body MRI provides superior marrow-based disease detection and avoids ionizing radiation, favoring its selection for multiple myeloma, cancer predisposition surveillance, and pediatric applications.

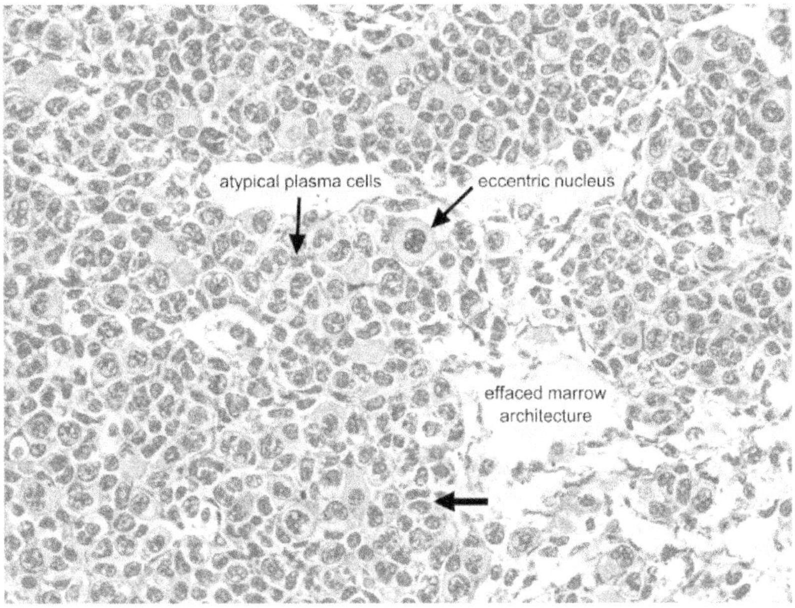

Patient Education and Counseling for Whole-Body MRI Surveillance

Counseling a patient beginning structured cancer predisposition syndrome surveillance benefits from proactive discussion of the high expected incidental finding rate this comprehensive whole-body examination characteristically generates, since a patient unprepared for this expectation may experience substantial anxiety when the radiology report lists several incidental observations even when each is individually categorized as benign or probably benign under the structured framework discussed throughout this chapter, and framing this expectation clearly before the first surveillance examination, together with clear explanation of the structured categorization system itself, supports a more measured, sustainable long-term relationship with a surveillance program the patient may continue for decades. For a patient undergoing whole-body MRI for multiple myeloma staging or metastatic disease assessment, clear communication that a persistent, non-enhancing marrow lesion following successful treatment does not indicate treatment failure, discussed earlier in this chapter, similarly supports realistic expectations and reduces unnecessary anxiety when a structurally persistent but biologically inactive lesion remains visible on follow-up imaging despite genuine, confirmed clinical remission.

Clinical Case Presentations

Case 1. A 64-year-old man with new back pain and anemia undergoes whole-body MRI demonstrating numerous discrete, diffusion-restricting lesions throughout the axial skeleton and proximal long bones with markedly reduced T1 signal replacing normal marrow fat, exceeding the threshold number of focal lesions used within the contemporary diagnostic criteria. The radiologist categorizes the findings as consistent with symptomatic multiple myeloma, and this imaging finding alone, together with confirmatory laboratory evaluation, establishes the diagnosis and treatment indication.

Case 2. A 34-year-old competitive endurance athlete undergoes whole-body MRI for an unrelated indication, incidentally demonstrating diffuse, mild diffusion restriction throughout the axial skeleton and proximal femora with preserved, though somewhat diminished, T1 fat signal in an expected proximal-to-distal reconversion distribution. The radiologist categorizes the findings as benign red marrow reconversion related to the patient's athletic training history, correlating the distribution pattern and preserved fat signal with this benign physiologic explanation rather than pursuing further malignancy-focused workup.

Case 3. A 19-year-old woman with confirmed Li-Fraumeni syndrome undergoes annual structured whole-body MRI surveillance, incidentally demonstrating a small, well-circumscribed, simple-appearing renal cyst and a subcentimeter, nonspecific pulmonary nodule. The radiologist categorizes the renal cyst as benign, no follow-up needed, and the pulmonary nodule as probably benign given its small size and smooth margins, recommending routine-interval follow-up rather than immediate biopsy for either finding, applying the structured categorization framework to avoid unnecessary additional workup.

Case 4. A 58-year-old man with metastatic prostate cancer undergoing systemic therapy has a follow-up whole-body MRI demonstrating increased sclerotic change within several previously identified skeletal lesions relative to the baseline examination, together with resolved diffusion restriction and rising apparent diffusion coefficient values at these same locations. The radiologist categorizes the findings as a favorable treatment response with a flare-type sclerotic healing pattern rather than disease progression, correlating the resolving diffusion characteristics with the treatment response interpretation despite the increasing sclerotic appearance.

Case 5. A 45-year-old woman with newly diagnosed breast carcinoma undergoes whole-body MRI for skeletal metastatic staging given a contraindication to the intravenous radiotracer used for conventional bone scintigraphy, demonstrating a single, small, diffusion-restricting lesion in the left iliac bone with markedly reduced T1 signal. Given the solitary nature of the finding and its atypical location for the most common benign marrow lesion mimics, the radiologist categorizes it as suspicious for a solitary skeletal metastasis and recommends targeted biopsy to confirm before finalizing the patient's overall stage and treatment plan.

Case 6. A 52-year-old man with longstanding myelofibrosis undergoes whole-body MRI performed for an unrelated indication, demonstrating diffuse, low T1 signal marrow replacement throughout the axial and proximal appendicular skeleton without discrete focal lesions or corresponding diffusion restriction. The radiologist correlates the diffuse, non-focal pattern and absent diffusion restriction with the patient's known myelofibrosis diagnosis, distinguishing this expected disease-related marrow appearance from a diffuse infiltrative malignant process and avoiding an unnecessary additional hematologic workup.

Case 7. A 29-year-old pregnant woman at 22 weeks gestation presents with new cervical lymphadenopathy and constitutional symptoms, and non-contrast whole-body MRI demonstrates extensive diffusion-restricting cervical, mediastinal, and para-aortic lymphadenopathy without hepatic or splenic involvement. The radiologist stages the findings as consistent with widespread lymphoma without evidence of extranodal organ involvement, and the radiation-free staging examination allows the multidisciplinary team to proceed with treatment planning while avoiding fetal radiation exposure during her ongoing pregnancy.

THE SIGNAL-TO-CATEGORY DECISION SYSTEM — Whole-Body Signal Correlation Arc

The Signal Pattern: This chapter's patterns share a whole-body, multi-sequence correlation structure, from diffusion-versus-T1 correlation distinguishing benign marrow change from tumor infiltration, to structured categorization of every surveillance finding across an entire high-risk patient's anatomic coverage.

Category Signature: Marrow findings are categorized benign red marrow reconversion or suspicious tumor infiltration based on correlated diffusion and T1 fat signal; surveillance findings are categorized benign, probably benign, or indeterminate-suspicious using a standardized structured framework.

The Decision: Category assignment in this chapter ranges from no further workup for benign marrow reconversion or a definitively benign surveillance finding to biopsy or focused additional imaging for suspicious marrow infiltration or an indeterminate surveillance finding.

The Trap Logic: Both patterns in this chapter share a common trap: relying on a single feature in isolation, diffusion signal alone or an individual finding's appearance without a structured framework, in a whole-body context characteristically producing numerous benign mimics and incidental findings that a single-feature approach cannot reliably sort.

Pattern Anchor: Correlate multiple sequences and apply a structured, standardized categorization framework across the entire whole-body dataset in both patterns this chapter describes; a whole-body examination's sheer anatomic scope makes single-feature, unstructured interpretation particularly prone to both under- and over-triage.

Summary and Key Concepts

Whole-body MRI combines T1-weighted, fat-suppressed T2-weighted, and diffusion-weighted imaging with background suppression across sequential stations for comprehensive skeletal and soft tissue coverage.

Contemporary multiple myeloma diagnostic criteria recognize a defined threshold number of focal marrow lesions on MRI as sufficient to establish symptomatic disease requiring treatment.

Benign red marrow reconversion can mimic diffuse marrow infiltrative disease on diffusion imaging; correlating T1 fat signal and distribution pattern distinguishes the two.

Cancer predisposition syndrome surveillance, most notably for Li-Fraumeni syndrome, relies on structured, standardized reporting to categorize the high volume of incidental findings this application generates.

Whole-body MRI provides comparably early skeletal metastatic detection to bone scintigraphy while avoiding ionizing radiation, an advantage particularly relevant for prostate cancer staging and pediatric applications.

A sclerotic flare response following successful skeletal metastatic treatment can mimic progression on conventional imaging; resolving diffusion restriction and rising apparent diffusion coefficient values support a genuine response interpretation.

Whole-body MRI and PET-CT are complementary modalities; PET-CT generally offers superior whole-body metabolic staging sensitivity while whole-body MRI offers superior marrow-based detection without ionizing radiation.

CHAPTER 23: BODY MRI IN PEDIATRIC AND PREGNANT PATIENTS

Learning Objectives

1. Describe technical adaptations for pediatric body MRI, including sedation and motion-reduction strategies.
2. Distinguish the major pediatric abdominal and pelvic oncologic masses using organ-of-origin and imaging feature criteria.
3. Recognize pediatric genitourinary congenital anomalies and their imaging features.
4. Apply MRI safety principles specific to pregnancy, including gadolinium contrast avoidance.
5. Recognize the role of fetal MRI in characterizing suspected congenital anomalies identified on obstetric ultrasound.

Clinical Overview

Pediatric and pregnancy-related body MRI share a foundational unifying principle running throughout this chapter, that imaging in these two populations, distinct as they are clinically, both demand deliberate technical adaptation and heightened attention to radiation avoidance and safety beyond the standard adult body MRI approach discussed throughout the remainder of this book. This chapter proceeds from pediatric body MRI technique, through pediatric abdominal and pelvic oncologic imaging, pediatric genitourinary congenital anomalies, MRI safety and technique in pregnancy, and closes with fetal MRI and placental imaging.

Two instances of the Signal-to-Category Decision System are applied in this chapter, the first to pediatric renal and adrenal mass categorization distinguishing Wilms tumor from neuroblastoma, and the second to fetal MRI anomaly categorization, reflecting this chapter's two most diagnostically consequential pediatric and prenatal categorization tasks.

Pediatric Body MRI Technique and Sedation Considerations

Sedation, Feed-and-Wrap, and Motion Reduction Strategies

Successful pediatric body MRI depends fundamentally on age-appropriate strategies for achieving the sustained immobility a diagnostically adequate examination requires, ranging from the feed-and-wrap technique, in which a young infant is fed immediately before the examination and then swaddled to encourage natural sleep through the acquisition, effective for infants generally under approximately three to six months of age, through structured child life specialist-supported preparation and practice for an older, cooperative child capable of understanding and following breath-hold and stillness instructions, to procedural sedation or general anesthesia for a child in the intermediate age range who can neither reliably sleep through feed-and-wrap nor cooperate with awake instruction. The decision to pursue sedation or general anesthesia carries genuine risk-benefit considerations beyond simple sedation-related risk itself, including the resource and scheduling demands of an anesthesia-supported examination and, increasingly recognized, questions regarding potential neurodevelopmental effects of repeated early-childhood anesthesia exposure, considerations that have driven substantial institutional investment in child life specialist programs, mock scanner practice sessions, and other awake-imaging optimization strategies specifically to reduce reliance on sedation and anesthesia wherever a technically adequate awake examination can reasonably be achieved.

Accelerated and Motion-Robust Sequence Techniques

Beyond behavioral and pharmacologic strategies, technical sequence adaptations play an increasingly important complementary role in pediatric body MRI, with accelerated acquisition techniques, including parallel imaging and compressed sensing reconstruction, substantially reducing total scan time and therefore the duration over which sustained stillness or sedation must be maintained, and motion-robust sequence variants, including radial k-space filling techniques less sensitive to the periodic respiratory and bulk motion artifact that would otherwise substantially degrade image quality in a non-breath-holding young child, providing genuine diagnostic salvage capability for an examination that might otherwise require sedation or repeat imaging. Free-breathing acquisition strategies, whether respiratory-triggered or the motion-robust radial techniques discussed above, have become particularly valuable for the youngest pediatric patients who cannot reliably perform breath-hold instructions regardless of cooperative intent, and the growing sophistication and clinical availability of these motion-robust techniques has meaningfully expanded the population of young children who can complete a diagnostically adequate body MRI examination without sedation, a genuinely significant advance given the risk-benefit considerations discussed in the preceding paragraph.

Feature	Wilms Tumor	Neuroblastoma
Organ of origin	Intrarenal	Extrarenal, adrenal or paraspinal
Renal interface	Claw sign	Displacement without claw sign
Calcification	Uncommon	Common
Vascular relationship	Displacement	Frequent encasement
Midline crossing	Uncommon	Common
Typical age	2 to 5 years	Under 2 years typical

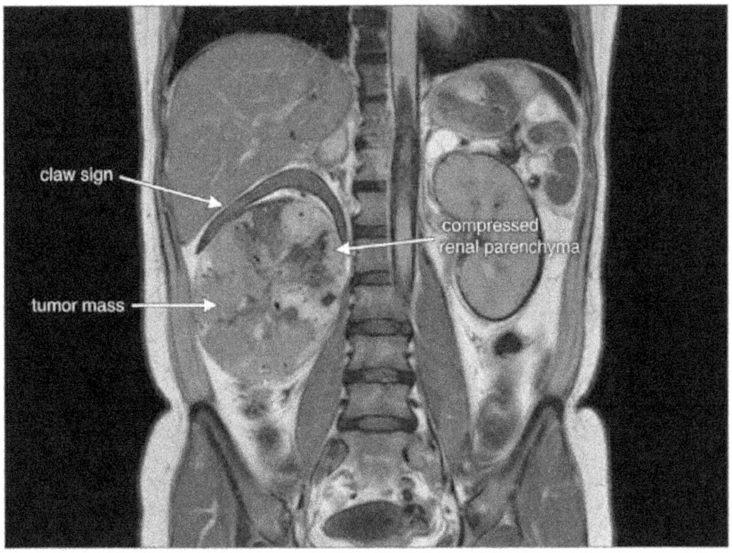

Figure 23.1: Wilms Tumor with Claw Sign on Pediatric Abdominal MRI

Contrast Agent Use and Dosing Considerations in Pediatric Patients

Gadolinium-based contrast agent administration in pediatric patients follows weight-based dosing principles paralleling adult practice, though with particular attention to the substantially wider weight range this population spans, from a several-kilogram neonate to an adolescent approaching adult body size, making accurate, current weight documentation immediately before contrast administration essential to safe, appropriately dosed pediatric contrast use, a consideration of greater practical significance in this population than in the comparatively narrower and more stable weight range typical of the adult patients discussed throughout most of this book. Gadolinium-based contrast agents are generally considered safe for use in pediatric patients beyond the neonatal period, with the same macrocyclic agent preference discussed in earlier chapters regarding nephrogenic systemic fibrosis risk minimization applying equally to this population, and renal function assessment before contrast administration, while relevant across all ages, carries particular importance in a pediatric patient with known or suspected renal impairment, whether from a congenital anomaly discussed elsewhere in this chapter or an acquired renal condition, given this population's comparatively limited physiologic reserve relative to a typical adult patient.

Pediatric Abdominal and Pelvic Oncologic Imaging

Epidemiology of Pediatric Abdominal Malignancy

Wilms tumor, or nephroblastoma, and neuroblastoma together represent the two most common pediatric abdominal malignancies, with Wilms tumor typically presenting in early childhood, most commonly between two and five years of age, as an incidentally discovered or parent-noted abdominal mass in an otherwise well-appearing child, and neuroblastoma, arising from primitive neural crest tissue and most commonly originating within the adrenal medulla or paraspinal sympathetic chain, demonstrating a somewhat younger typical age of presentation and a comparatively more frequent association with systemic symptoms, including fever, irritability, and, for a subset of cases with catecholamine-secreting tumor tissue, hypertension, reflecting this tumor's distinct neuroendocrine biology relative to the renal epithelial origin of Wilms tumor. Both entities carry recognized, though distinct, syndromic associations, Wilms tumor with several defined overgrowth and genitourinary anomaly syndromes including WAGR syndrome and Beckwith-Wiedemann syndrome, and neuroblastoma with a smaller subset of familial predisposition syndromes, associations that inform both individual patient counseling and, for a subset of syndromically predisposed children, structured surveillance imaging protocols paralleling the cancer predisposition syndrome surveillance principles discussed in the preceding chapter.

Wilms Tumor Versus Neuroblastoma: Organ of Origin and Imaging Distinction

Distinguishing Wilms tumor from neuroblastoma represents the single most clinically consequential categorization task in pediatric abdominal oncologic imaging, given the substantially different staging systems, treatment sequencing, whether upfront nephrectomy for many Wilms tumor presentations versus neoadjuvant chemotherapy before surgical resection favored for higher-risk neuroblastoma, and overall prognosis each entity carries, and this distinction relies fundamentally on establishing the tumor's organ of origin, intrarenal for Wilms tumor, producing the claw sign in which a thin rim of compressed but preserved normal renal parenchyma is visible at the tumor's margin, confirming the mass's origin from within, rather than adjacent to, the kidney, against the characteristically extrarenal, adrenal or paraspinal origin of neuroblastoma, which instead displaces rather than arises from the kidney, producing a distinct displacement rather than claw sign pattern at the renal interface.

Figure 23.2: Retroperitoneal Sympathetic Chain and Adrenal Anatomy in the Child.

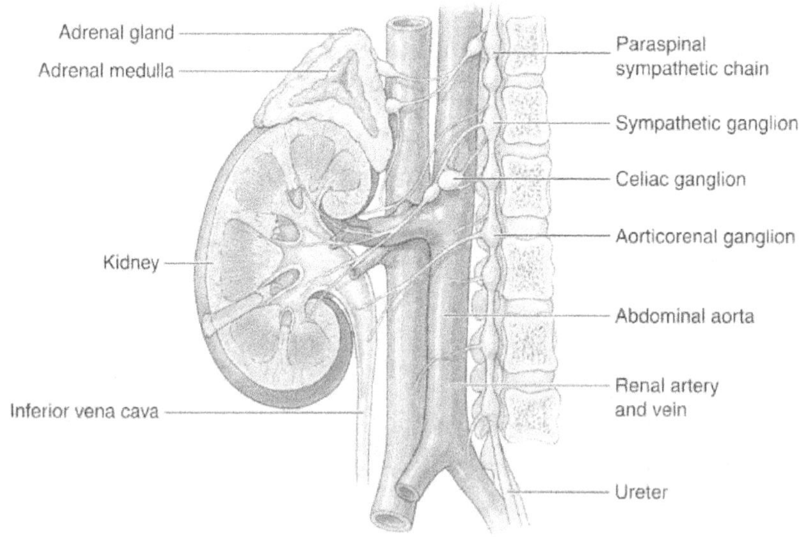

Additional distinguishing features include neuroblastoma's characteristic tendency toward calcification, encasement rather than simple displacement of adjacent major vessels including the aorta and its branches, a pattern reflecting this tumor's more infiltrative growth relative to the more expansile, well-circumscribed growth pattern typical of Wilms tumor, and frequent crossing of the midline, a pattern less characteristic of the more typically unilateral, renal-confined Wilms tumor presentation, together providing a constellation of features that, combined with the fundamental organ-of-origin determination, support confident preoperative categorization in the great majority of cases.

THE SIGNAL-TO-CATEGORY DECISION SYSTEM — Pediatric Renal and Adrenal Mass Categorization

---

The Signal Pattern: A pediatric abdominal mass is identified on MRI, and the reader must determine the mass's organ of origin and characterize its relationship to the kidney, adjacent vasculature, and midline.

Category Signature: An intrarenal mass with a claw sign of compressed but preserved renal parenchyma, well-circumscribed margins, and vessel displacement without encasement is categorized as consistent with Wilms tumor; an extrarenal, adrenal or paraspinal mass displacing rather than arising from the kidney, with calcification, vascular encasement, and frequent midline crossing, is categorized as consistent with neuroblastoma.

The Decision: A Wilms tumor categorization generally supports staging evaluation and, per current risk-adapted protocols, either upfront nephrectomy or neoadjuvant chemotherapy depending on specific staging and imaging criteria; a neuroblastoma categorization prompts assessment of image-defined risk factors, most notably vascular encasement, directly informing whether neoadjuvant chemotherapy before surgical resection is favored over upfront surgery.

Trap Logic: A very large tumor, of either origin, can produce sufficient mass effect and architectural distortion that the fundamental organ-of-origin distinction becomes genuinely difficult to establish with confidence, since a massively enlarged Wilms tumor can efface the claw sign through sheer bulk, and a massively enlarged neuroblastoma can produce a comparably confusing renal interface; the discriminating step is searching specifically and deliberately for any preserved claw sign remnant, however subtle, and for vascular encasement versus displacement, rather than relying on overall gestalt tumor size or general appearance when the mass is large enough to distort the more straightforward smaller-tumor pattern.

Pattern Anchor: Establish organ of origin through the claw sign and vessel displacement-versus-encasement pattern, not overall tumor gestalt; this distinction directly determines staging system, treatment sequencing, and prognosis.

CLINICAL PEARL: The claw sign, a thin rim of compressed but preserved normal renal parenchyma at a mass's margin, confirms intrarenal origin and favors Wilms tumor; its absence, together with vascular encasement and midline crossing, favors an extrarenal neuroblastoma origin instead.

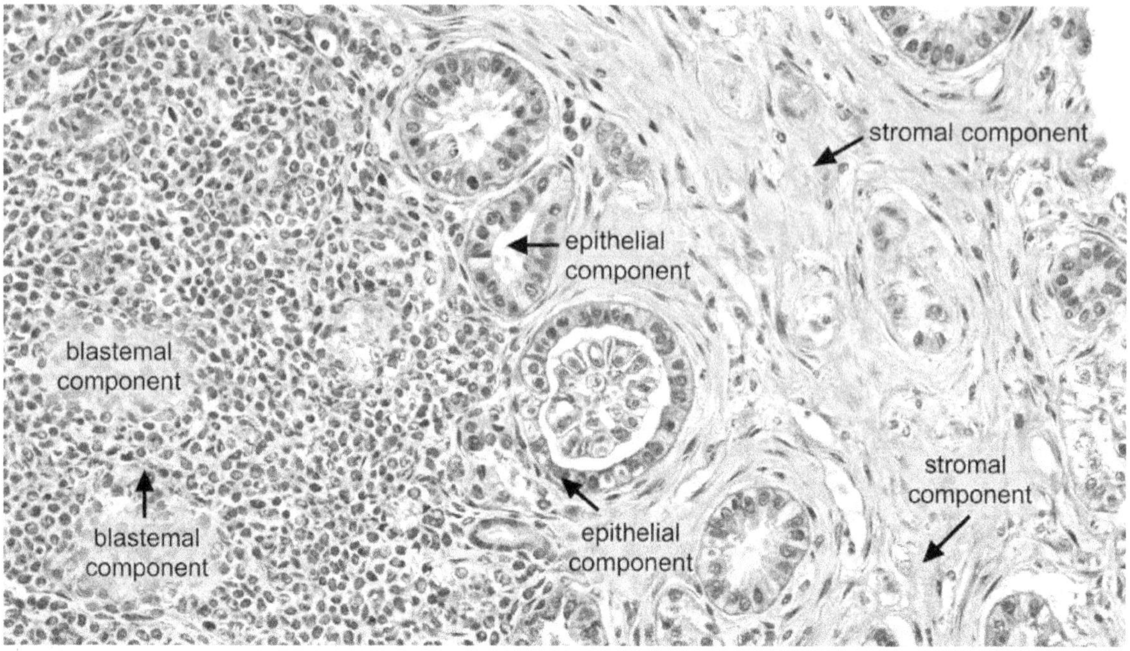

Hepatoblastoma and Other Pediatric Abdominal Tumors

Hepatoblastoma, the most common primary pediatric liver malignancy, typically presents in early childhood, most commonly under three years of age, as a heterogeneous, often multinodular hepatic mass with variable enhancement and, in a substantial proportion of cases, markedly elevated serum alpha-fetoprotein, a tumor marker whose degree of elevation and trend over treatment provides valuable complementary information to the imaging staging framework this chapter's principles otherwise emphasize, applying the PRETEXT staging system, which characterizes tumor extent by the number of liver segments free of disease, directly analogous in structural logic to the organ-segment-based staging approaches discussed for adult hepatic malignancy in earlier chapters of this book. Rhabdomyosarcoma, the most common pediatric soft tissue sarcoma, can arise from a genitourinary primary site, most notably the bladder or prostate in a young child, producing a botryoid, grape-like mass pattern when arising within a hollow, mucosa-lined structure, a distinctive morphologic pattern reflecting this specific tumor subtype's polypoid growth pattern along a mucosal surface, and recognizing this specific pattern, together with the patient's age and the tumor's genitourinary location, supports appropriate diagnostic consideration and staging evaluation distinct from the renal and adrenal mass differential this chapter's primary rhythm framework addresses.

Pediatric Genitourinary and Congenital Anomalies

Complications and Prognosis in Wilms Tumor and Neuroblastoma

Prognosis for Wilms tumor is generally favorable, with contemporary risk-adapted multimodal treatment achieving high overall survival rates for favorable-histology, localized disease, though anaplastic histology and higher-stage or bilateral disease carry meaningfully reduced survival relative to this favorable baseline, considerations that reinforce the direct prognostic significance of the accurate preoperative staging and imaging characterization this chapter's framework addresses, including deliberate evaluation for bilateral involvement and for the venous tumor thrombus extension into the renal vein or inferior vena cava that a subset of Wilms tumor cases demonstrate, a finding carrying direct surgical planning significance analogous to the venous tumor thrombus assessment discussed for adult renal cell carcinoma in an earlier chapter of this book. Neuroblastoma prognosis demonstrates substantially greater heterogeneity than Wilms tumor, ranging from a favorable, sometimes spontaneously regressing pattern in a very young infant with low-stage, favorable-biology disease to a considerably more guarded prognosis for older children with high-risk, unfavorable-biology, or metastatic disease at presentation, and this prognostic heterogeneity is informed by a combination of imaging-defined risk factors discussed throughout this chapter, patient age, and tumor biology and genetic markers assessed through tissue sampling, together forming the comprehensive risk stratification framework that guides treatment intensity selection for this biologically diverse malignancy.

Renal Congenital Anomalies

Congenital renal anomalies encountered on pediatric body MRI span a broad spectrum, including renal agenesis, complete absence of one kidney, generally identified incidentally or during workup of a contralateral compensatory hypertrophied kidney, horseshoe kidney, in which the two kidneys are fused, most commonly at their lower poles, across the midline anterior to the great vessels, a fusion anomaly carrying modestly elevated risk for both urinary tract obstruction and Wilms tumor relative to the general population, and duplicated collecting system, in which a single kidney demonstrates two distinct collecting systems and ureters, an anomaly whose clinical significance depends substantially on whether the duplication is uncomplicated or is instead associated with ureteral ectopia or ureterocele producing obstruction or reflux. Multicystic dysplastic kidney, a distinct entity from the polycystic kidney disease processes discussed in earlier chapters of this book, represents a congenital malformation in which the affected kidney is replaced by a cluster of non-communicating cysts without functioning renal parenchyma, generally identified on prenatal or early postnatal imaging and typically managed with conservative observation given this entity's characteristic tendency toward spontaneous involution over time, in contrast to the more assertive intervention that a genuinely obstructive uropathy would warrant.

Posterior Urethral Valves and Obstructive Uropathy

Posterior urethral valves, obstructing membranous folds within the male posterior urethra representing the most common cause of lower urinary tract obstruction in male infants, produce a characteristic upstream effect cascade, bladder wall thickening and trabeculation from chronic outlet obstruction, bilateral hydroureteronephrosis, and, in more severe or earlier-onset cases, renal parenchymal dysplasia from the sustained back-pressure effect on developing renal tissue, and this cascade's severity and the degree of associated renal dysplasia carry direct prognostic significance for eventual renal function, making comprehensive anatomic and functional characterization, whether by MRI or, more commonly in this specific application, ultrasound and voiding cystourethrography, essential to both diagnosis and longitudinal management planning. MRI's role in this specific pediatric genitourinary context is generally more prominent for characterizing associated renal parenchymal change and, particularly, for surgical planning in a more complex or ambiguous anatomic presentation, than for primary posterior urethral valve diagnosis itself, which relies predominantly on the fluoroscopic and ultrasound techniques better suited to this specific anatomic region's dynamic functional assessment, reinforcing that MRI functions as one component within a broader, multimodality pediatric genitourinary imaging armamentarium rather than a universal first-line tool for every pediatric genitourinary indication.

Pediatric Ovarian and Testicular Considerations

Pediatric ovarian masses, most commonly mature cystic teratoma paralleling the adult entity discussed in an earlier chapter of this book, warrant particular attention to ovarian torsion given the elevated torsion risk in this age group discussed in this book's adnexal masses chapter, and MRI, when performed for a pediatric adnexal finding, applies largely the same imaging principles established for the adult population, with the important caveat that a normal, structurally unremarkable ovary in a prepubertal or peripubertal girl can itself torse without a predisposing mass, a pattern this book's earlier discussion specifically flagged as disproportionately represented in this younger population, reinforcing that a normal-appearing ovary on imaging in a child with acute pelvic pain does not exclude this specific diagnosis. Pediatric testicular and scrotal imaging, while more commonly performed with ultrasound given its excellent resolution and lack of sedation requirement for this comparatively superficial, readily accessible anatomic region, occasionally benefits from MRI as a problem-solving tool for an indeterminate testicular or paratesticular mass, applying the same signal characterization principles, including the fat-suppression technique for confirming a teratoma's fat content, discussed throughout this book's genitourinary imaging chapters, adapted to this specific pediatric anatomic and clinical context.

PATIENT EDUCATION: Preparing a child and family for MRI benefits from age-appropriate explanation, child life specialist involvement where available, and, for an older cooperative child, a practice or mock scan session; clear communication about the examination's noise, duration, and the importance of stillness supports successful completion and reduces the likelihood that sedation or anesthesia becomes necessary.

MRI Safety and Technique in Pregnancy

Gadolinium Contrast Avoidance in Pregnancy

Gadolinium-based contrast agents are generally avoided during pregnancy given demonstrated placental crossing and animal-model evidence of free gadolinium ion deposition in fetal tissue with uncertain, though theoretically concerning, long-term developmental implications, a precautionary avoidance principle referenced throughout several earlier chapters of this book in the context of pregnancy-specific imaging protocols, and this avoidance generally applies across essentially the entire gestational period rather than being confined to a specific trimester, reflecting the genuinely uncertain and inadequately characterized nature of the theoretical risk rather than a risk understood to be confined to a specific, more vulnerable developmental window. When gadolinium contrast administration is judged genuinely necessary despite this general avoidance principle, generally reserved for a clinical scenario where the diagnostic information gained is considered to meaningfully outweigh the theoretical fetal risk, this decision warrants explicit multidisciplinary discussion and documented informed consent reflecting the genuinely individualized risk-benefit calculation this uncommon scenario requires, rather than a routine, unreflective contrast administration decision as would apply in the non-pregnant population.

Maternal Positioning and Sequence Optimization

MRI performed during pregnancy benefits from several technical and positioning adaptations beyond the contrast avoidance principle discussed above, including left lateral decubitus positioning, particularly in the later second and third trimester, to avoid aortocaval compression from the gravid uterus that supine positioning can produce, a physiologic consideration paralleling standard obstetric care positioning recommendations more broadly, and single-shot, rapid acquisition sequence techniques, including single-shot fast spin echo and similar rapid T2-weighted approaches, which substantially reduce sensitivity to fetal motion, an inherent and unavoidable consideration given the fetus's own spontaneous movement throughout the examination that no maternal cooperation or stillness can control. Specific absorption rate monitoring and management, ensuring the radiofrequency energy deposition throughout the examination remains within established safety limits, receives particular attention in the pregnancy context, and most major professional imaging societies have published specific pregnancy-adapted safety and technique guidance addressing these considerations, guidance the interpreting radiologist and technologist team should actively consult and apply when performing MRI in a pregnant patient rather than defaulting to a standard, non-pregnancy-adapted protocol.

Fetal MRI and Placental Imaging

EVIDENCE: Comparative studies of fetal MRI against postnatal outcome have demonstrated meaningful diagnostic accuracy improvement over ultrasound alone for central nervous system anomaly characterization specifically, supporting fetal MRI's established role as a problem-solving adjunct for this indication rather than a routine, universal addition to standard obstetric ultrasound screening.

Indications and Technique for Fetal MRI

Fetal MRI serves as a valuable problem-solving adjunct to obstetric ultrasound, the primary and first-line prenatal imaging modality, when ultrasound identifies a suspected anomaly requiring more detailed anatomic characterization than ultrasound's inherent technical limitations, including maternal body habitus, fetal positioning, and oligohydramnios reducing the acoustic window available for ultrasound assessment, can reliably provide, with central nervous system anomalies representing the single most common indication for fetal MRI referral, given MRI's superior soft tissue contrast for detailed brain and spinal cord characterization relative to ultrasound, followed by thoracic anomalies, including congenital diaphragmatic hernia and congenital pulmonary airway malformation, and select complex genitourinary and gastrointestinal anomalies where detailed anatomic delineation meaningfully informs prenatal counseling and delivery planning. Fetal MRI technique relies predominantly on the same rapid, motion-robust single-shot sequences discussed in the preceding maternal safety section, applied specifically to characterize fetal anatomy despite the fetus's own spontaneous, uncontrollable movement throughout the examination, and maternal, rather than fetal, sedation is generally avoided given both its own risk profile and its limited efficacy at controlling fetal movement specifically, reinforcing the central importance of these rapid acquisition techniques as the primary technical strategy for achieving diagnostically adequate fetal imaging despite this fundamental, unavoidable motion challenge.

Figure 23.3: Fetal MRI Guided Prenatal Counseling Session

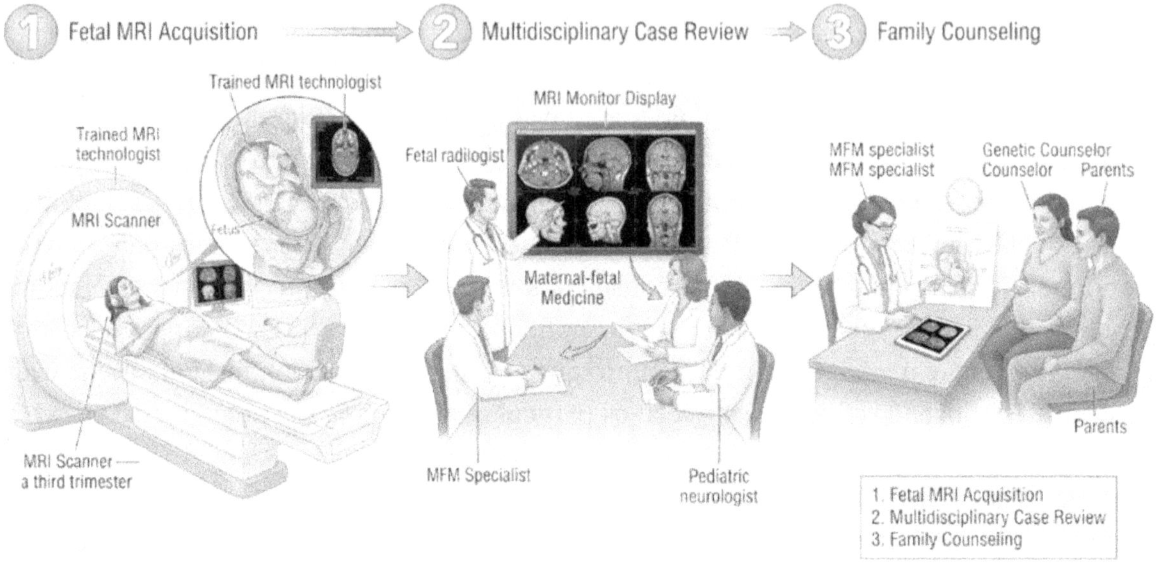

Special Populations: Multiple Gestation and Postpartum MRI Considerations

Fetal MRI in a multiple gestation pregnancy carries additional technical and interpretive complexity beyond the singleton considerations discussed throughout this chapter, given the need to clearly identify and independently characterize each fetus, particularly important in a monochorionic multiple gestation where twin-twin transfusion syndrome and its associated discordant fetal growth, amniotic fluid volume, and, in more severe cases, brain injury from hemodynamic instability require careful independent assessment of each twin rather than a single, undifferentiated overall impression, and clear, unambiguous labeling of each fetus's position and laterality throughout the report supports accurate communication with the obstetric and maternal-fetal medicine team managing this complex pregnancy. MRI performed in the immediate postpartum period, whether for a suspected retained placental fragment, postpartum hemorrhage evaluation, or another indication, benefits from awareness of expected normal postpartum uterine involution changes, including transient uterine enlargement and heterogeneous endometrial signal in the immediate postpartum window, changes that should not be mistaken for a pathologic process, paralleling the postsurgical change recognition principle emphasized throughout several other chapters of this book, and correlation with the specific delivery date and clinical presentation supports accurate distinction between expected postpartum change and a genuinely concerning finding requiring further intervention.

Placental Imaging and Placenta Accreta Spectrum

Placental imaging, most notably for suspected placenta accreta spectrum, abnormal placental invasion into or through the myometrium carrying substantial hemorrhagic risk at delivery, represents a distinct and increasingly important fetal and maternal MRI application, with MRI serving as a problem-solving adjunct to ultrasound, the first-line modality for this indication, particularly for posterior placental location where ultrasound's acoustic window is comparatively more limited, or when the depth and lateral extent of placental invasion requires more detailed characterization for surgical planning than ultrasound alone can reliably provide. MRI findings suggestive of placenta accreta spectrum include loss of the normal retroplacental T2 dark line representing the myometrial-placental interface, uterine bulging beyond the expected contour, and, for the more severe percreta subtype, frank placental tissue extension through the myometrium and serosa with potential bladder or other adjacent organ involvement, and accurate preoperative characterization of the specific depth and extent of this invasion directly informs the multidisciplinary delivery planning, including surgical team composition, blood product availability, and delivery location, essential to safely managing this high-risk obstetric scenario given the substantial hemorrhagic risk placenta accreta spectrum carries at the time of attempted placental separation.

Congenital Diaphragmatic Hernia and Thoracic Anomalies

Congenital diaphragmatic hernia, herniation of abdominal contents into the thoracic cavity through a diaphragmatic defect, represents one of the more common and clinically significant thoracic indications for fetal MRI referral, with fetal lung volume measurement, whether expressed as absolute total fetal lung volume or as the observed-to-expected lung volume ratio accounting for gestational age, providing essential prognostic information regarding the pulmonary hypoplasia this condition characteristically produces through the mass effect and disrupted normal lung development that herniated abdominal viscera impose upon the developing fetal thorax throughout gestation. Liver herniation into the thoracic cavity, when present alongside the more commonly herniated bowel and stomach, carries additional prognostic significance beyond lung volume alone, generally associated with more severe pulmonary hypoplasia and a more complex postnatal surgical repair, and this comprehensive fetal MRI characterization, lung volume, liver position, and herniated content, directly informs prenatal counseling regarding expected postnatal severity and, for the most severely affected cases, discussion of specialized delivery planning at a center equipped for immediate postnatal surgical and respiratory support this condition's most severe presentations require.

THE SIGNAL-TO-CATEGORY DECISION SYSTEM — Fetal MRI Anomaly Categorization

The Signal Pattern: Fetal MRI is performed for a suspected anomaly identified on obstetric ultrasound, and the reader must characterize the finding relative to gestational-age-appropriate normative developmental reference values before determining clinical significance.

Category Signature: A finding within the expected range of normal developmental variation for the fetus's gestational age is categorized as a normal variant; a finding outside this expected range, with a specific, recognized anomaly pattern, is categorized as a confirmed structural anomaly, further characterized by organ system and severity.

The Decision: A normal variant categorization supports reassurance and standard obstetric care without additional intervention; a confirmed anomaly prompts multidisciplinary counseling addressing prognosis, potential in-utero or postnatal intervention options, and delivery planning tailored to the specific anomaly identified.

Trap Logic: Several normal fetal developmental variants, including transient mild ventriculomegaly and cavum septum pellucidum variation, can superficially resemble pathology if the reader is not specifically familiar with gestational-age-appropriate normative reference values, risking unnecessary parental anxiety and inappropriate additional workup from a finding that represents normal developmental variation rather than a genuine structural anomaly; the discriminating step is correlating every finding against specific gestational-age-matched normative data before categorizing it as abnormal.

Pattern Anchor: Correlate every fetal MRI finding against gestational-age-appropriate normative reference values before categorizing it as abnormal; normal developmental variants are a recognized and important source of false-positive anomaly categorization in fetal imaging.

CAUTION: Fetal ventricular measurement and other developmental parameters must be interpreted against gestational-age-specific normative reference ranges rather than fixed adult or general pediatric thresholds; a measurement appropriate for one gestational age may represent a genuine abnormality at an earlier gestational age or a normal variant at a later one.

Clinical Case Presentations

Case 1. A 3-year-old boy with an incidentally palpated abdominal mass undergoes MRI without sedation using a motion-robust free-breathing protocol, demonstrating a large intrarenal mass with a preserved claw sign of compressed renal parenchyma at its margin and vessel displacement without encasement. The radiologist categorizes the findings as consistent with Wilms tumor, and the patient proceeds to nephron-sparing surgical evaluation per current risk-adapted staging protocols.

Case 2. A 14-month-old girl with irritability and new hypertension undergoes MRI under general anesthesia, demonstrating a calcified, extrarenal left adrenal mass displacing the kidney inferiorly and encasing the adjacent renal artery, with extension across the midline. The radiologist categorizes the findings as consistent with neuroblastoma with image-defined risk factors given the vascular encasement, and the patient proceeds to neoadjuvant chemotherapy before surgical resection is attempted.

Case 3. A newborn boy with prenatally identified bilateral hydronephrosis undergoes postnatal MRI demonstrating bilateral hydroureteronephrosis with a markedly thickened, trabeculated bladder wall and a dilated posterior urethra. The findings, correlated with subsequent voiding cystourethrography confirming posterior urethral valves, prompt urologic evaluation for valve ablation given the obstructive uropathy pattern and its risk to long-term renal function.

Case 4. A 32-year-old pregnant woman at 28 weeks gestation with suspected appendicitis undergoes non-contrast MRI in left lateral decubitus positioning, demonstrating a dilated, fluid-filled, blind-ending tubular structure in the right lower quadrant with surrounding fat stranding. The radiologist categorizes the findings as consistent with acute appendicitis, and the patient proceeds to surgical management with the diagnosis established without ionizing radiation exposure to the fetus.

Case 5. A fetus at 24 weeks gestation with ventriculomegaly identified on obstetric ultrasound undergoes fetal MRI demonstrating mild, symmetric lateral ventricular enlargement measuring within one to two millimeters of the upper limit of the gestational-age-appropriate normal range, without associated cortical malformation or other structural anomaly. The radiologist categorizes the findings as within the spectrum of a normal developmental variant given the borderline measurement and absence of associated findings, and the family is counseled accordingly with continued routine obstetric surveillance rather than additional invasive workup.

Case 6. A 34-year-old pregnant woman at 32 weeks gestation with a known posterior, low-lying placenta and two prior cesarean deliveries undergoes MRI demonstrating loss of the normal retroplacental T2 dark line with focal uterine bulging and placental tissue extending to but not clearly through the myometrium overlying the prior cesarean scar. The radiologist categorizes the findings as consistent with placenta accreta spectrum, and the multidisciplinary team proceeds with coordinated delivery planning at a facility equipped for the associated hemorrhagic risk this diagnosis carries.

Case 7. A 9-year-old girl with acute pelvic pain undergoes MRI demonstrating a normal-appearing, non-enlarged right ovary without a predisposing mass, but with absent enhancement relative to the contralateral side and a whirlpool configuration of the adnexal pedicle. The radiologist recognizes that torsion of a structurally normal ovary occurs disproportionately in this age group and categorizes the findings as ovarian torsion despite the absence of a predisposing mass, prompting urgent surgical detorsion.

THE SIGNAL-TO-CATEGORY DECISION SYSTEM — Developmental Signal Correlation Arc

The Signal Pattern: This chapter's patterns share a developmental correlation structure, from organ-of-origin determination for pediatric abdominal masses to gestational-age-matched normative correlation for fetal anomaly assessment.

Category Signature: Pediatric masses are categorized by organ of origin, claw sign versus displacement, and vascular relationship; fetal findings are categorized as normal developmental variant or confirmed structural anomaly based on gestational-age-matched reference values.

The Decision: Category assignment in this chapter ranges from nephron-sparing surgery for favorable Wilms tumor to neoadjuvant chemotherapy for neuroblastoma with image-defined risk factors, and from reassurance for a normal fetal variant to multidisciplinary counseling and delivery planning for a confirmed anomaly.

The Trap Logic: Both patterns in this chapter share a common trap: a large or ambiguous finding that obscures the specific discriminating feature, claw sign remnant or gestational-age-matched normative comparison, the framework requires, risking miscategorization if the reader relies on overall gestalt rather than the specific discriminating criterion.

Pattern Anchor: Search specifically for the discriminating feature, claw sign and vascular relationship, or gestational-age-matched normative correlation, in both patterns this chapter describes, rather than relying on overall size or gestalt appearance alone.

Summary and Key Concepts

Pediatric body MRI relies on age-appropriate immobility strategies, feed-and-wrap for infants, cooperative awake imaging for older children, and sedation or anesthesia for the intermediate age range, together with motion-robust accelerated sequence techniques.

The claw sign, compressed but preserved renal parenchyma at a mass margin, confirms intrarenal Wilms tumor origin, while vascular encasement and midline crossing favor extrarenal neuroblastoma.

Common pediatric renal congenital anomalies include renal agenesis, horseshoe kidney, duplicated collecting system, and multicystic dysplastic kidney, each with distinct clinical and management implications.

Posterior urethral valves produce a characteristic obstructive cascade of bladder wall thickening, bilateral hydroureteronephrosis, and renal dysplasia, with severity carrying direct prognostic significance.

Gadolinium contrast is generally avoided throughout pregnancy given placental crossing and uncertain fetal deposition effects; left lateral decubitus positioning and rapid single-shot sequences optimize pregnancy MRI technique.

Fetal MRI serves as a problem-solving adjunct to ultrasound, most commonly for suspected central nervous system anomalies, using rapid motion-robust sequences to overcome inherent fetal movement.

Fetal MRI findings must be correlated against gestational-age-appropriate normative reference values, since several normal developmental variants can mimic pathology if this correlation is not applied.

CHAPTER 24: CARDIAC AND THORACIC APPLICATIONS OF BODY MRI

Learning Objectives

1. Describe cardiac MRI technique, including cine imaging, late gadolinium enhancement, and parametric mapping.
2. Distinguish ischemic from non-ischemic late gadolinium enhancement patterns and correlate with specific cardiomyopathy diagnoses.
3. Apply transmural extent quantification to assess myocardial viability and predict functional recovery after revascularization.
4. Recognize pericardial disease patterns, including constrictive pericarditis and pericardial effusion.
5. Recognize mediastinal and chest wall mass characteristics relevant to thoracic body MRI applications.

Clinical Overview

Cardiac and thoracic MRI represent a natural closing application for this textbook's body MRI framework, extending the mural and tissue characterization principles developed throughout the preceding chapters, active-versus-fibrotic bowel wall change, tumor regression grading, marrow infiltration assessment, to the myocardium itself, where the fundamental question of viable versus scarred, or ischemic versus non-ischemic, tissue carries comparably direct treatment-pathway consequences. This chapter proceeds from cardiac MRI technique, through cardiomyopathy characterization, myocardial viability and ischemic heart disease, pericardial disease, and closes with thoracic mediastinal and chest wall applications.

Two instances of the Signal-to-Category Decision System are applied in this chapter, the first to late gadolinium enhancement pattern categorization distinguishing ischemic from non-ischemic distribution, and the second to myocardial viability categorization based on transmural scar extent, reflecting this chapter's two most treatment-consequential cardiac MRI categorization tasks.

Cardiac MRI Technique and Sequence Fundamentals

Cine Imaging and Functional Assessment

Cine cardiac MRI, acquired using balanced steady-state free precession sequences across the cardiac cycle and synchronized to the electrocardiographic signal, provides the foundational functional assessment anchoring the remainder of the cardiac MRI examination, generating a dynamic, beating-heart dataset from which left and right ventricular volumes, ejection fraction, and regional wall motion are directly measured with a reproducibility and accuracy widely regarded as the reference standard against which other cardiac imaging modalities, including echocardiography, are validated. Standard cine imaging planes include the vertical and horizontal long-axis views and a contiguous short-axis stack spanning the ventricles from base to apex, this short-axis stack specifically enabling the volumetric, slice-by-slice summation method used for the precise ejection fraction and chamber volume quantification that represents cardiac MRI's principal functional assessment contribution, a measurement precision particularly valuable for serial monitoring of a patient undergoing cardiotoxic chemotherapy or another condition requiring reproducible longitudinal ejection fraction tracking.

Late Gadolinium Enhancement Technique

Late gadolinium enhancement imaging, acquired approximately ten to fifteen minutes following contrast administration using an inversion recovery-prepared sequence specifically timed, or nulled, to suppress signal from normal myocardium, exploits the differential gadolinium washout kinetics between normal and abnormal myocardial tissue, with fibrotic or scarred myocardium retaining contrast longer than normal tissue given its expanded extracellular space, producing a bright, hyperenhancing signal against the nulled, dark normal myocardial background, a technique that has become the single most important sequence for the tissue characterization framework this chapter's discussion emphasizes throughout the following sections. Accurate inversion time selection, adjusted individually for each patient based on the specific contrast washout kinetics observed during a preparatory sequence, represents a critical technical requirement for reliable late gadolinium enhancement interpretation, since inadequate or excessive nulling of normal myocardium can respectively obscure genuine enhancement or produce a falsely diffuse hyperenhancing appearance that does not reflect the true, focal pattern of underlying disease, reinforcing why this sequence, despite its apparent technical simplicity, benefits substantially from careful, patient-specific optimization rather than a fixed, one-size-fits-all inversion time applied uniformly across all patients.

Parametric Mapping: T1, T2, and Extracellular Volume

Parametric mapping techniques, generating pixel-by-pixel quantitative T1 and T2 relaxation time maps of the myocardium, have substantially expanded cardiac MRI's tissue characterization capability beyond the late gadolinium enhancement technique discussed above, with native, precontrast T1 mapping providing sensitivity to both diffuse fibrotic processes that late gadolinium enhancement's normal-myocardium-nulling approach can systematically underdetect, given diffuse disease's tendency to elevate the nulling threshold for the entire myocardium rather than producing the focal contrast this technique is optimized to detect, and to specific myocardial infiltrative or storage processes, including amyloid and iron overload, each producing a characteristic, diagnostically distinctive native T1 signature. Extracellular volume fraction, calculated by combining pre- and postcontrast T1 mapping measurements with the patient's hematocrit, provides a further quantitative refinement specifically estimating the proportion of myocardial tissue occupied by extracellular space, a measurement directly reflecting diffuse fibrotic burden with a precision and reproducibility that has established this parameter as an increasingly important complementary tool alongside the late gadolinium enhancement pattern categorization this chapter's rhythm framework addresses, particularly valuable for the diffuse, non-focal fibrotic processes that late gadolinium enhancement alone can incompletely characterize.

Stress Perfusion Imaging and Flow Quantification

Stress perfusion cardiac MRI, acquired during pharmacologic vasodilator stress, most commonly with adenosine or regadenoson, and compared against a rest perfusion acquisition, assesses regional myocardial blood flow by tracking first-pass gadolinium contrast transit through the myocardium, with a region of relatively reduced signal intensity or delayed contrast arrival during stress relative to the corresponding rest acquisition and relative to adjacent, normally perfused myocardium indicating a flow-limiting coronary stenosis in that vascular territory, a technique providing a direct, non-invasive functional correlate to the anatomic coronary stenosis that invasive angiography or CT coronary angiography would otherwise characterize without this same functional flow information. Quantitative flow imaging, using phase-contrast velocity-encoded sequences, provides complementary assessment of valvular regurgitant fraction, shunt quantification for a congenital cardiac anomaly, and great vessel flow measurement, extending cardiac MRI's functional assessment capability beyond the myocardial perfusion and viability framework this chapter's primary discussion emphasizes into the valvular and congenital heart disease domains, applications that, while beyond this chapter's primary scope, illustrate the broader versatility this single imaging modality provides across the full spectrum of structural and functional cardiac assessment.

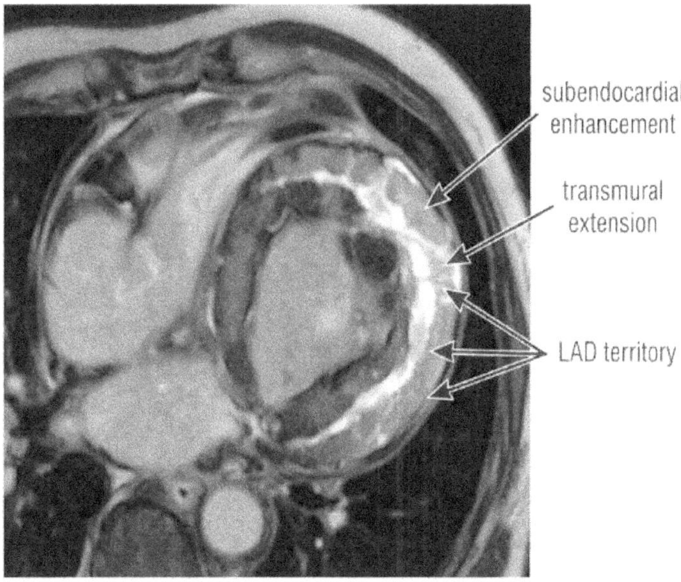

Figure 24.1: Late Gadolinium Enhancement in Ischemic Cardiomyopathy

Cardiomyopathy Characterization

Cardiomyopathy	Typical LGE Distribution	Key Complementary Finding
Ischemic disease	Subendocardial to transmural, coronary territory	Wall motion abnormality matching territory
Hypertrophic cardiomyopathy	Patchy mid-wall, RV insertion points	Asymmetric septal hypertrophy
Dilated cardiomyopathy	Mid-wall, septal-predominant, or absent	LV dilation, reduced ejection fraction
Acute myocarditis	Subepicardial or mid-wall, inferolateral	Myocardial edema on T2 mapping
Cardiac amyloidosis	Diffuse, subendocardial, global	Elevated native T1, poor nulling

Epidemiology and Genetic Basis of Hypertrophic Cardiomyopathy

Hypertrophic cardiomyopathy represents the most common inherited cardiomyopathy, affecting a meaningful proportion of the general population when assessed by contemporary genetic and imaging screening criteria, with autosomal dominant inheritance of a sarcomeric protein-encoding gene mutation, most commonly involving beta-myosin heavy chain or myosin-binding protein C, identified in a substantial proportion of cases, though genetic testing fails to identify a causative mutation in a meaningful minority, reflecting the condition's genetic heterogeneity and the ongoing discovery of additional contributing genetic variants. First-degree relative cascade screening, whether through genetic testing when a causative familial mutation has been identified or through periodic clinical and imaging screening when genetic testing is uninformative, represents standard practice following a new hypertrophic cardiomyopathy diagnosis, given this condition's autosomal dominant inheritance pattern and the substantial clinical value early identification provides for a relative who may otherwise remain asymptomatic until a potentially catastrophic sudden cardiac death event, reinforcing why hypertrophic cardiomyopathy diagnosis in an index patient carries family-wide, not merely individual, clinical significance.

Hypertrophic Cardiomyopathy

Hypertrophic cardiomyopathy, a genetically heterogeneous condition of sarcomeric protein mutation producing asymmetric or, less commonly, symmetric left ventricular hypertrophy without an identifiable secondary cause such as hypertension or aortic stenosis, demonstrates a characteristic mid-wall, patchy late gadolinium enhancement pattern, most pronounced at the right ventricular insertion points and within the most hypertrophied myocardial segments, a fibrotic pattern distinct from the subendocardial or transmural, coronary territory-respecting pattern characteristic of ischemic disease discussed later in this chapter, and this fibrotic burden, quantified through the late gadolinium enhancement extent and complemented by extracellular volume fraction measurement discussed in the preceding technique section, carries direct prognostic significance for sudden cardiac death risk, a risk stratification consideration of particular clinical importance in this specific cardiomyopathy given its recognized association with sudden cardiac death, including in young, otherwise asymptomatic patients and athletes. Cardiac MRI additionally provides precise, reproducible septal wall thickness measurement and, through dedicated flow imaging sequences, quantification of any associated left ventricular outflow tract obstruction from systolic anterior motion of the mitral valve apparatus, measurements that directly inform both risk stratification and, for a patient with substantial outflow obstruction, treatment planning regarding septal reduction therapy, whether surgical myectomy or catheter-based alcohol septal ablation.

Dilated Cardiomyopathy and Myocarditis

Dilated cardiomyopathy, characterized by left ventricular dilation and systolic dysfunction without a coronary or valvular etiology sufficient to explain the degree of dysfunction observed, demonstrates a variable late gadolinium enhancement pattern on cardiac MRI, with a substantial proportion of cases showing no late gadolinium enhancement at all and others demonstrating a mid-wall, linear, septal-predominant pattern distinct from both the ischemic pattern and the more diffusely patchy hypertrophic cardiomyopathy pattern discussed above, and the presence and extent of this mid-wall enhancement, when present, carries independent prognostic significance for both arrhythmic risk and overall mortality beyond ejection fraction alone. Acute myocarditis, inflammatory myocardial injury most commonly related to a preceding viral illness, demonstrates a characteristic combination of findings applying the updated Lake Louise criteria framework, myocardial edema on T2-weighted or T2 mapping sequences, and non-ischemic, typically subepicardial or mid-wall, late gadolinium enhancement, most commonly involving the inferolateral wall, a combination of edema and non-ischemic-pattern fibrosis that together support this diagnosis with substantially greater confidence than either finding in isolation, and cardiac MRI has become an essential diagnostic tool for myocarditis given both its non-invasive nature relative to endomyocardial biopsy and its superior sensitivity relative to the comparatively nonspecific findings biopsy of a patchy, sometimes missed inflammatory process can otherwise provide.

THE SIGNAL-TO-CATEGORY DECISION SYSTEM — Late Gadolinium Enhancement Pattern Categorization

---

The Signal Pattern: Late gadolinium enhancement is identified on cardiac MRI, and the reader must characterize its distribution, subendocardial versus mid-wall versus subepicardial, and determine whether it respects a specific coronary artery vascular territory.

Category Signature: Subendocardial or transmural enhancement respecting a single coronary artery territory is categorized as an ischemic pattern; mid-wall, subepicardial, or patchy enhancement not respecting a coronary territory is categorized as a non-ischemic pattern, further characterized by its specific distribution, septal mid-wall, right ventricular insertion point, or inferolateral subepicardial, to suggest a specific underlying cardiomyopathy.

The Decision: An ischemic pattern supports coronary artery evaluation and consideration of revascularization, with viability assessment discussed in the following section further refining this decision; a non-ischemic pattern supports the specific cardiomyopathy-directed workup suggested by its distribution, whether hypertrophic cardiomyopathy, myocarditis, sarcoidosis, or another non-ischemic entity.

Trap Logic: Diffuse or extensive disease can obscure the subendocardial-versus-mid-wall distinction this categorization fundamentally depends upon, since severe, confluent enhancement spanning the full myocardial thickness can appear similar regardless of its true point of origin, and partial volume averaging from an insufficiently thin imaging slice can further blur this distinction; the discriminating step is correlating the enhancement's overall distribution across multiple myocardial segments and slices with expected coronary territory anatomy, rather than assessing a single segment's transmural extent in isolation.

Pattern Anchor: Correlate late gadolinium enhancement distribution with coronary artery territory anatomy across multiple segments before categorizing as ischemic or non-ischemic; enhancement that does not respect a vascular territory favors a non-ischemic etiology regardless of its transmural extent within any single segment.

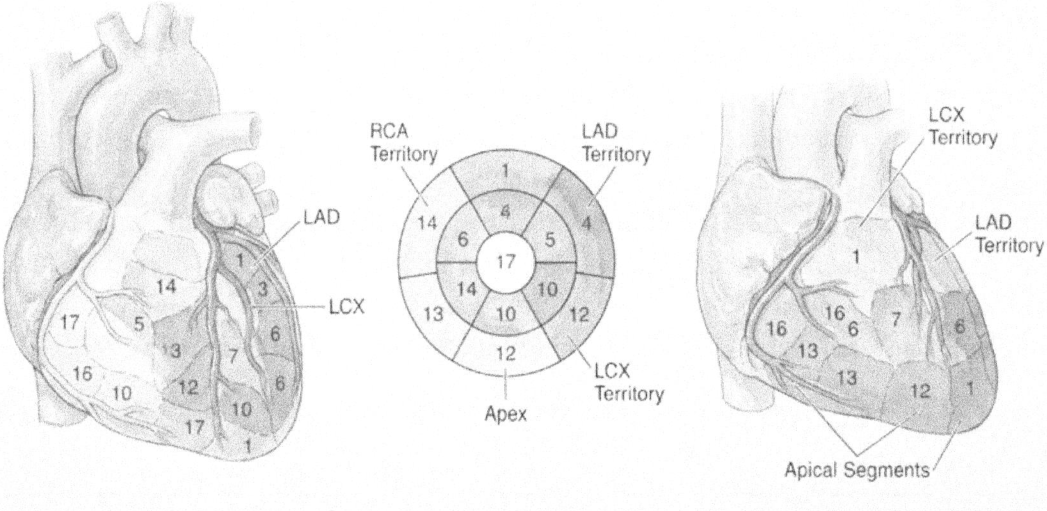

Figure 24.2 — Coronary Artery Territory and Myocardial Segment Anatomy

CLINICAL PEARL: Late gadolinium enhancement distribution, not extent within a single segment, is the primary discriminator between ischemic and non-ischemic disease; enhancement crossing multiple coronary territories or confined to the mid-wall or subepicardium favors a non-ischemic cardiomyopathy regardless of how extensive the enhancement appears.

CAUTION: A nulling difficulty during late gadolinium enhancement imaging, in which normal myocardium cannot be adequately suppressed relative to the blood pool, is itself a diagnostic clue suggesting diffuse infiltrative disease such as cardiac amyloidosis, and should prompt native T1 mapping correlation rather than being dismissed as a technical failure alone.

Cardiac Amyloidosis and Infiltrative Cardiomyopathy

Cardiac amyloidosis, myocardial infiltration by misfolded amyloid protein, most commonly transthyretin-related or light chain-related in etiology, produces a characteristic diffuse, global, predominantly subendocardial late gadolinium enhancement pattern often accompanied by a distinctive nulling difficulty in which the normal myocardium and blood pool null at a similar inversion time, reflecting the diffuse gadolinium retention throughout the amyloid-infiltrated myocardium, a pattern distinct from both the ischemic and the other non-ischemic patterns discussed throughout this chapter and one that native T1 mapping, discussed in this chapter's technique section, characteristically confirms through markedly elevated native T1 values reflecting the expanded extracellular space this infiltrative process produces. Distinguishing transthyretin from light chain amyloidosis, a distinction carrying substantial treatment and prognostic significance given each subtype's distinct underlying mechanism and available disease-specific therapy, relies on a combination of imaging pattern, patient demographic and clinical context, most notably older age and, for transthyretin amyloidosis, a wild-type or hereditary genetic basis, and dedicated nuclear medicine bone scintigraphy, which demonstrates a characteristic cardiac radiotracer uptake pattern specific to transthyretin amyloidosis, together with serum and urine testing for the abnormal light chain protein characteristic of the light chain subtype, illustrating cardiac MRI's role as one essential component within a broader, multimodality diagnostic pathway for this specific infiltrative cardiomyopathy rather than a fully standalone diagnostic tool.

Myocardial Viability and Ischemic Heart Disease

Transmural Extent Quantification and Functional Recovery Prediction

Myocardial viability assessment, determining whether a hypokinetic or akinetic myocardial segment retains the potential for functional recovery following revascularization, relies on quantifying the transmural extent of late gadolinium enhancement within each affected segment, applying the well-established principle that a segment with limited transmural scar extent, generally under 50 percent of wall thickness, retains substantial viable myocardium and a correspondingly favorable likelihood of functional recovery following successful revascularization, while a segment with extensive transmural scar, generally exceeding 50 percent of wall thickness, is unlikely to demonstrate meaningful functional recovery even if blood flow is successfully restored, since the scarred, non-viable tissue itself cannot regain contractile function regardless of its perfusion status. This segment-by-segment transmural extent quantification, applied systematically across the standard seventeen-segment left ventricular model referenced in this chapter's coronary territory figure, provides the cardiology and cardiac surgery team with a detailed, spatially specific viability map directly informing the revascularization strategy, since a patient with extensive non-viable segments throughout a broad myocardial territory may derive limited benefit from an aggressive revascularization approach relative to a patient with a more limited scar burden and substantial viable, potentially recoverable myocardium.

Microvascular Obstruction and Acute Infarction

Microvascular obstruction, a no-reflow phenomenon in which the microvasculature within the infarct core remains obstructed despite successful restoration of epicardial coronary artery flow, appears on early, first-pass or early postcontrast imaging as a dark, non-enhancing core within the otherwise hyperenhancing infarct territory, a finding requiring specifically timed early imaging to reliably detect given this phenomenon's tendency to fill in and become less conspicuous, or entirely obscured, on the standard, later-timed late gadolinium enhancement acquisition discussed throughout this chapter's technique section. Recognition of microvascular obstruction carries independent prognostic significance beyond infarct size and transmural extent alone, associated with adverse left ventricular remodeling and increased major adverse cardiac event risk following acute myocardial infarction, and this finding's detection specifically requires the interpreting radiologist or cardiologist to deliberately acquire and review early postcontrast imaging in the acute infarction setting, rather than relying solely on the standard-timing late gadolinium enhancement sequence that this specific early-phase finding can be substantially underrepresented or entirely missed on.

Figure 24.3 — Procedural Diagram: Percutaneous Coronary Intervention

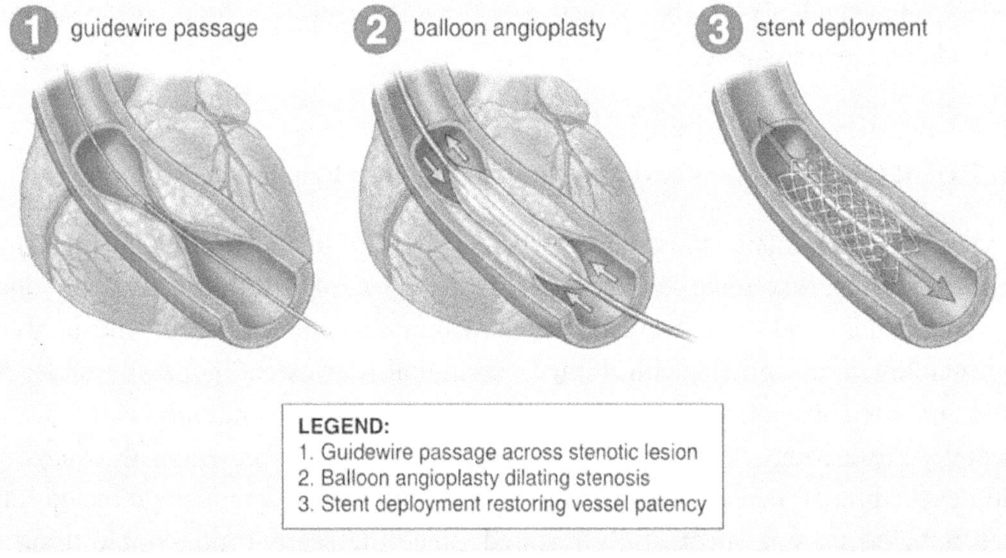

THE SIGNAL-TO-CATEGORY DECISION SYSTEM — Myocardial Viability Segmental Assessment

The Signal Pattern: A hypokinetic or akinetic myocardial segment is identified in a patient with known coronary artery disease being considered for revascularization, and the reader must quantify the transmural extent of late gadolinium enhancement within that specific segment.

Category Signature: A segment with transmural late gadolinium enhancement extent under 50 percent of wall thickness is categorized as viable; a segment with transmural extent of 50 percent or greater is categorized as non-viable, applied and reported individually across every affected segment using the standard seventeen-segment model.

The Decision: Predominantly viable segments support proceeding with revascularization given the favorable likelihood of functional recovery; predominantly non-viable segments support a more conservative approach, since revascularization is unlikely to meaningfully improve function in myocardium that has already progressed to extensive transmural scarring.

Trap Logic: Microvascular obstruction within an acute infarct core can be substantially underrepresented on standard-timing late gadolinium enhancement imaging if early postcontrast imaging is not specifically acquired, risking an incomplete acute prognostic assessment that fails to capture this independently significant adverse finding; the discriminating step is deliberately acquiring and reviewing early postcontrast imaging in the acute infarction setting specifically to assess for microvascular obstruction, rather than relying on standard-timing imaging alone.

Pattern Anchor: Quantify transmural extent segment by segment using the standard model, not a single global impression, to predict functional recovery; in the acute setting, specifically assess early postcontrast imaging for microvascular obstruction, a finding standard-timing imaging alone can miss.

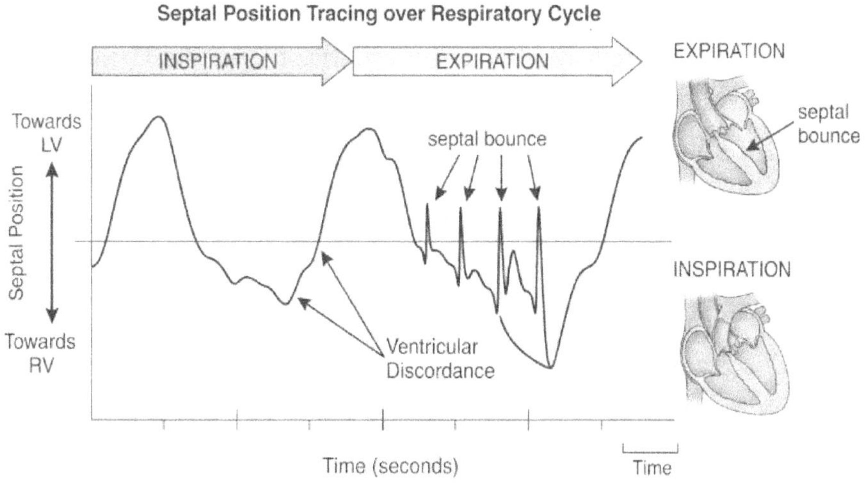

Figure 24.4: Real-Time Cine Septal Bounce Tracing in Constrictive Pericarditis

Pericardial Disease

Epidemiology and Etiology of Pericardial Disease

Pericardial disease spans a broad etiologic spectrum, with idiopathic or presumed viral pericarditis representing the most common cause of acute pericarditis and associated effusion in most clinical populations, and malignant pericardial effusion, most commonly from lung, breast, or hematologic malignancy metastatic to the pericardium, representing a distinct and clinically important etiology given both its generally more guarded prognosis and its frequent association with recurrent, symptomatic effusion requiring more assertive management than the typically self-limited idiopathic or viral presentation. Constrictive pericarditis, discussed in greater technical detail in the following section, most commonly arises following cardiac surgery, radiation therapy to the chest, or, in regions with higher tuberculosis prevalence, tuberculous pericarditis, and this etiologic context carries direct relevance to pretest diagnostic probability when a patient presents with the clinical syndrome of diastolic dysfunction and systemic venous congestion this condition characteristically produces, supporting a higher index of suspicion for constrictive disease specifically in a patient with a compatible surgical, radiation, or tuberculosis exposure history.

Pericardial Effusion and Tamponade

Pericardial effusion, fluid accumulation within the pericardial space, is readily identified on cardiac MRI as fluid signal, variable in T1 and T2 characteristics depending on the effusion's protein content and any hemorrhagic component, separating the visceral and parietal pericardial layers, and while echocardiography remains the primary, first-line modality for pericardial effusion assessment given its rapid, bedside availability, cardiac MRI provides valuable complementary characterization for a loculated or complex effusion, for distinguishing hemorrhagic from simple effusion based on signal characteristics, and for identifying associated pericardial thickening or nodularity that might suggest an underlying malignant or inflammatory process rather than a simple, idiopathic effusion. Cardiac tamponade, hemodynamically significant compression of the cardiac chambers from pericardial fluid accumulation, represents a clinical diagnosis primarily established through physical examination and echocardiographic hemodynamic assessment rather than MRI-specific criteria, though MRI-identified findings including right ventricular diastolic collapse and exaggerated respiratory septal motion, when present, corroborate this diagnosis and, together with the effusion characterization discussed above, contribute to the comprehensive imaging picture supporting the urgent pericardiocentesis this diagnosis generally requires.

Constrictive Pericarditis

Constrictive pericarditis, a fibrotic, thickened, and often calcified pericardium restricting normal diastolic ventricular filling, produces a distinct hemodynamic pattern requiring careful distinction from restrictive cardiomyopathy, a myocardial rather than pericardial process producing a superficially similar clinical presentation of diastolic dysfunction and systemic venous congestion, and cardiac MRI contributes both direct morphologic assessment of pericardial thickness, generally exceeding 4 millimeters in constrictive disease though notably present in only a subset of confirmed cases, making pericardial thickness alone an imperfect discriminator, and dynamic, real-time cine imaging demonstrating the characteristic septal bounce, an abrupt, early-diastolic septal motion abnormality reflecting the discordant respiratory filling pattern between the ventricles characteristic of constrictive physiology. This constrictive-versus-restrictive distinction carries substantial treatment significance, since constrictive pericarditis is a potentially surgically curable condition through pericardiectomy, while restrictive cardiomyopathy generally requires medical management directed at the underlying myocardial process, making the combination of morphologic pericardial assessment and the dynamic, functional cine imaging findings discussed above, rather than either category of finding in isolation, essential to confident, actionable distinction between these two conditions with such divergent treatment implications.

Practical Considerations: Cardiac Devices and MRI Safety

Cardiac implantable electronic devices, including pacemakers and implantable cardioverter-defibrillators, historically represented an absolute contraindication to MRI given concerns regarding lead heating, device malfunction, and inappropriate device therapy delivery in the scanner's magnetic and radiofrequency environment, but the development and now widespread availability of MRI-conditional device systems, together with established protocols for safely scanning even a subset of legacy, non-conditional devices under appropriate monitoring and device reprogramming precautions, has substantially expanded MRI access for the many patients who both require cardiac device therapy and would benefit from the cardiac or other body MRI applications discussed throughout this book. Confirming a specific device's MRI conditional status, together with adherence to the device-specific scanning protocol, including any required preprocedural device interrogation and reprogramming and postprocedural device function verification, represents an essential safety prerequisite before proceeding with any MRI examination in a patient with a cardiac implantable electronic device, and close coordination between the radiology and cardiology or electrophysiology teams, following the specific institutional protocol developed for this patient population, supports safe examination completion without the device-related complications this specific safety consideration is designed to prevent.

Thoracic Applications: Mediastinal and Chest Wall Imaging

Mediastinal Mass Characterization

Mediastinal mass characterization on MRI applies a compartmental localization framework, anterior, middle, and posterior mediastinum, directly analogous in organizing principle to the compartment-based frameworks applied throughout this book's pelvic floor and other anatomically compartmentalized chapters, with the anterior mediastinum characteristically harboring thymoma, lymphoma, germ cell tumor, and thyroid-related masses, the middle mediastinum harboring lymphadenopathy and foregut duplication cysts, and the posterior mediastinum harboring neurogenic tumors, paralleling the neuroblastoma and related entities discussed in the preceding pediatric chapter for their thoracic paraspinal counterpart presentation in this specific compartment. MRI's particular value for mediastinal mass characterization lies in its superior soft tissue contrast for distinguishing a cystic from a solid mass, relevant given the substantially different differential diagnosis and management implications this distinction carries, and in its capability for direct assessment of great vessel or cardiac invasion for a locally advanced anterior or middle mediastinal malignancy, a surgical planning consideration for which MRI's multiplanar capability and superior soft tissue contrast offer genuine advantages over CT for the specific subset of cases where this invasion assessment proves genuinely ambiguous on CT alone.

Chest Wall Mass and Brachial Plexus Considerations

Chest wall mass evaluation, whether for a soft tissue sarcoma, a metastatic deposit, or a benign entity including a rib-based lesion or peripheral nerve sheath tumor, benefits from MRI's superior soft tissue characterization for determining the specific tissue plane of origin and the relationship to adjacent critical structures, including the brachial plexus for a mass in the thoracic inlet or axillary region, an anatomic relationship carrying direct surgical planning significance given the functional consequences that inadvertent brachial plexus injury during resection would produce. Pancoast tumor, a superior sulcus lung malignancy characteristically invading the brachial plexus, subclavian vessels, and adjacent vertebral structures, represents a specific and clinically important application of this thoracic inlet imaging principle, with MRI's detailed characterization of the specific structures invaded, whether the lower brachial plexus trunks alone or more extensive vertebral or vascular involvement, directly informing surgical resectability assessment and, for a tumor with more extensive invasion, the decision to pursue neoadjuvant chemoradiation before any surgical resection is attempted, paralleling the neoadjuvant-therapy-before-surgery treatment sequencing principle this book has emphasized across several other anatomically challenging oncologic staging contexts.

Clinical Case Presentations

Case 1. A 58-year-old man with a remote myocardial infarction and reduced ejection fraction undergoes viability assessment, demonstrating subendocardial late gadolinium enhancement with transmural extent under 50 percent in the mid-anterior and anteroseptal segments, corresponding to a hypokinetic left anterior descending territory. The radiologist categorizes these segments as viable, and the patient proceeds to revascularization with subsequent functional improvement confirmed on follow-up imaging.

Case 2. A 34-year-old man with a recent febrile illness presents with chest pain and elevated cardiac biomarkers without significant coronary stenosis on angiography, and cardiac MRI demonstrates myocardial edema on T2 mapping together with subepicardial, non-coronary-territory late gadolinium enhancement in the inferolateral wall. The radiologist categorizes the findings as consistent with acute myocarditis per the Lake Louise criteria, correlating the non-ischemic distribution pattern with the clinical presentation to establish this diagnosis without requiring endomyocardial biopsy.

Case 3. A 45-year-old competitive athlete with a family history of sudden cardiac death undergoes cardiac MRI demonstrating asymmetric septal hypertrophy measuring 22 millimeters with patchy, mid-wall late gadolinium enhancement at the right ventricular insertion points, and no significant left ventricular outflow tract obstruction on flow imaging. The radiologist categorizes the findings as hypertrophic cardiomyopathy with a moderate fibrotic burden, and the quantified enhancement extent contributes to the patient's overall sudden cardiac death risk stratification and subsequent implantable defibrillator discussion.

Case 4. A 62-year-old woman with progressive dyspnea, hepatomegaly, and systemic venous congestion undergoes cardiac MRI demonstrating pericardial thickening measuring 6 millimeters with associated calcification and a characteristic septal bounce on real-time cine imaging during respiration. The radiologist categorizes the findings as constrictive pericarditis rather than restrictive cardiomyopathy, correlating the morphologic thickening with the dynamic septal bounce finding, and the patient proceeds to surgical pericardiectomy evaluation.

Case 5. A 51-year-old man with a superior sulcus lung mass undergoes dedicated thoracic inlet MRI demonstrating tumor invasion of the lower brachial plexus trunks and adjacent subclavian artery without vertebral body invasion. The radiologist categorizes the findings as a Pancoast tumor with brachial plexus and vascular invasion, and the multidisciplinary team recommends neoadjuvant chemoradiation before surgical resection is attempted, given the extent of invasion identified.

Case 6. A 71-year-old man with heart failure with preserved ejection fraction and bilateral carpal tunnel syndrome undergoes cardiac MRI demonstrating diffuse, global subendocardial late gadolinium enhancement with a nulling difficulty in which normal myocardium and blood pool null at a similar inversion time, together with markedly elevated native T1 values. The radiologist categorizes the findings as consistent with cardiac amyloidosis, and given his age and the absence of a monoclonal protein on subsequent laboratory testing, confirmatory bone scintigraphy supports a diagnosis of transthyretin, rather than light chain, amyloidosis, directing him toward transthyretin-specific therapy.

Case 7. A 39-year-old woman with a pacemaker implanted for complete heart block requires cardiac MRI for evaluation of new heart failure symptoms, and after confirming her device is MRI-conditional and completing the required preprocedural device interrogation and reprogramming per institutional protocol, the examination proceeds without complication, demonstrating a non-ischemic, mid-wall septal late gadolinium enhancement pattern. Postprocedural device interrogation confirms normal device function, and the findings support a non-ischemic dilated cardiomyopathy diagnosis with independent prognostic significance from the mid-wall enhancement identified.

THE SIGNAL-TO-CATEGORY DECISION SYSTEM — Myocardial Tissue Characterization Arc

The Signal Pattern: This chapter's patterns share a tissue characterization structure anchored by late gadolinium enhancement, from distribution-based ischemic-versus-non-ischemic categorization to segment-by-segment transmural extent quantification for viability.

Category Signature: Enhancement is categorized ischemic or non-ischemic based on coronary territory correlation; viability is categorized viable or non-viable per segment based on transmural extent relative to the 50 percent threshold.

The Decision: Category assignment in this chapter ranges from cardiomyopathy-specific workup for a non-ischemic pattern to coronary evaluation for an ischemic pattern, and from revascularization for predominantly viable myocardium to conservative management for predominantly non-viable, scarred myocardium.

The Trap Logic: Both patterns in this chapter share a common trap: an incomplete or improperly timed assessment, diffuse disease obscuring distribution pattern, or standard-timing imaging missing microvascular obstruction, that produces a category assignment not reflecting the complete underlying tissue state.

Pattern Anchor: Correlate enhancement distribution with coronary anatomy across multiple segments, and quantify transmural extent segment by segment with deliberate early-phase imaging in the acute setting, before finalizing either category in this chapter; incomplete technique or assessment risks a management decision the true myocardial tissue state does not support.

Summary and Key Concepts

Cine cardiac MRI provides the reference-standard measurement of ventricular volumes, ejection fraction, and regional wall motion using electrocardiographically gated balanced steady-state free precession imaging.

Late gadolinium enhancement distinguishes ischemic, subendocardial or transmural and coronary territory-respecting, from non-ischemic, mid-wall or subepicardial, fibrotic patterns, directly guiding cardiomyopathy-specific workup.

Hypertrophic cardiomyopathy shows patchy mid-wall enhancement at right ventricular insertion points; acute myocarditis shows combined T2 edema and non-ischemic subepicardial enhancement per the Lake Louise criteria.

Myocardial viability is determined by segment-by-segment transmural late gadolinium enhancement extent, with under 50 percent supporting functional recovery potential following revascularization.

Microvascular obstruction, a no-reflow phenomenon within an acute infarct core, requires deliberate early postcontrast imaging for detection and carries independent adverse prognostic significance.

Constrictive pericarditis is distinguished from restrictive cardiomyopathy through pericardial thickening together with the dynamic septal bounce finding on real-time cine imaging, a distinction carrying major treatment implications.

Mediastinal mass compartmental localization, anterior, middle, and posterior, directs the differential diagnosis, and MRI provides superior soft tissue contrast for assessing great vessel, cardiac, and brachial plexus invasion.

THE SIGNAL-TO-CATEGORY MASTER INDEX

The Signal-to-Category Master Index consolidates every Signal-to-Category Decision System instance introduced throughout this textbook into a single, indexed, cross-referenced reference navigator. Each entry restates the pattern's name, its Category Signature, its governing Decision, and its Pattern Anchor, the single discriminating step that prevents the most common categorization error for that pattern, organized by the same seven-part organ-system structure used throughout the book's table of contents and cross-referenced to its originating chapter. This index is designed for rapid consultation during clinical practice, on call, in a multidisciplinary tumor board, or during case preparation, functioning as a scannable structural reference rather than a narrative retelling of chapter content. A closing alphabetical Quick-Lookup Index and a Named-Framework Cross-Reference table provide two additional pathways into the same underlying pattern set, by pattern name and by established diagnostic framework respectively.

How to Use This Master Index

Three navigation pathways are provided, each suited to a different lookup scenario. A reader who recalls the relevant organ system or anatomic region, adrenal, hepatobiliary, gynecologic, should proceed directly to the corresponding Part below, where every pattern from that organ system's chapters is tabulated together regardless of which specific chapter it originated in. A reader who recalls a specific standardized diagnostic framework by name, Bosniak, PI-RADS, O-RADS, and needs to locate the corresponding pattern and chapter should proceed to the Named-Framework Cross-Reference table. A reader who recalls a pattern's name but not its organ system, or who is scanning for a specific keyword within a pattern title, should proceed to the closing Quick-Lookup Alphabetical Index, which lists every pattern in this textbook by name with its chapter of origin. Each table entry's Category Signature and Pattern Anchor columns are deliberately condensed relative to the full Rhythm Layer discussion in the originating chapter, distilled specifically to the single categorization rule and single discriminating trap most essential to safe, confident application, and a reader requiring the complete clinical reasoning, evidence base, trap logic discussion, and management detail behind any entry should consult the cited chapter directly.

Part I: Foundations — Physics, Protocol, Safety, and Artifact

The four foundational patterns in this part share a common structural theme: distinguishing a genuine finding from a technical artifact or a safety-relevant signal, the discriminating skill that underlies confident interpretation throughout the remainder of this textbook.

Pattern (Chapter)	Category Signature	Pattern Anchor
Chemical Shift Artifact and the Lipid-Poor Adenoma Trap (Ch. 1)	Intravoxel signal drop-out is lipid and diagnostic; a peripheral dark line alone is artifact only	Signal loss inside the lesion means lipid; a dark line only at its edge means nothing

Susceptibility Artifact from Metallic Hardware (Ch. 1)	Round or linear geometry matching known hardware history is artifact, not pathology	Switch to wide-bandwidth fast spin-echo before concluding an area cannot be assessed
Respiratory Misregistration and the Pseudo-Lesion Trap (Ch. 2)	A finding that follows the diaphragmatic contour and vanishes on an adjacent sequence is misregistration	A subcapsular finding that changes or disappears across breath-hold depths is misregistration, not pathology
Incomplete Bowel Distension Mimicking Wall Thickening (Ch. 2)	Apparent thickening confined to a collapsed loop that normalizes on another sequence is distension-related	Never characterize wall thickening on a single sequence without confirming adequate distension
Grading the Acute Contrast Reaction (Ch. 3)	Cutaneous findings alone are mild; bronchospasm or facial edema without airway compromise is moderate; airway or hemodynamic compromise is severe	Hypotension with tachycardia points to true reaction; hypotension with bradycardia points to a vasovagal event
Screening the Implanted Cardiac Device (Ch. 3)	A device verified MR-conditional at the intended field strength with requirements met is safe to proceed	No device proceeds on verbal report alone; verify the specific model against current labeling every time
Aortic Pulsation Ghosting Mimicking a Lesion (Ch. 4)	Findings aligned with the phase-encoding direction, recurring as evenly spaced fainter foci, are ghosting	Any focal finding along the phase-encoding direction from the aorta is presumed ghosting until proven otherwise
Dielectric Shading Mimicking Diffuse Disease (Ch. 4)	A geographic signal alteration ignoring organ boundaries, worse centrally at 3 tesla, is dielectric shading	A geographic abnormality ignoring organ boundaries in a large-habitus 3-tesla patient is presumed dielectric artifact

Part II: Hepatobiliary and Pancreatic

This part's patterns govern the liver, biliary tree, and pancreas, spanning diffuse parenchymal quantification, focal lesion characterization, ductal filling defects, and pancreatic mass and cyst triage.

Pattern (Chapter)	Category Signature	Pattern Anchor
Iron-Confounded Fat Quantification (Ch. 5)	A discordant fat fraction with elevated R2-star reflects coexistent iron and requires cautious interpretation	Never finalize a fat fraction grade without checking R2-star or T2-star for confounding iron
Elastography Stiffness Confounded by Inflammation (Ch. 5)	Elevated stiffness with acute transaminase elevation or venous congestion is confounded, not true fibrosis	Elevated stiffness with acute hepatitis or heart failure warrants deferral, not immediate fibrosis staging
Flash-Filling Hemangioma Mimicking Malignancy (Ch. 6)	Sustained enhancement matched to blood pool through delayed phase, without washout, is flash-filling hemangioma	Never diagnose flash-filling hemangioma from the arterial phase alone; confirm sustained matched enhancement through delayed phase
LI-RADS Category Assignment and the Pseudocapsule Trap (Ch. 6)	A smooth, complete, uniformly enhancing rim in the at-risk population is a true capsule favoring LR-5	Confirm capsule timing, completeness, and population before applying this category
True Ductal Calculus versus Pneumobilia (Ch. 7)	A dependently layering, faceted, blooming defect is calculus; a nondependent, non-blooming defect is gas	Check for blooming on gradient-echo and correlate with sphincterotomy history before diagnosing calculus
Malignant versus Post-Inflammatory Benign Stricture (Ch. 7)	A short, smooth, tapering stricture without an enhancing mass at a plausible benign site favors benign	Base categorization on the presence of an associated enhancing soft tissue component when history is discordant
IPMN Risk Stratification (Ch. 8)	A branch-duct cyst under 3 cm without a mural nodule or main duct dilation is low-risk	Never categorize a mural nodule as high-risk without confirming genuine enhancement relative to a precontrast baseline
Adenocarcinoma versus Mass-Forming Pancreatitis (Ch. 8)	Ill-defined, duct-penetrating morphology favors adenocarcinoma; duct-penetrating sign favors pancreatitis	The duct-penetrating sign favors pancreatitis but should not be treated as absolutely excluding malignancy

Part III: Splenic, Adrenal, and Retroperitoneal

This part's patterns address the spleen, adrenal gland, and retroperitoneal and peritoneal compartments, three anatomic regions unified by a shared emphasis on confirming true enhancement and biochemical safety before proceeding to biopsy.

Pattern (Chapter)	Category Signature	Pattern Anchor
Cystic versus Solid Splenic Lesion Triage (Ch. 9)	Simple T2-hyperintense signal without any postcontrast enhancement is cystic; any measurable enhancement is solid	The cystic-versus-solid branch point is decided by postcontrast enhancement alone, not precontrast signal complexity
Diffuse Splenic Infiltration versus Reactive Splenomegaly (Ch. 9)	A discrete mass or miliary nodular pattern favors infiltration; homogeneous signal favors reactive change	Splenic size alone is unreliable; integrate parenchymal signal homogeneity before assigning category
Chemical-Shift Signal Drop Adenoma Triage (Ch. 10)	Signal drop exceeding the validated threshold is lipid-rich adenoma; macroscopic fat is myelolipoma	A negative chemical-shift result does not exclude malignancy in a lipid-poor lesion
Indeterminate Adrenal Mass versus Pheochromocytoma Safety Check (Ch. 10)	Marked T2 hyperintensity with avid enhancement and no signal drop is suspicious for pheochromocytoma	Biochemical screening, not imaging phenotype, is the definitive safety gate before biopsy
Fat-Containing Retroperitoneal Mass Triage (Ch. 11)	Homogeneous uncomplicated fat without septation favors lipoma; nodular septation or a non-fatty component favors liposarcoma	In the retroperitoneum, a fat-containing mass is treated as liposarcoma until proven otherwise
Peritoneal Nodularity: Benign versus Carcinomatosis (Ch. 11)	Smooth, thin, uniform enhancement with a plausible benign cause favors reactive change; nodularity favors carcinomatosis	Nodular peritoneal thickening is not synonymous with carcinomatosis; granulomatous disease can mimic this pattern

Part IV: Genitourinary

This part's patterns anchor renal, prostate, bladder, and scrotal mass characterization, including three of the book's standardized categorical frameworks, Bosniak, PI-RADS, and VI-RADS, each cross-referenced again in the Named-Framework table below.

Pattern (Chapter)	Category Signature	Pattern Anchor
Bosniak Category Assignment (Ch. 12)	Septation number, thickness, and confirmed enhancement determine category I through IV	Category assignment hinges on confirmed true enhancement and convex nodular morphology at the III-versus-IV boundary
Angiomyolipoma versus Fat-Poor RCC Trap (Ch. 12)	Unambiguous macroscopic fat without calcification is classic angiomyolipoma; fat with calcification is not	Confirm fat is genuinely intralesional before applying the reassuring angiomyolipoma category
Acute Pyelonephritis versus Renal Abscess Triage (Ch. 13)	Wedge-shaped reduced enhancement without a discrete collection is pyelonephritis; a rim-enhancing collection is abscess	A discrete, rim-enhancing, non-enhancing-center collection mandates drainage
Urothelial Tumor versus Stone or Clot Trap (Ch. 13)	A filling defect with measurable soft tissue enhancement favors tumor; a non-enhancing defect favors stone or clot	True enhancement, not the presence of a filling defect alone, distinguishes tumor from stone or clot
PI-RADS Category Assignment (Ch. 14)	Peripheral zone category follows diffusion and ADC appearance; transition zone category follows T2 morphology	Confirm the lesion's zone of origin before applying category criteria; the dominant sequence differs by zone
Transition Zone Cancer versus BPH Nodule (Ch. 14)	A well-circumscribed, encapsulated, heterogeneous nodule favors benign hyperplasia; a lenticular, homogeneous lesion favors cancer	Margin and encapsulation, not signal intensity alone, distinguish benign nodule from transition zone cancer
VI-RADS Category Assignment (Ch. 15)	An intact, continuous low-signal muscularis propria layer is VI-RADS 1 or 2; disruption raises category	Assess muscularis propria integrity, not lesion size, as the primary category-determining feature

Intratesticular versus Extratesticular Scrotal Mass Triage (Ch. 15)	A mass clearly distinct from normal testicular parenchyma is extratesticular; a mass distorting the testis is intratesticular	An intratesticular solid mass in an adult defaults to malignant and proceeds to orchiectomy, not biopsy

Part V: Gynecologic and Female Pelvic

This part's patterns span uterine, adnexal, and pelvic floor imaging, including the O-RADS framework and the compartment-based logic shared by pelvic organ prolapse grading and deep infiltrating endometriosis mapping.

Pattern (Chapter)	Category Signature	Pattern Anchor
Leiomyoma versus Leiomyosarcoma Triage (Ch. 16)	Well-defined, homogeneously low T2 signal without diffusion restriction favors leiomyoma; ill-defined margins with restriction favor sarcoma	No single feature excludes leiomyosarcoma; integrate margin, diffusion, and growth trajectory together
Myometrial Invasion Depth Assessment (Ch. 16)	Inner-half invasion versus outer-half invasion determines lymphadenectomy extent in endometrial carcinoma	Distinguish true invasive extension from mechanical thinning by an exophytic mass using dynamic enhancement
O-RADS Category Assignment (Ch. 17)	Composition, septation, and confirmed solid component enhancement kinetics assign category 1 through 5	Confirm true enhancement of any apparent solid component; clotted blood commonly mimics a solid nodule
Ovarian Torsion Surgical Urgency Triage (Ch. 17)	Preserved enhancement supports urgent detorsion with salvage potential; absent enhancement suggests compromised viability	Assess perfusion, not size, to inform urgency; intermittent torsion can produce a falsely reassuring single examination
Pelvic Organ Prolapse Compartment Grading (Ch. 18)	Descent under 1 cm is mild, 1 to 3 cm is moderate, over 3 cm is severe, per compartment	Confirm genuine maximal straining effort; report all three compartments independently
Deep Infiltrating Endometriosis Compartment Mapping (Ch. 18)	Infiltration beyond 5 mm below the peritoneal surface into a named structure is deep infiltrating disease	Search each compartment individually; a fused, adhesion-distorted pelvis most often conceals a missed nodule

Part VI: Gastrointestinal and Mesenteric

This part's patterns govern inflammatory bowel disease activity, rectal cancer staging, and peritoneal and mesenteric vascular disease, unified by the shared distinction between active or viable tissue and its fibrotic, scarred, or necrotic counterpart.

Pattern (Chapter)	Category Signature	Pattern Anchor
Crohn Disease Mural Activity Assessment (Ch. 19)	Stratified hyperenhancement with restricted diffusion is active disease; homogeneous mild enhancement with low T2 signal is fibrotic	Characterize enhancement pattern and diffusion signal together, not wall thickness alone
Perianal Fistula Sphincter Classification (Ch. 19)	Tract course relative to the internal and external sphincter assigns intersphincteric through extrasphincteric category	Trace the complete tract including secondary extensions before finalizing classification
Mesorectal Fascia Threat Assessment (Ch. 20)	Measured tumor-to-fascia distance assigns clear, threatened, or involved anticipated margin	Measure the shortest tumor-to-fascia distance including deposits and nodes, not T-stage alone
Post-Neoadjuvant Response Categorization (Ch. 20)	Fibrosis without residual signal or diffusion restriction is complete response; persistent signal with restriction is poor response	Correlate T2 fibrosis morphology with diffusion signal together before assigning regression grade
Peritoneal Cancer Index Regional Scoring (Ch. 21)	Thirteen regions scored 0 to 3 by lesion size sum to a composite index guiding cytoreductive candidacy	Score all regions systematically; small bowel and mesenteric regions carry the greatest imaging-surgical discordance risk
Mesenteric Ischemia Vascular Territory Assessment (Ch. 21)	Preserved mural enhancement despite vessel occlusion is viable bowel; absent enhancement is non-viable, infarcted bowel	Correlate enhancement with vessel patency and collateral status; absent enhancement mandates resection regardless of intervention

Part VII: Oncologic, Whole-Body, and Advanced Applications

This part's patterns close the book with whole-body, pediatric, prenatal, and cardiac applications, each extending the same tissue-characterization discipline established in Part I to progressively more specialized clinical contexts.

Pattern (Chapter)	Category Signature	Pattern Anchor
Diffusion Whole-Body Lesion Categorization (Ch. 22)	Diffuse restriction with preserved T1 fat signal is benign marrow reconversion; a focal lesion with replaced fat signal is suspicious	Correlate diffusion restriction with T1 fat signal and distribution before categorizing as suspicious
Cancer Predisposition Surveillance Finding Categorization (Ch. 22)	Findings are categorized benign, probably benign, or indeterminate-suspicious using a standardized structured framework	Apply the structured categorization framework to every finding, expected and incidental alike
Pediatric Renal and Adrenal Mass Categorization (Ch. 23)	An intrarenal claw sign favors Wilms tumor; an extrarenal mass with encasement and calcification favors neuroblastoma	Establish organ of origin through the claw sign and vessel relationship, not overall tumor gestalt
Fetal MRI Anomaly Categorization (Ch. 23)	A finding within gestational-age-appropriate normative range is a variant; outside this range is a confirmed anomaly	Correlate every finding against gestational-age-matched normative values before categorizing as abnormal
Late Gadolinium Enhancement Pattern Categorization (Ch. 24)	Enhancement respecting a coronary territory is ischemic; enhancement not respecting a territory is non-ischemic	Correlate enhancement distribution with coronary anatomy across multiple segments before categorizing
Myocardial Viability Segmental Assessment (Ch. 24)	Transmural extent under 50 percent is viable; 50 percent or greater is non-viable, scored per segment	Quantify transmural extent segment by segment; assess early postcontrast imaging for microvascular obstruction in the acute setting

Named-Framework Cross-Reference

Several patterns in this index implement a widely recognized, externally standardized diagnostic framework rather than a system unique to this textbook. This cross-reference identifies each such framework, the pattern that applies it, and its chapter location, for the reader specifically seeking the standardized-framework application rather than browsing by organ system.

Standardized Framework	Applying Pattern	Chapter
LI-RADS	LI-RADS Category Assignment and the Pseudocapsule Trap	6
Bosniak Classification (2019, MRI-specific)	Bosniak Category Assignment	12
PI-RADS	PI-RADS Category Assignment	14
VI-RADS	VI-RADS Category Assignment	15
O-RADS	O-RADS Category Assignment	17
Peritoneal Cancer Index	Peritoneal Cancer Index Regional Scoring	21
MRI Tumor Regression Grade	Post-Neoadjuvant Response Categorization	20

Quick-Lookup Alphabetical Index

Every Signal-to-Category Decision System pattern introduced in this textbook, listed alphabetically by pattern name with its chapter of origin, for rapid lookup when the reader recalls a pattern name but not its organ system or part.

Peritoneal Nodularity: Benign versus Carcinomatosis	11
PI-RADS Category Assignment	14
Post-Neoadjuvant Response Categorization	20
Respiratory Misregistration and the Pseudo-Lesion Trap	2
Screening the Implanted Cardiac Device	3
Susceptibility Artifact from Metallic Hardware	1
Transition Zone Cancer versus BPH Nodule	14
True Ductal Calculus versus Pneumobilia	7
VI-RADS Category Assignment	15

Chapter-End Signal Synthesis Recap Index

Every chapter in this textbook closes with a Signal Synthesis Recap, a third-layer consolidation distinct from the two chapter-embedded Rhythm Layer instances indexed throughout the tables above, synthesizing that chapter's shared categorization theme into a single closing arc. This table lists each chapter's Recap arc name for direct navigation to the chapter-end synthesis when a broader, whole-chapter thematic summary, rather than a single pattern entry, is what the reader is seeking.

Chapter	Signal Synthesis Recap Arc
1	Foundational Artifact Recognition Arc
2	Protocol Quality-Control Arc
3	Contrast and Device Safety Arc
4	Artifact Troubleshooting Arc
5	Diffuse Liver Disease Quantification Arc
6	Focal Liver Lesion Characterization Arc
7	Biliary Tract Characterization Arc
8	Pancreatic Lesion Triage Arc
9	Splenic Lesion Triage Arc
10	Adrenal Mass Triage Arc

11	Retroperitoneal and Peritoneal Triage Arc
12	Renal Mass Triage Arc
13	Renal Parenchymal and Collecting System Triage Arc
14	Prostate Lesion Triage Arc
15	Bladder and Male Pelvic Triage Arc
16	Uterine Mass and Staging Triage Arc
17	Adnexal Mass Triage Arc
18	Pelvic Floor and Endometriosis Compartment Arc
19	Inflammatory Bowel Disease Structural Arc
20	Rectal Cancer Treatment Pathway Arc
21	Mesenteric and Peritoneal Triage Arc
22	Whole-Body Signal Correlation Arc
23	Developmental Signal Correlation Arc
24	Myocardial Tissue Characterization Arc

This Master Index reflects the complete Signal-to-Category Decision System as built into the forty-eight Rhythm Layer instances and twenty-four chapter-end Signal Synthesis Recaps distributed throughout this textbook's core chapters. It is intended as a return-to reference, not a substitute for the fuller clinical reasoning, evidence base, and management context each pattern's originating chapter provides, and the reader is encouraged to consult the relevant chapter directly whenever a specific clinical scenario warrants the complete discussion this condensed index summarizes.

CONCLUSION

This textbook began with the physics of fat and water precessing slightly out of phase with one another, a phenomenon subtle enough to be mistaken for artifact by an unpracticed eye, and closed with the transmural extent of scar tissue within a single myocardial segment determining whether a patient returns to the catheterization laboratory or is spared it. Between those two points lies the full anatomic range of body MRI: the liver and biliary tree, the pancreas and spleen, the adrenal gland and retroperitoneum, the kidney and prostate and bladder, the uterus and adnexa and pelvic floor, the bowel and mesentery and peritoneum, and, in closing, the whole body considered at once, in the pediatric patient, in the pregnant patient, and in the beating heart. Read end to end, the distance traveled is considerable. Read as a single argument, however, the distance collapses, because the same reasoning discipline reappears at every stop along the way.

That discipline is what the Signal-to-Category Decision System, threaded through every chapter of this book, was built to make explicit. A signal is identified, whether a region of restricted diffusion, a septation within a cyst, a stricture's enhancement pattern, or a fascial distance measured in millimeters. That signal is then tested against a specific, named criterion, not a general impression, before it is permitted to determine a category. The category, once assigned, drives a specific next step, surveillance or referral, medical therapy or surgery, reassurance or urgent intervention, and the step is never taken until the trap most likely to produce a wrong category for that specific pattern has been deliberately checked and ruled out. Chemical shift artifact and a genuine lipid-poor lesion, a hemorrhagic cyst and a true enhancing nodule, red marrow reconversion and marrow infiltration, dense fibrosis and residual viable tumor: each pair recurs throughout this book in a different anatomic costume, and each pair is resolved the same way, by confirming the discriminating feature before committing to the diagnosis it would otherwise support.

Much of the specific content in the preceding chapters will be superseded. Numeric thresholds will be revised as evidence accumulates, staging systems will be updated, named frameworks will enter new editions, and sequences considered advanced at the time of this writing will become routine, replaced in turn by techniques not yet developed. This is the ordinary condition of a field built on continuously accumulating evidence, and no textbook, however current at publication, is exempt from it. What should outlast any individual threshold or criterion is the underlying habit of mind this book has tried to model throughout: read the image for what it actually shows rather than for what a differential diagnosis expects it to show, confirm a suspicious finding against its specific discriminating feature before naming it, and state the resulting uncertainty honestly when the discriminating feature cannot be confirmed rather than resolving that uncertainty by assumption.

The chapters of this book are written to be returned to, not read once and set aside. A resident preparing for an unfamiliar case, a radiologist encountering an indeterminate adrenal mass at two in the morning, a clinician trying to understand why a mesorectal fascia distance of four millimeters changed a patient's treatment sequence, each is better served by the specific chapter addressing that specific problem than by a general recollection of having read the book once. The Signal-to-Category Master Index exists for exactly this purpose, offering three paths back into the same material, by organ system, by named framework, and by pattern name, so that the return visit costs a minute rather than a search.

KEY POINT: The specific numbers in this book will age. The discipline of confirming a signal against its discriminating feature before assigning it a category, and of stating uncertainty plainly when that confirmation cannot be made, does not.

Body MRI, more than most imaging modalities, rewards exactly this kind of patience. Its tissue contrast is rich enough to answer questions other modalities cannot ask, and rich enough, in the same measure, to mislead a reader who moves too quickly from signal to conclusion. The chapters of this book have tried to show, case after case and organ after organ, what it looks like to move at the right speed. The rest belongs to the reader, and to the patients whose care depends on getting it right.

www.ingramcontent.com/pod-product-compliance
Lightning Source LLC
LaVergne TN
LVHW062034101126
852251LV00025B/329
* 9 7 8 1 1 0 5 0 4 5 3 9 4 *